PSYCHOLOGY LIBRARY EDITIONS:
NEUROPSYCHOLOGY

Volume 12

COGNITIVE REHABILITATION IN PERSPECTIVE

COGNITIVE REHABILITATION IN PERSPECTIVE

Edited by
RODGER LL. WOOD AND IAN FUSSEY

Routledge
Taylor & Francis Group
LONDON AND NEW YORK

First published in 1990 by Taylor & Francis, reprinted in 1994 by Lawrence Erbaum Associates Ltd.

This edition first published in 2019
by Routledge
2 Park Square, Milton Park, Abingdon, Oxon OX14 4RN

and by Routledge
711 Third Avenue, New York, NY 10017

Routledge is an imprint of the Taylor & Francis Group, an informa business

British Library Cataloguing in Publication Data
A catalogue record for this book is available from the British Library

ISBN: 978-1-138-48894-6 (Set)
ISBN: 978-0-429-45935-1 (Set) (ebk)
ISBN: 978-1-138-59230-8 (Volume 12) (hbk)
ISBN: 978-0-429-49008-8 (Volume 12) (ebk)

Publisher's Note
The publisher has gone to great lengths to ensure the quality of this reprint but points out that some imperfections in the original copies may be apparent.

Disclaimer
The publisher has made every effort to trace copyright holders and would welcome correspondence from those they have been unable to trace.

Cognitive Rehabilitation in Perspective

edited by

Rodger Ll. Wood

Clinical Director of the Brain Injury Rehabilitation Trust, Milton Keynes

Ian Fussey

Consultant Psychologist at the BUPA Hospital, Leicester

LAWRENCE ERLBAUM ASSOCIATES, PUBLISHERS
Hove (UK) Hillsdale (USA)

First published by Taylor & Francis 1990
Reprinted by Lawrence Erlbaum Associates 1994

Lawrence Erlbaum Associates Ltd., Publishers
27 Palmeira Mansions
Church Road
Hove
East Sussex, BN3 2FA
U.K.

British Library Cataloguing in Publication Data

A catalogue record for this book is available from the British Library

ISBN 0-86377-193-9 (Pbk)

Printed and bound by BPC Wheatons Ltd, Exeter, UK

Contents

Acknowledgements

We would like to express our gratitude to Vivien Pegg and Liz Trundle for their continued good humour and tolerance through the many draft revisions imposed upon them. We particularly appreciated the stoical way in which they have organized both data and correspondence, acting as the 'frontal lobes' to the editors of this volume.

List of Contributors

Nick Alderman, M.App. Sci.
St. Andrew's Hospital, Billing Road, Northampton, UK.

Sverre Andresen, Cand.Psychol.
Sunnaas Rehabilitation Hospital, 1450 Nesoddtangen, Oslo, Norway.

Ina J. Berg, Ph.D.
Department of Neuropsychology, University Hospital, University of Groningen, Oostersingel 59, 9713 EZ, Groningen, The Netherlands.

Paul W. Burgess, B.A.
M.R.C. Applied Psychology Unit, University of Cambridge, Cambridge, CB2 2EF, UK.

William H. Burke, Ph.D.
New Medico Highwatch Rehabilitation Center, PO Box 99, Center Ossipee, New Hampshire 03814, USA.

Betto G. Deelman, Ph.D.
Department of Neuropsychology, University Hospital, University of Groningen, Oostersingel 59, 9713 EZ, Groningen, The Netherlands.

Azriel Evyatar, Ph.D.
Teaching Institute of Technology, Department of Science and Technology Education, Haifa, Israel.

Arnstein Finset, Ph.D.
Sunnaas Rehabilitation Hospital, 1450 Nesoddtangen, Oslo, Norway.

Ian Fussey, M.Sc., C.Psychol.
BUPA Hospital, Gartree Road, Oadby, Leicester, LE2 2FF, UK.

John M. Gray, Ph.D.
Astlie Ainslie Hospital, Grange Loan, Edinburgh, EH9 2HL, UK.

Zeev Groswasser, M.D.
Loewenstein Rehabilitation Hospital, Department of Head Injuries, 278 Ahuza Street, Ra'anana, POB3, 43100 Israel.

C. Alan Hopewell, Ph.D.
Dallas Neuropsychological Institute, 2435 W. Northwest Highway, Suite 109, Dallas, Texas, 75220, USA.

Marthe Koning-Haanstra, Ph.D.
Department of Neuropsychology, University Hospital, University of Groningen, Oostersingel 59, 9713 EZ, Groningen, The Netherlands.

Catherine A. Mateer, Ph.D.
Good Samaritan Center for Cognitive Rehabilitation, Puyallup, Washington 98372, USA.

Gabriele Matthes-von Cramon, Ph.D.
Munich Neuropsychological Department, City Hospital, Munchen-Bogenhausen, West Germany.

Jennie Ponsford, Ph.D.
Bethesda Hospital, 30 Erin Street, Richmond, Victoria 3121, Australia.

Margalit Schem-Tov, Ph.D.
Psychiatric Hospital, NessZiona, Israel.

McKay Moore Sohlberg
Good Samaritan Center for Cognitive Rehabilitation, Puyallup, Washington 98372, USA.

Max J. Stern, Ph.D.
Loewenstein Rehabilitation Hospital, Department of Head Injuries, 278 Ahuza Street, Ra'anana, POB3, 43100 Israel.

Detlev Yves von Cramon, M.D.
Munich Neuropsychological Department, City Hospital, Munchen-Bogenhausen, West Germany.

Michael Wesolowski, Ph.D.
New Medico Highwatch Rehabilitation Center, PO Box 99, Center Ossipee, New Hampshire 03814, USA.

Rodger Ll. Wood, Ph.D. C.Psychol.
The Devonshire Hospital, 29–31 Devonshire Street, London, W1N 1RF, UK.

Patricia K. Youngman
Good Samaritan Center for Cognitive Rehabilitation, Puyallup, Washington 98372, USA.

Richard Zawlocki, Ed.D.
New Medico Highwatch Rehabilitation Center, PO Box 99, Center Ossipee, New Hampshire 03814, USA.

Preface

Brain injury rehabilitation has experienced many changes in its short history. Some of the naive notions that passed as 'therapy' ten years ago would now be challenged on the basis that the techniques used lack an acceptable theoretical foundation and are difficult to evaluate in terms of outcome criteria which have some meaning as far as community independence is concerned. Hart and Hayden (1985) recommended that training must be relevant to the individual's life and be capable of generalization to actual life skills. During rehabilitation, therefore, patients must have an opportunity to apply, in real life situations, the skills learned in therapy to help them consolidate and generalize. The aim should be to help new skills acquire the properties of a 'habit' because habits have enduring qualities which survive changes of environment and therefore do not alter when the patient has been discharged from treatment.

The report of the Medical Disability Society *The Management of Traumatic Brain Injury* (1988) pointed out that despite the emphasis given to physical disability, cognitive and behavioural defects produce the major morbidity following brain damage and impair the capacity of individuals to return to work or maintain social activities. Five years after injury, deficits in memory, complex information processing, organizational thinking and planning are still evident and contribute to various forms of psychological instability, often preventing social reentry (Brooks *et al.*, 1986). The report further pointed out that participation in rehabilitation therapy can be adversely affected by cognitive deficits and recommended that therapists working with the brain injured develop an understanding of cognitive dysfunction and its impact on compliance, effort and tolerance. Cognitive rehabilitation is indicated as a method of helping patients and families 'come to terms with, manage, by-pass or reduce acquired cognitive deficits' (p. 13).

The methods of cognitive rehabilitation offered by the Society's report include modifying the environment, finding alternative solutions through functional adaptation and the effective utilization of skills that have been retained. These recommendations offer an operational perspective for cognitive rehabilitation but fail to provide a conceptual foundation from which principles of retraining cognitive skills can be developed. It would appear that the minimal criteria for any clinical discipline of cognitive rehabilitation must include the following components in order for the practice to acquire scientific respectability:

1 A theoretical or conceptual model which unites clinical procedures with mechanisms of dysfunction.
2 An appreciation of how cognitive dysfunction after brain injury can be interpreted in terms of abilities of daily living which are significant for personal or community independence.
3 A set of procedures, individually or collectively designed, to remediate specific cognitive disabilities and different levels of dysfunction (i.e. from basic cognitive processes — attention, memory, etc. to the utilization of those abilities in terms of adaptive social behaviour).
4 Methods for evaluating recovery of cognitive abilities in terms, not only of clinical recovery, but also with respect to social or functional change. These measures should be capable of establishing a treatment-effect in order to unequivocally relate cognitive-behaviour change to specific methods of remediation.

The chapters in this book attempt to conform to these criteria, but, unlike most of the existing texts devoted to cognitive rehabilitation, this book is not restricted to a review of the field, primarily because the field, as such, does not exist! There are few published studies in the area of cognitive rehabilitation, which include the criteria mentioned above, to explain the rationale of training procedures, neither are there clear indications of the value of cognitive rehabilitation as judged by social outcome (as opposed to the narrow and often artificial measures of ability adopted by some psychologists to support the value of their procedures). This book is an attempt to correct the imbalance between the large number of words written about cognitive rehabilitation and the few controlled or systematic studies evaluating the effect of cognitive rehabilitation. The following chapters provide a collection of clinical procedures, each of which has a conceptual basis to explain the training methods, as well as attempting to evaluate the success of training. Success is determined not only by improvement on narrowly defined clinical criteria but also with respect to behavioural changes that reflect improved social outcome.

The areas of cognitive impairment represented in this book were not selected according to any preference on the part of the editors or contributing authors but reflect those areas of cognitive rehabilitation which are receiving increasing attention by clinicians working in brain injury rehabilitation, who recognize their importance to social behaviour and functional independence. Attention, for example, is regarded by many rehabilitation experts as one of the keys to adaptive social behaviour, memory and learning ability (see Wood, Chapter 1). This introductory chapter also attempts to outline the various ingredients of cognitive rehabilitation and examine their contribution to a clinical model that offers both a theoretical framework and an operational perspective for restoring cognitive ability.

The remainder of the book provides a selection of clinical procedures designed to improve those aspects of behaviour and functional ability that depend upon an intact or integrated cognitive system. The first section addresses attentiveness and information processing. Alternative training strategies are presented, each capable of addressing different attentional problems imposed by various clinical conditions. Gray describes procedures which can improve attentiveness, in order to improve visual scanning of the environment, as well as the information-processing aspects of attention that form the pre-requisites of thinking and memory. Ponsford both reviews the use of computers as training aids and also describes procedures which utilize this form of technology. Mateer and her colleagues consider the importance of attentional training following mild head injury, completing the spectrum of procedures and applications of this important cognitive training area.

The next section considers strategies for dealing with the social and behavioural problems resulting from memory impairment. Instead of the traditional and clinically dubious procedures traditionally used to retrain memory itself, the approach adopted by Finset and Andresen, and Deelman, Berg and Koning-Haanstra, focuses on strategies that ameliorate the social handicap imposed by memory problems. Neither approach is conceptually difficult. Finset and Andresen adopt a training procedure that helps the development of utilization behaviour based on a diary concept to structure and regulate activities. Deelman and his colleagues adopt a procedure similar to cognitive-behavioural training, using language as a mediator to regulate thinking and impose structure on daily activities.

The third section attempts to provide strategies for improving the organizational thinking, planning and reasoning that follow in the wake of frontal brain injury. These cognitive problems represent the most pervasive and intractable of all cognitive disabilities. They require an innovative form of training that provides opportunities for patients to test hypotheses, exercise reasoning and make judgements on the outcome of intended action. This is not easily achieved within the existing clinical framework, but Evyatar and his colleagues and von Cramon and Matthes-von Cramon provide interesting perspectives that can be tested in the context of a neuropsychological 'laboratory', possibly as a preparation to exposing the patient to environmental activities which demand the kind of cognitive adaptability normally mediated by the frontal structures. The first approach utilizes computers to provide structured feedback that allows hypothesis testing to take place. The second is another combination of cognitive and behavioural methods to reduce complex ideas and actions to components which are more easily construed and manipulated in terms of adaptive behaviour.

The final clinical section addresses the problems of behaviour which many would argue impose the greatest constraint upon community reentry and social acceptability. Experience is beginning to show the limitations of a purely behavioural approach to regulating emotional dyscontrol and conduct disorders. The chapters by Burgess and Alderman show how a patient's cognitive status determines their response to changing environmental conditions. The first chapter in this section (Burgess and Alderman) provides a cognitive model which is both capable of explaining many kinds of maladaptive behaviour as well as addressing such behaviour from a cognitive-behavioural perspective. The second chapter (Alderman and Burgess) emphasizes the role of language as a mediator of cognitive awareness in the control of behaviour. The last clinical chapter, by Hopewell *et al.*, shows how prosocial behaviour depends largely upon recognizing social cues that call for certain styles of interpersonal behaviour and emotional regulation.

While the reader will appreciate that every effort has been made to link theory with method to achieve results which have both clinical utility and social relevance, further effort is required to properly validate techniques of cognitive rehabilitation in order for them to become established as a central component of brain injury rehabilitation. We feel, however, that the chapters contained in this volume represent the 'state of the art' in the sense that they provide a collection of verifiable cognitive rehabilitation procedures which is unparalleled in the clinical literature, offering an approach to changing cognitive behaviour in ways which are both clinically and socially relevant.

R. Ll. Wood
I. Fussey 1989

References

BROOKS, N., CAMPSIE, L., SYMINGTON, C., BEATTIE, A. and MCKINLAY, W., 1986, 'The five year outcome of severe blunt head injury: A relative's view.' *Journal of Neurology, Neurosurgery and Psychiatry*, **49**, 764–70.

HART, T. and HAYDEN, M. E., 1985, 'The current status of head injury rehabilitation'. In M. E. Milner and K. Wagner (Eds.), *Neurotrauma, treatment, rehabilitation and related issues* (Boston: Butterworths).

MEDICAL DISABILITY SOCIETY 1988, *Report of the working party on the management of traumatic brain injury*, Royal College of Physicians, London.

WOOD, R. Ll., 1989, 'Salient factors in brain injury rehabilitation'. In R. Ll. Wood and P. G. Eames (Eds.), *Models of brain injury rehabilitation* (London: Chapman Hall).

PART 1
INTRODUCTION

Chapter 1

Towards a Model of Cognitive Rehabilitation

R. Ll. Wood

Introduction

Cognitive or neuropsychological rehabilitation utilizes an assortment of procedures to improve or restore a diverse collection of abilities and skills. However, there is an absence of rules that inform the cognitive rehabilitation therapist which procedures to apply and under what circumstances. Consequently, many of the training tasks used by practitioners of cognitive rehabilitation to restore cognitive or functional abilities owe more to a dogmatic belief that the methods work than to any scientific formula which links the training task to a cognitive theory of information processing, on the one hand, and a neuropsychological system of analysis and retraining, on the other. The result of this apparently heuristic approach to conceptualizing a clinical model of cognitive rehabilitation is an unnecessary and undesirable variation in the quality of procedures employed to represent cognitive rehabilitation and a very limited fund of reliable information that will allow practitioners to evaluate the clinical utility of the methods used.

To some extent the pot pourri of methods, procedures and techniques that represent cognitive rehabilitation can be explained by the lack of a clear conceptual basis of what 'cognition' means and, *parri passu*, what cognitive rehabilitation should be attempting to do. There is no common frame of reference to describe cognitive rehabilitation procedures themselves or the rationale upon which they are based. Some practitioners adopt a psychometric perspective to training, while others use a behavioral (conditioning) paradigm, or a psychotherapeutic approach to improve awareness, understanding and, by implication, social or functional adaptivity.

Traditionally, psychologists have avoided intangible and nebulous processes such as 'thinking' because they were seen as mentalistic and, therefore, unscientific by the behaviorally dominated psychology of the 1940s and 50s. Cognitive events, such as memory and perception, were addressed as relatively circumscribed phenomena, distinct from each other and separate from behavior. Consequently, recent efforts at restoring higher cortical functions in man following brain injury have suffered from the absence of a conceptual framework. The notion of cognition has, in many cases, been over-simplified and practitioners of cognitive rehabilitation have dissected and compartmentalized fragments of the cognitive process, working on those fragments as though they were ends in themselves rather than simply a means to an end ('cogs' in the vastly more complex cognitive system).

Perhaps part of the solution to this dilemma can be found by considering what the terms 'cognition' and 'rehabilitation' mean. The dictionary definition of cognition is 'a mental act or process by which knowledge is acquired', while rehabilitation is defined as 'helping people who are physically or mentally disabled, readapt to society'. Using the terms 'cognition' and 'rehabilitation' in tandem implies, therefore, that a clinical procedure is being used to train individuals to acquire knowledge which can be utilized to help them readapt to society!

Establishing definitions is a simple but useful exercise because it provides a perspective on what cognitive training procedures are intended to do. They are not intended to invest individuals with artificial capabilities, the value of which is to change a score on some psychometric scale of ability. On the contrary, they are intended as a method for changing behavior by reducing the social handicap imposed by cognitive disability. During their short occupational history, most cognitive rehabilitation therapists have come to realize that there is little merit in training patients on artificial cognitive tasks, such as how to complete block design assemblies or learn word lists, unless these activities lead to some meaningful improvement in functional skills, self-initiation of cognitive strategies, or greater spontaneity and organization of behavior. This greater awareness of the social impact of cognitive impairment has influenced current approaches to the remediation of memory problems. The chapters by Finset and Andresen (Chapter 5) and Deelman, Berg and Koning-Haanstra (Chapter 6) reflect this move away from attempts to train some assumed memory process in favor of the development of behavioral strategies that obviate the problems of memory.

Diller (1987) suggests that the early focus on artificial aspects of cognitive recovery may have been a consequence of the different backgrounds and methods that have traditionally surrounded neuropsychologists and rehabilitation therapists. The former have been pre-occupied with an analysis of impairment, identified by responses to standardized tests, while the latter have primarily been concerned with disability and the limitations imposed by that disability on acts of daily living. Diller points out that there are no data which relate cognitive impairment to cognitive disability and, because of their traditional laboratory and experimental approach, neuropsychologists have problems 'translating the language of impairment into a language of disability without a complex chain of assumptions' (Diller, 1987, p. 4).

Ironically, the growing awareness of what cognitive rehabilitation is not (the development of artificial intellectual skills) has perplexed many cognitive rehabilitation therapists; an enormous conceptual gulf exists between devising training tasks for artificial abilities, compared to improving those intangible cognitive processes such as reasoning, judgement and insight that are the cognitive fabric of human behavior. The efforts of Evyatar *et al.* (Chapter 8) and von Cramon and Matthes-von Cramon (Chapter 7) represent a step forward in the development of a systematic approach to help promote concept formation, hypothesis testing and reasoning ability which many would regard as the pre-requisites of judgement and social adaptability. It is possible to argue, however, that the strategies forming part of these training procedures are simply an extension of sophisticated computer games software on one hand and the skills that form the basis of certain behavioral procedures (shaping and chaining) on another. The key to successful rehabilitation of such intangible cognitive functions is whether or not the concepts can be translated into actions which improve social adaptability. In many respects this represents the antithesis between declarative and procedural approaches to learning and rehabilitation discussed by Wood (1990b).

Consequently, while cognitive rehabilitation is regarded by many as an important component of brain injury rehabilitation, it still lacks a coherent scientific framework to integrate treatment methods and direct therapy activities towards the achievement of realistic treatment goals. This lack of a clear perspective for cognitive rehabilitation seems to underlie Diller's thoughtful and provocative comment in the introduction to *Neuropsychological Rehabilitation* (Diller, 1987). He stated that some neuropsychologists are sceptical about the theoretical or scientific basis of cognitive remediation and supports attempts to 'create a clinical discipline where none now exists' (p. 9). The scepticism of cognitive rehabilitation comes not only from the ranks of neuropsychologists but from other health-care professionals (c.f. Butler and Namerow, 1988). These concerns cannot be ignored, and in order for cognitive rehabilitation to find its proper place in brain-injury rehabilitation, some attempt must be made to provide it with a clinical perspective which has a sound conceptual foundation upon which to base treatment procedures.

The Search for a Model

The term 'model' has been used loosely in the clinical literature on cognitive rehabilitation. It has been applied to a collection of procedures used to restore cognitive function (e.g. Gianutsos and Gianutsos, 1979; Bracy, 1983; Wilson, 1987) and again to describe specific milieus is which combinations of procedures are applied, usually in the context of a psychotherapeutic frame of reference (Ben-Yishay and Diller, 1983; Prigatano, 1986). In other cases, efforts have been made to devize treatment methods in relation to underlying mechanisms of cognitive dysfunction (Sohlberg and Mateer, 1987), and finally, attempts have been made to integrate the milieu approach with a systems approach under the banner of neurobehavioral techniques which try to relate injury characteristics to learning disabilities that interfere with progress in rehabilitation and prejudice social outcome (Wood, 1989).

Another way of approaching cognitive rehabilitation has been provided by Diller and Gordon (1981). They offered three alternative ways of analysing rehabilitation problems in order to address their consequences: (1) the psychometric model, (2) the biologist's model and (3) the engineer's model. The psychometrist analyses the components of cognitive disability in relation to specific tasks by means of neuropsychological tests. The biologist employs a hypothesis-testing approach which seeks to elicit what aspects of the task cause a patient difficulty and then develops hypotheses about the cause of the defect by observing other tasks or situations where the same pattern of difficulty is displayed. The engineer employs an ergonometric approach to understand how the interaction between the person and task produces difficulties, in order to establish which features of the environment are rewarding or punishing to the person. The difference between the biologist and engineer is that the former tries to educate the person as to the nature of their deficit and ways to overcome it (c.f. Ben-Yishay and Diller, 1983; Prigatano, 1986), while the latter changes the environment, manipulates stimuli and focuses on reinforcement to accelerate learning or reduce the frequency of inappropriate social habits (c.f. Malec, 1983; Wood, 1987).

This way of formulating how cognitive deficits impact behavior helps provide a rationale for different treatment approaches. The 'neurobehavioral approach', for example, is a combination of the biological and engineering models while the Bracy, Gianutsos and Wilson methods appear to subscribe to the psychometry model. The educational focus of the Ben-Yishay and Diller and Prigatano approaches, helping patients to become more aware of their problems and hence control or adapt to them more effectively, is closely related to Diller's biological model, except that a biologist would adopt a more rigorous functional analysis of the cognitive problem than appears to be reflected in the various forms of milieu therapy. In this respect, the attention-performance training methods described by Sohlberg and Mateer (1987) are more in line with a biological approach.

Another perspective for cognitive rehabilitation has been provided by Gross and Schutz (1986) who presented a hierarchical model which takes account of the learning difficulties presented by patients with different forms of brain injury. At the lowest level of the hierarchy, Gross and Schutz recommend an environmental control model, similar to Diller's engineer. The next stage, described as a stimulus-reinforcement conditioning model, is even more behavioral in character and is similar to the neurobehavioral approach applied by Wood (1987) in which complex behaviors are reduced to their component parts. A higher level of training involves the application of basic cognitive and social skills in a realistic setting. This stage, called the skills-training model, assumes that adaptive functional and social skills can be obtained through practice, very much of the spirit of the procedural learning tradition proposed by Dickinson (1980) and Wood (1990a). The final step in their hierarchy is described as a strategy-substitution model, which is designed to ameliorate the problems imposed by cognitive disability and corresponds closely to the recommendation of Miller (1984) who regarded amelioration as a 'much more sensible and potentially attainable goal than restitution' (p. 79).

Wilson (1988) also considered cognitive models used in rehabilitation. She remarked on the potential of a procedural learning model in cognitive rehabilitation, citing the work of Baddeley (1982) and Schacter and Glisky (1986) as examples where this operates in a memory-retraining context. However, while acknowledging the contribution of behavioral psychology in generating a technology of learning, Wilson expressed doubts about the relevance of its underlying theory. She recommended that a model for cognitive rehabilitation should combine the principles and technologies of cognitive psychology, neuropsychology and behavioral psychology, rather than be limited to any one tradition or theoretical perspective.

Wilson used the analogy of the sinfonia hemispherical model, derived from the work of Buffery and Burton (1982). This compares the brain to an orchestra and brain damage to a situation which might arise should several of the strings section die just before the concert. Four strategies are offered to explain how the orchestra could deal with this problem. They include (1) recruiting new members (the substitution or regeneration argument), (2) changing the repertoire so that the missing musicians are not required (the engineer or environmental control argument), (3) asking other musicians to learn the violin (the plasticity or reorganizational argument) and (4) asking other instrument sections to play the violin parts (another variant of functional adaptation which stresses the achievement of goals without giving too much thought to the mechanisms by which the goals are achieved). The value of this approach is difficult to assess because the different models lack a central scheme linking training to underlying mechanisms presumed to produce cognitive dysfunction. As such the model would more realistically be described as a set of procedures based on different theories of neuronal recovery rather than a coherent approach to the retraining of cognitive processes presumed to underlie behavior.

In order to combine these often disparate approaches into a model which has both scientific respectability and clinical utility, we need to adopt an operational perspective on the role of cognition in behavior and recognize how information-processing systems mediate learning. The role of attention also needs to be considered because this is clearly important to any formulation of brain-behavior relationships. Attention seems to integrate the physiological mechanisms responsible for arousal and drive, with the psychological mechanisms related to motivation, awareness and recognition. Language also integrates thought and behavior because it helps focus attention and sequentially organize actions.

The approach to this chapter, however, is not to propose one model as such but to consider the different components which underlie any system of cognitive rehabilitation. The purpose is to help practitioners appreciate how the chapters in this book all subscribe to a common understanding of cognitive theory and a need for conceptually driven approaches to restoring cognitively mediated behavior as a basis for independent living.

Understanding Cognition

One of the problems facing psychologists attempting to understand cognition is that we can never witness the process of thinking. All we see is its product — behavior. The act of cognition is therefore inferred from the behavior an individual displays in relation to some problem. Dickinson (1980) made the point that 'there is no reason why mental processes should not be inferred from behavior'. Attempts to rehabilitate thinking ability may best be considered within some form of behavioral framework. As Davey (1988) stated, 'An important goal in human operant theory is to understand the processes by which humans come to learn about the relationships between behavior and its consequences, and how they translate this knowledge into behavior' (p. 9). There are, however, a number of problems related to restricting oneself entirely to the external or phenomenological aspects of thinking because while behavior itself may be the end product of thinking, cognition is a response to both internal and external stimuli. This dilemma forms the basis of the work carried out by Burgess and Alderman on emotional regulation and behavioral change (Chapters 9 and 10). They have attempted to integrate cognition and behavior within a cognitive-neuropsychological framework in a bid to increase a patient's awareness of his or her inappropriate behavior, leading to more effective self-control under conditions where external control has failed.

Dickinson proposed that the way in which we characterize the role of cognition in learning depends very much upon what exactly we wish to study. The focus can either be the behavioral change itself (presumed to reflect learning) or the learning process assumed to underlie behavioral change. If our aim is limited to simply describing behavioral change, then the terminology provided by conditioning theory is adequate to explain increments and decrements in a specific response. However, the nomenclature of conditioning theory lacks a conceptual framework to explain how cognitive representations of the environment change during a learning experience. These changing representations are not simply a consequence of S-R associations but involve changing perceptions, attitudes and expectations, each of which can alter the motivational system. Bolles (1979) considered the role of cognition in behavioral change and suggested that a cognitive psychologist has two alternative ways to describe such change. One utilizes the theoretical language of hypothetical constructs (e.g. expectancy, perception, memory), while the second adopts a procedural language, containing terms like 'prediction' and 'information', which operationalize the process of behavioral change and can be applied in the context of conditioning procedures.

For example, why did Pavlov's dog salivate when it heard the bell? Answer, the bell predicted food! A cognitive explanation would be that the dog salivated because it expected food (see Bolles, 1979). In many ways the concept of expectation provides a deeper interpretation than offered by the notion of prediction because saying that the response was conditioned (predicted) by the bell seems to omit the role of memory as a mediator of behavior. In this example, the bell initiates processes which arouse a representation (some image) of food. This is not an isolated image, however, because in turn, the memory of food elicits another process, the anticipation of eating food. Bolles pointed out that both the conditioning and cognitive explanations are tautologous, one is just as basic as the other but each provides a different conception of how the process of learning can be explained; one involving a set of ideas, expectations and associated reactions, the other a basic operational transfer which conveys nothing about the mechanism of learning and behavior change. The former approximates a declarative explanation of thinking and behavior, the latter a procedural explanation of how knowledge is employed.

Dickinson argued that something must alter during learning. He considers this alteration to be a modification of some internal cognitive structure. Brain injury, however, produces changes to neural processes that may prevent such cognitive restructuring, for example, preventing the relationship between S and R becoming established (see Wood, 1988). Consequently, we need to understand the characteristics of learning in terms of processes controlling the formation of cognitive systems. This may allow us to predict how the learning system operates, both in terms of the mechanisms reponsible for the identification of stimuli relevant to current behavior and also which stimuli elicit which responses in order to discover what properties of a stimulus elicit a response (and why). It may then become possible to enhance these properties (increase cue salience) to improve learning.

The Role of Attention in Cognition

Rehabilitation is essentially about learning, some forms of which are didactic while others are incidental or observational. Whatever the learning mode one thing is essential, the ability of a person to direct attention to the source of information and then maintain a focus of attention upon the relevant task parameters (see Gray, Chapter 2). What this requires is a continuous reciprocal interaction between a person and the environment, without which information is not processed properly and learning, if it takes place at all, is slow and unreliable.

The concept of attention has grown in importance as a major cognitive variable since neuropsychologists recognized its role in mediating and integrating information from the internal and external environment. This is seen as part of a continuous 'cybernistic' process which starts with a perception of a stimulus followed by an analysis of its component parts. In turn, this leads to some kind of response being selected, one appropriate to the environmental changes created by the stimulus. The final stage in the sequence is an evaluation of the response in order that future responses can be refined or adjusted according to the previous information or chain of cognitive events that initiated the first response.

This continuous feedback system allows our interactions with the environment to be initiated, monitored and changed; in other words, regulated. For this reason attention has been described as 'a controlled process that enables the individual to select, from a number of alternatives, the tasks he will perform or the stimulus he will process and the cognitive strategy he will adopt to carry out these operations' (Moscovitch, 1979, p. 422). Consequently, any model of cognitive rehabilitation must incorporate mechanisms of information processing and provide techniques to improve processing abilities in ways which produce changes in behavioral adaptability. As Posner and Rafal (1987) suggested, 'cognitive rehabilitation is best guided by a sophisticated knowledge of the underlying mechanisms involved in the process of attention' (p. 182).

The components of attention and their neuropsychological correlates have been described by Posner (1980), Posner and Boies (1971), Stuss and Benson (1986) and Posner and Rafal (1987), while others have discussed some of the phenomena associated with disorders of attention (van Zomeren *et al.*, 1984; Sohlberg and Mateer, 1987, 1989; Wood, 1987, 1988, 1990a). In the context of cognitive rehabilitation, however, there may be greater value in considering how attention is involved in the process of learning, rather than simply reiterating the components of attention or describing the phenomenology of attentional disorders in relation to their underlying cognitive mechanisms. The reason for this is that all the authors referred to above implicitly acknowledge that attention mediates learning, but none seem to forcefully echo the statement of William James on the importance of attention to learning: 'My experience is what I attend to. Only those items that I notice shape my mind — without selective interest, experience is an utter chaos.' (James, 1890, p. 87).

Learning, therefore, relies on the efficient processing of information which, in turn, depends upon the following factors: (1) The quality of stimulus input: (2) the cerebral structures needed to perform the mental operations necessary for processing stimulus input (this includes a level of mental effort or stamina to maintain a focus of attention long enough for the new information to be analysed); and (3) a processing system which has the capacity to absorb sufficient information for learning to occur.

In a rehabilitation context, one cannot guarantee the quality of stimulus input (see Wood, 1989) while the brain injury itself compromises the processing capacity of the cognitive system, meaning that the essential requirements for learning are neither always available or operational, as the following sections indicate.

Attending to stimulus input

The quality of stimulus input depends firstly on the nature of the training task and the type of environment in which training takes place. If the training task is complex (for a person with a damaged brain) then the components of the task need to be reduced to a number of small units of learning. As Malec (1983) stated, 'persons with severe cognitive difficulties can relearn self-management skills if these skills are broken down into simple components' (p. 129). The reason for this is to help a person discriminate between stimuli which are important for learning and those which are not (e.g. noise).

A major factor in social learning is the ability to discriminate relevant cues from a background containing multiple stimuli. It obviously helps the discrimination process if the salient stimulus variables are identifiable to the learner. Some studies of normal individuals suggest that learning can take place without awareness of the stimulus cue (see Keehn, 1967), but Bandura (1969) argued that 'simply exposing an individual to repeated stimuli does not guarantee that he will select from the total stimulus complex those cues necessary for learning to occur' (p. 132).

Malec (1983) reported on a head-injured patient who did not make progress in rehabilitation because she failed to attend to many important stimuli (pp. 133–135). Wood (1987) also gave an example of a patient who failed to control inappropriate conversational themes because she was not aware of (could not discriminate between) selective reinforcement procedures applied in an effort to 'cue' alternative forms of conversation (p. 82). Consequently, to ensure that environmental cues are attended to, their cue salience should be increased, or some form of training should take place, similar to that offered by Mateer, Sohlberg and Youngman (Chapter 4), to help a patient attend to relevant cues.

Cerebral control in attention

The ability to direct attention towards goal-orientated activities is acquired (learned) during an individual's development and matures into a largely automatic process, the complexity of which is easy to overlook until the automatic character of an action is lost or diminished as a result of injury. Luria (1973) was aware of the dual nature of attention and tried to distinguish involuntary attention (orientation), which has an elementary biological basis, from voluntary (directed and sustained) attention which he interprets as a social act; voluntary attention is unrelated to biological maturation, being instead the product of selective mental activity.

Most forms of brain injury, especially those involving damage to the frontal lobes, interfere with the process of voluntary attention and create the phenomena of inattention (short attention span and distractibility). Luria (1973) commented on the essential role of the frontal structures mediating voluntary attention. However, most forms of brain injury (and virtually all decelerative traumatic brain injuries) affect the integrity of the frontal structures or their connections. Consequently, the ability of the undamaged brain to inhibit responses to irrelevant stimuli and preserve goal-directed behavior does not necessarily apply after head trauma. Luria felt that the loss or reduction of this inhibitor mechanism could cause a 'severe disturbance of goal-directed or selective behavior and leads to a disinhibition of impulsive responses to irrelevant stimuli' (distractibility) (Luria, 1973, p. 189).

The inability to maintain a focus of attention is due to a different cognitive failure. It is important to distinguish between distractibility and short attention span because a patient with an attention span of only five minutes may still prove to be distractible within that time, even if engaged on an enjoyable task. Attention span has more to do with vigilance and the effort components of attention, both of which are susceptible to many forms of brain injury. In such cases an internal (organic) constraint is an inability to maintain a focus of attention, while the external factor imposing that constraint is the length of a therapy session and/or the amount of information presented to a patient during that period. This is such a simple point but one which seems to be continually overlooked by therapy staff of all disciplines and at every stage of rehabilitation.

Processing capacity

Attention is involved in behavior to different degrees depending upon the level of skill that has been attained. In a new task, for example, one needs to pay close attention to the consequences of one's action in order to achieve certain goals (van Zomeren, 1981; Reason, 1984). With increasing practice, however, the sequence of actions of behaviors becomes more automatic and requires less conscious attention. Some action sequences can become so fluent and automatic that giving too much attention to them can actually disrupt the smooth flow of motor output (e.g. trying to think about where to place one's feet when running up or down stairs, a form of cognitive interference over an automatic motor sequence that almost inevitably precipitates a fall).

A possible problem for rehabilitation therapists is that much of human behavior exists at an automatic level. Some of the basic requirements for independent living are all present as automatic action sequences, e.g. putting food to one's mouth; getting washed, dressed, walking, etc. In many cases of serious brain injury, these automatic behaviors are disabled and patients have to revert to a conscious mode of operation. This requires a major behavioral and attitudinal adjustment because suddenly it becomes necessary for individuals to think about the performance of certain behaviors that previously were conducted without conscious attention. For many individuals the greater effort needed to operate in this way is defeated by the limitations imposed on their attentional system by brain injury, but even when this obstacle is overcome, the habitual nature of automatic response patterns may prevent a person controlling the focus of attention long enough for learning to take place. As James (1890) stated,

'Habit diminishes the conscious attention with which our acts are performed' (p. 101). Cognitive rehabilitation, therefore, needs to consider the relationship between attention and skilled performance, recognizing, of course, that skill is something fundamental to even the most routine activities of daily living but may be masked by the overlearned nature of the activity.

Cognition, Behavior and Performance

Burgess and Alderman (Chapter 9) utilize a cognitive a model proposed by Shallice (1982, 1988) which explains some aspects of the complex relationship between thinking and behavior. They apply this model in a rehabilitation context to modify behavior by helping patients with frontal injury increase awareness of certain aspects of the environment which control their responses. Briefly, the model conceptualizes different levels of organization, comprising basic cognitive units which are specific neuropsychological functions that form the basis of different types of behavior (e.g. attention, memory, perception, etc.), and schemas, which represent a combination of cognitive units that activate overlearned skills, some of which are performed automatically (walking, eating, drinking, etc.), while others require varying degrees of thought and coordination (such as driving). The act of problem solving or response selection relies upon what Shallice (1982, 1988) described as 'contention scheduling'. This is a process of selecting schemas appropriate to the demands of a task. In many respects, contention scheduling is the cognitive process that provides our thinking with the flexibility that permits social adaptation, a process invariably diminished by frontal brain injury (Luria, 1966, 1973).

The operation of this cognitive process relies on the attentional system to select, from the internal or external environment, those stimuli which are relevant to ongoing behavior. Shallice (1982) described this as the 'Supervisory Attentional System' (SAS). Its role is to deal with stimuli present in unfamiliar situations and to monitor actions in response to stimuli. In some ways the SAS provides the cybernistic function referred to earlier, regulating responses according to the nature or amount of stimulus input. Shallice's model offers an extension of the Shiffrin and Schneider (1977) concept of controlled information processing which has served as a very useful model for explaining how attention and information-processing systems regulate behavior and learning in a rehabilitation context. Both are devoted to explaining how the cognitive system processes information in routine and unfamiliar tasks, but the Shallice model has yet to be fully tested in a rehabilitation framework.

Current cognitive rehabilitation methods rely heavily on the Shiffrin and Schneider notion of focused attention deficits to explain why habit responses often conflict with the process of acquiring new responses and divided attentional deficits to explain the slow performance times on tasks which are unfamiliar or where new learning is required (see van Zomeren, 1981; van Zomeren *et al.*, 1984; van Zomeren and Brouwer, 1987; Wood, 1987, 1990b; Sohlberg and Mateer, 1989). The potential of Shallice's model to cognitive rehabilitation is considerable however. Stuss and Benson (1986) have already remarked upon its ability to explain many real-life situations, while Sohlberg and Mateer (1989) and Wood (1990a) have referred to it as an advanced form of analysis capable of linking cognitive theory to observable aspects of behavior.

Attentional processes, therefore, influence the speed and efficiency of learning and selecting information from the environment and processing such information through sensory channels into short-term memory. This was recognized by the exponents of information-processing models of memory (Atkinson and Shiffrin, 1968, Craik and Lockhart, 1972) and by Baddeley (1982) who proposed the concept of a 'central executive' as a hypothetical construct which allows information to be held in temporary storage while attention is temporarily shifted to other stimuli. As such, working memory (that most frequently impaired following traumatic brain injury) relies heavily on attention. The memory deficit reflected by most individuals after trauma is forgetfulness or absent-mindedness, the nature of which conforms closely to Reason's description of memory failures which are caused by lapses of attention (Reason, 1984). The overwhelming influence of attention in learning and memory led Wood (1984) to suggest that there may be greater merit in attempting to rehabilitate attention, as opposed to memory disorders, if the aim of treatment is to restore greater independence and social adaptivity to individuals.

From a neuropsychological perspective, attention training would have to involve at least seven cognitive operations which form part of the information-processing continuum. These include:

1 Perceptual scanning — to locate the source of the visual or auditory stimulus.
2 Discriminative perception — to identify and isolate salient cues from the mass of sensory information available (selective attention).
3 Vigilance — the ability to maintain a state of readiness to detect and respond to small changes occurring at random time intervals in the environment (Mackworth, 1957).
4 Sustained attention — the ability to maintain a focus of attention over a period of time to detect and respond to changes in stimulus patterns (the effort component of attention). In this continuum, vigilance is largely dependent upon sustained attention.
5 Alternating attention — to shift the focus of attention from one task component to another in order to maintain a fluent style of behavior (i.e. the capacity for mental flexibility (Sohlberg and Mateer, 1989).
6 Attentional capacity — to maintain a sufficient amount of information at a level of awareness alongside other (competing) information in order that an

individual can select which items of information are most important for current behavior and act upon them (the concept of a central executive) (Baddeley, 1982).

7 Divided attention — to allow new information to be processed without slowing down or interfering with current behavior which requires spontaneous processing (speed of information processing).

The Role of Language in Cognitive Rehabilitation

Language has given man a unique opportunity to create his own subjective environment. This special ability has allowed human behavior to become independent of its physical environment making it possible to regulate behavior on the basis of some 'private' process. During the 1920s, Russian psychology placed great emphasis on investigating the reorganization of mental processes which takes place under the influences of speech, and one of the first psychologists to express the view that speech plays a decisive role in the formulation of mental processes was Vygotsky (Vygotsky and Luria, 1929; Vygotsky, 1962). His investigations were almost entirely directed to an analysis of children's cognitive development but, as Gelb and Goldstein (1920) and Head (1926) showed, the concepts provide a valuable basis for explaining the nature of cognitive impairment after acquired brain injury.

More recently, the work of Luria (1973) has offered insights into how verbally mediated aspects of behavior influence rehabilitation and the acquisition of complex skills. Luria's studies trace the self-regulatory function of language from dependence on environmental cues, or feedback from one's own motor responses (which indicates a concrete style of thinking and behavior), through stages of partial self-control in which initiation or inhibition gradually shift from control by sensory cues to control by verbal cues and responses. The final stage is inner speech, which allows an abstract style of thinking to develop and where problems and their solutions can be considered in the absence of actual events themselves. Such verbally regulated behavior is highly dependent upon (but also contributes to) memory and allows prospective organization of thinking and behavior.

Luria and Yudovich (1972) suggested that words 'have an indiscernible but decisively important influence on the foundation of mental processes' (p. 30). They felt that words influenced perception by isolating the essential features of an object, investing it with a function. In some ways, therefore, words enhance discriminative perception by isolating the salient qualities of the stimulus while simultaneously inhibiting the less essential properties. In addition, by associating an object or activity with a word, we give it a permanence and help the process of generalization. Luria and Yudovich (1971) attributed to Goldstein, Gelb and Head the opinion that 'Speech allows man to rise above direct visual perception to an analysis of data, relating perceived objects to certain categories, so enabling him to organise his behaviour, not according to the visually perceived situation, but according to a deeper "categorised" reflection of the world' (p. 31).

Of more direct relevance to rehabilitation is the role of speech as a regulator of behavior. Vygotsky and Luria (1929) showed how children, when faced with a complex problem, used 'external speech' to regulate their actions and help focus attention on those ideas and responses that allowed progress towards task completion. Luria and Yudovich (1971) emphasized that Vygotsky and Luria were not referring to 'egocentric speech' (Piaget, 1928) but 'overt speech' as a way of mediating behavior by 'mobilising verbal connections to solve a difficult problem' (p. 32). Vygotsky's observations showed that children first regulate their actions by speaking aloud to themselves, but then speech gradually dies away, passing into a whisper, finally becoming internal speech. During this progression, the actions under the control of speech become more fluent and require less conscious effort to maintain.

Luria (1961, 1969) proposed three developmental stages by which the initiation and inhibition of voluntary motor behavior comes under verbal control:

Stage 1. External control by others which directs and regulates a person's behavior.
Stage 2. A person's own overt speech regulates behavior.
Stage 3. Covert or inner speech assumes a self-regulatory role.

The process will be obvious to anyone who remembers learning to drive. In order to help focus attention on the task requirements, we tend to talk ourselves through each stage of a complex sequence, emphasizing or repeating certain words that are associated with specific actions, giving them prominence and helping us focus attention upon them in order to avoid errors. Words, therefore, help isolate a particular event or observation and serve as a signal for a particular action. As such, words become regulators of behavior, freeing us from simple S-R action sequences, allowing what Pavlov (1927) referred to as an 'analysis and synthesis of stimuli which gives man an infinite capacity for orientation and self-regulation' (p. 27). Pavlov considered this to be the essential peculiarity of man's higher nervous activity. Much human thought and activity is evoked by anticipating the consequences of an action. Luria felt that intentions and plans were consciously generated and reflected a social motivation that depends initially upon external, but ultimately upon internal, speech. Speech allows us to formulate intentions, define goals and commence a program of action leading to the attainment of the goal.

The effect of brain injury on verbal mediation

Luria and Yudovich (1971) stated that the participation of speech in the formulation of new ideas can be seriously disturbed by injuries to the brain. Possibly the reason for this disturbance, as far as head injury is concerned, lies in the nature of the injury and the particular brain structures and mechanisms involved. Most forms of concussion (and all acceleration/deceleration injuries) inflict damage either to the structures or mechanisms of the frontal regions of the brain (Teasdale and Mendelow, 1984; Levin *et al.*, 1983). The frontal lobes regulate most aspects of human behavior (Luria, 1973; Stuss and Benson, 1986), therefore, most patients who sustain serious closed-head injury lack the organizational ability that allows economical use of time, sequential ordering of activities or the anticipation of consequences to display sophisticated and adaptive human behavior.

One of the principal results of frontal brain injury was, according to Luria (1973), a disturbance of speech-based activation. A major feature of such damage is 'a loss of the selectivity of mental processes affecting all spheres of mental activity' (Luria and Homskya, 1969, p. 32). Luria (1973) later refined his opinion, however, suggesting that extensive frontal damage disturbs only complex forms of regulated conscious activity, in particular, behavior which is based on motives, formulated with the aid of speech. This can lead to complex programs of activity disintegrating and being replaced by simple, stereotyped or concrete forms of behavior. Following a review of the electrophysiological changes seen in frontal patients, Luria (1973) concluded, 'lesions of the frontal lobe disturb only the higher cortical forms of activation brought about by the aid of speech' (p. 195). He inferred from this that voluntary attention (focused attention and concentration), which is so important to learning and skilled performance, is disturbed in the absence of any impairment to involuntary attention (orientating responses or distractibility). This system not only remains intact but may even, by default, be actually enhanced (causing distractibility).

One interesting factor in these situations is the apparent dislocation between a patient's ability to verbalize the components of a task directly yet fail to translate this apparent knowledge to direct-task performance. Many frontal patients can explain quite well, and in correct sequence, the activities necessary to make a cup of tea but, when actually executing the behavior, they appear disorganized and task performance takes on a fragmented quality with no apparent concept of the proper sequence of behavior. Often, this situation can be complicated by a patient not appreciating the nature or extent of the difficulties observed by others, meaning that 'they not only lose control over their actions but also the ability to check their results' (Luria, 1973, p. 210).

If, as Luria (1973) claimed, language is a primary cognitive mechanism for behavioral self-regulation, the loss or reduction in this ability will lead to changes in a person's ability to regulate emotional behavior under certain conditions. Some support for this has been provided in the clinical literature. Lishman (1968) noted a consistent relationship between psychiatric disorder and the presence of dysphasia in brain-injured patients. Weinstein and Lyerly (1968) also found that language disorders were associated with social maladjustment later in recovery. More recently, a study by Levin and Grossman (1978) found that a large number of brain-injured patients with severely agitated behavior also displayed forms of dysphasia. The examples of behavior problems provided by Burgess and Alderman (Chapters 9 and 10) strongly suggest that a breakdown in certain language-related abilities prevented their patients conceptualizing their environment in terms that helped them adjust to changing situations and utilize verbal regulation to control emotional expression.

Using verbal regulation in rehabilitation

Luria (1973) stated that 'attempts to incorporate the patient's own speech as a means of regulating behaviour do not give the required results' (p. 202). However, Craine (1982) suggested that 'overt verbal mediation' is a useful method for improving self-regulatory behavior in cases of frontal lobe dysfunction. The technique he described involves training patients to memorize cues which initiate, sequence and time poorly regulated behaviors. A method similar to this was described by Kanfer and Phillips (1970) who applied verbal regulation to several brain-injured patients to whom they taught verbal mediation to improve motor performance. Training employed a shaping procedure, fading external verbal cues and self-instructions as motor skills improved. Kanfer and Phillips found that this method helped patients acquire skills and execute simple tasks.

The use of verbal regulation has also been employed in cognitive-behavioral treatment approaches (Beck *et al.*, 1979; Meichenbaum, 1979) where 'self-talk' has been used as a means of promoting behavior change. Malec (1983) suggested that self-monitoring can be prompted by verbal modelling of correct and incorrect performance. In this way Malec felt stimulus-response-outcome relationships could be linguistically coded as behavioral rules, helping individuals to predict the outcome of a particular response and improve the regulation of behavior. He successfully applied these ideas to a number of brain-injured patients who had difficulty monitoring and controlling behavioral responses and found that the improvement in predictive ability and self-monitoring ability generalized beyond the training procedures themselves, increasing the patient's response repertoire and improving their social acceptability. Stuss *et al.* (1987) also found that the performance of individuals could be improved through the use of 'self-talk'. During a motor impersistence task they found that when verbal regulation was used to train one procedure, the action generalized to other procedures. Generalization was also found by Wood (1987) who utilized a conditioning paradigm to shape functionally adaptive behaviors by means of verbal regulation. It was found that the verbal mediation of movement could facilitate the forward sequencing in units of activity. In more severe cases, the verbal prompts were externally delivered (by a therapist) until the patient could remember (internalize) them and use them to regulate a complex action sequence.

Another example of external verbal cueing was given by Sohlberg *et al.* (1988) to train a patient with frontal damage who found initiating behavior difficult. This patient was taught to ask himself 'Am I initiating?' or to respond appropriately by asking 'Am I acknowledging other people talking?'. As the patient progressed, the cues were faded, allowing self-cueing to become established. This procedure successfully helped the patient monitor his behavior in several situations. (For other interventions using verbal mediation see the remarks of Gray, Chapter 2, and Alderman and Burgess, Chapter 10).

Cognitive Mediators in Motor Learning

The damage to the monitoring and regulatory systems of the brain following cerebral trauma makes the relearning of motor movement at least difficult and occasionally impossible. It is important for physical and occupational therapists to recognize that, in many cases, the reason for chronic, physical disability (even in cases of brain-stem injury) may be more to do with the patient being unable to learn (a cognitive constraint) than the complex and extensive nature of neurological and soft-tissue damage (a physical constraint).

Luria (1961) suggested that voluntary movements are controlled by a combination of goals and intentions. For example, a movement sequence begins with a goal ('comb my hair') which, in turn, initiates some intention ('pick up the comb') in order to execute an action (pulling comb through hair). In this respect, almost any motor act is preceded by a cognitive process which determines the nature of isolated motor acts, subroutines of motor patterns and combinations of motor patterns to achieve complex action sequences.

Luria (1961) argued that it was not the movement itself, but the goal of the movement that is represented in the motor cortex. The goal of a motor act constitutes a more complex notion than the movement itself, usually comprising several units of motor activity which have to be integrated sequentially and temporally if the goal is to be achieved. In a similar fashion, Bernstein (1967) argued that the human motor act is so varied that it cannot be explained in purely mechanical terms. He stated that 'every intelligent purposeful movement is made as an answer to a motor problem' (p. 16). In the process of solving such problems, movements change, both in terms of mechanical modifications to alter the trajectory of movement and qualitatively to re-organize motor patterns by changing successive elements and stages in the motor sequence. The combination of these changes eventually leads to new movement strategies being adopted to overcome some obstacle preventing mobility.

The arguments offered by Luria and Bernstein imply that the development of motor skills is directly linked to some problem-solving activity, emphasizing the central role of cognition as a mediator of motor performance. After serious brain injury, many patients lose the ability to execute discreet or localized motor actions, displaying instead stereotyped mass action patterns which occur as a result of damage to the inhibitory mechanisms that developed through maturation to control the reflex patterns present in the newborn and young infant. From a neuropsychological perspective, this problem can be explained as a lack of regulatory control normally provided by the complex network of interconnections between the frontal system (in its role as a coordinator of normal movement), the cerebral motor cortex and the midbrain structures that initiate movement and control the fine motor sequence (basal ganglia, cerebellum).

This is essentially a Lurian notion (Luria, 1973), but one which has influenced western thinking. For example, Stuss and Benson (1986) stated, 'Any learned movement is originally made up of independent isolated impulses. Practice results in a synthesis or fusion of the isolated impulses into the single integral component, sometimes called a "kinetic melody". With long practice, this complex movement becomes automatic. Instead of individual pulses initiating each section of a movement, one pulse is sufficient to trigger the entire complex' (p. 77). After head injury, one impulse may still initiate a sequence of nervous impulses but the synthesis and coordination of nervous activity is disrupted, resulting in the uncoordinated mass movement so frequently seen in spastic hemiplegia.

To reestablish a controlled pattern of motor activity it is necessary to isolate each unit of movement and sequentially link that unit to subsequent units that form a complex action sequence. Cognitive intervention can help by emphasizing how these movement sequences have to be structured in order to be learned and, also, to help physical therapists recognize how cognitive deficits can interfere with learning in physical therapy. The most obvious being: (1) Failure to understand the requirement of a task; (2) an inability to focus attention properly in order to rehearse motor patterns; (3) difficulty in carrying out movements in a sequentially correct manner; (4) remembering procedures from one training session to another; and (5) generalizing skills learned in one context to another.

Finally, it is important to remember that the greatest influence on motor learning is language (Vygotsky, 1962). Many adult motor skills are learned almost exclusively through verbal instruction, backed up by practice. Through practice individuals bring their movements under verbal control. Often this begins by 'talking' oneself through a task and repeating the phrases until performance becomes more fluent and less effortful; overt speech then becomes progressively more 'silent', assuming a less obvious, but still important, regulatory function until the skilled performance becomes so automatic that it appears to take place with no verbal mediation at all. By helping physical therapists and patients understand the value of verbal regulation during mobilization exercises, the cognitive rehabilitation therapist can improve concentration during therapy and increase the feedback opportunities important for motor learning.

Conclusions

In one of the earliest discussions of a model for cognitive rehabilitation, Diller (1976) stated that 'remediating cognitive deficit remains the greatest challenge to those concerned with the rehabilitation of the brain injured' (p. 13). At that time he felt that neuropsychology had 'contributed little to the problem of direct therapeutic intervention'. Little has changed over the last 14 years, and the progress that has been made in this aspect of rehabilitation owes more to the traditions of cognitive and behavioral psychology. Cognitive psychology has provided rehabilitation with a theoretical foundation from which remediation tasks could be developed. The actual relationship between many of these tasks and their presumed theoretical base does not always pass close inspection, but a new generation of training methods is being developed which stand firmly on the rock of scientific theory and promise great advances in the scope and reputation of cognitive rehabilitation (see Sohlberg and Mateer, 1989).

Behavioral psychology, so long the enemy of 'thinking' psychologists, has forced the practice of cognitive rehabilitation away from its narrow application in changing psychometric test performance, allowing a broader perspective to prevail — one which looks at skills training and the development of activities of daily living. In future, cognitive rehabilitation will need to address the motor, language and memory skills that are displayed in every day activities, recognizing that while it may be necessary to train the basic cognitive units of skilled behavior, the main thrust of training must be aimed at helping people utilize those skills in the context of social and functional behavior.

This chapter has tried, in a small way, to expand the conceptual horizons of those engaged in cognitive rehabilitation procedures by pointing to some of the main ingredients that comprise the cognitive rehabilitation pie. Without a clear exposition of the relationship between cognition and behavior, the clinical practitioner will find it difficult to understand the nature of cognitive impairment and its relationship to a particular kind of brain injury. Similarly, not recognizing the role of attention and information processing in determining the content of cognition may result in a neglect of certain factors important to learning. Finally, the role of language as a regulator of thinking and behavior and its potential to enhance stimulus cues during learning should never be underestimated, making it plausible to suggest that more treatment in brain injury rehabilitation should be redesigned to incorporate verbal mediation.

Language is critical to the reasoning process. The opportunity to analyse one's actions as they are performed may be lost or reduced following injury to the frontal structures. This can lead to inappropriate responses being made which cause embarrassment to onlookers without making any impression on the person displaying the behavior because the once automatic act of self-monitoring is no longer operating. Encouraging patients to verbalize their actions or to overtly question their intentions may increase their awareness of the consequences of their thinking and reduce impulsivity or inappropriate behavior.

The brain-damaged person has only a limited response repertoire and has difficulty selecting stimuli from the environment in order to choose the most appropriate response. Normal stimuli may lose their saliency or cue value making it necessary for treatment staff to devise strategies that will call attention to certain cues, making patients more aware of how behavior interacts with the environment. Unfortunately, therapy staff are not taught this during training and many neuropsychologists seem to forget the basic tenets of behavior and learning when given the option of choosing a test battery as opposed to structured observation as the basis for clinical evaluation of a patient. Perhaps what is needed is a new discipline — a 'cognitive rehabilitation therapist' free of the discipline-bound thinking that chains other therapists to narrow ideas and procedures, allowing use of those elements from other therapy disciplines that promote functional adaptation to be combined into one discipline.

References

ATKINSON, R. C. and SHIFFRIN, R. M., 1968, 'Human memory: A proposed system and its control processes'. In K. W. Spence and J. G. Spence (Eds) *The psychology of learning and motivation*, Vol. II (New York: Academic Press).

BADDELEY, A. D., 1982, 'Implications of neuropsychological evidence for theories of normal memory'. *Philosophical Transactions of the Royal Society of London*, **V, 298**, 59–72.

BANDURA, A., 1969, *Principles of behaviour modification* (New York: Holt, Reinhart and Winston).

BECK, A. T., RUSH, A. J., SHAW, B. F. and EMERGY, V., 1979, *Cognitive therapy of depression* (New York: Guilford).

BEN-YISHAY, Y. and DILLER, L., 1983, 'Cognitive rehabilitation'. In M. Rosenthal, E. R. Griffiths, M. R. Bond and J. D. Miller (Eds) *Rehabilitation of the head injured adult* (Philadelphia: F. A. Davies) pp. 367–78.

BERNSTEIN, N. A., 1967, *The co-ordination and regulation of movements* (Oxford: Pergamon Press).

BOLLES, R. C., 1979, *Learning Theory* (New York: Holt, Reinhart and Winston).

BRACY, O. L., 1983, 'Computer based cognitive rehabilitation'. *Cognitive Rehabilitation*, **1**, 7–9.

BUFFERY, W. H. and BURTON, A., 1982, 'Information processing and redevelopment: Towards a science of neuropsychological rehabilitation'. In A. Burton (Ed.) *The pathology and psychology of cognition* (London: Methuen).

BUTLER, R. W. and NAMEROW, N. S., 1988, 'Cognitive retraining in brain injury rehabilitation: A critical review'. *Journal of Neurological Rehabilitation* **2**, 97–101.

CRAIK, F. I. M. and LOCKHART, R. S., 1972, 'Levels of processing: A framework for memory research' *Journal of Learning and Verbal Behavior*, **11**, 671–84.

CRAINE, J. F., 1982, 'The retraining of frontal lobe dysfunction'. In L. E. Trexler (Ed.) *Cognitive rehabilitation: Conceptualisation and intervention* (New York: Plenum).

DAVEY, G., 1988, 'Trends in human operant theory'. In G. Davey and C. Cullen (Eds) *Human Operant Conditioning and Behavior Modification* (New York: Wiley).

DICKINSON, A., 1980, *Contemporary animal learning theory* (Cambridge: Cambridge University Press).

DILLER, L., 1976, 'A model for cognitive retraining in rehabilitation'. *Clinical Psychologist*, **29**, 13–6.

DILLER, L., 1987, 'Neuropsychological rehabilitation'. In M. J. Meier, A. L. Benton and L. Diller (Eds) *Neuropsychological rehabilitation*.

DILLER, L. and GORDON, W. A., 1981, 'Interventions for cognitive deficits in brain injured adults'. *Journal of Consulting and Clinical Psychology*, **49**, 822–34.

GELB, A. and GOLDSTEIN, K., 1920, 'A psychological analysis of neuropathological cases'. Referred to by A. R. Luria and F. Yudovich (Eds) *Speech and the development of mental processes in the child* (London: Penguin) 1972.

GIANUTSOS, R. and GIANUTSOS, J., 1979, 'Rehabilitating the verbal recall of brain injured patients by mnemonic training: An experimental demonstration using single-case design methodology'. *Journal of Clinical Neuropsychology*, **1**, 117–35.

GROSS, Y. and SCHUTZ, L. E., 1986, 'Intervention models in neuropsychology. In B. P. Uzzell and Y. Gross (Eds) *Clinical neuropsychology of intervention* (Boston: Martinus Nijhoff).

HEAD, H., 1926, *Aphasia and kindred disorders of speech* (London: Cambridge University Press).

JAMES, W., 1890, *The principles of psychology* (New York: Holt).

KANFER, F. H. and PHILLIPS, J. S. (1970) *Learning Foundations of Behavior Therapy* (New York: McGraw Hill).

KEEHN, A. E., 1967, 'Experimental studies of 'the unconscious', operant conditioning of unconscious eye-blinking'. *Behaviour Therapy*, **5**, 95–102.

LEVIN, H. S. and GROSSMAN, R. G., 1978, 'Behavioural sequelae of closed head injury: A quantitative study', *Archives of Neurology*, **35**, 720–7.

LEVIN, H. S., BENTON, A. L. and GROSSMAN, R. G., 1983, *Neurobehavioural consequences of closed head injury* (New York: Oxford University Press).

LISHMAN, W. A., 1986, 'Brain damage in relation to psychiatric disability after head injury', *British Journal of Psychiatry*. **116**, 377–410.

LURIA, A. R., 1961, *The role of speech and regulation of normal and abnormal behaviour* (London: Pergamon).

LURIA, A. R., 1963, *Restoration of function after brain injury* (New York: Pergamon).

LURIA, A. R., 1966, *Higher cortical functions in man* (New York: Basic Books).

LURIA, A. R., 1969, Frontal lobe syndromes. In P. J. Vinken and G. W. Bryun (Eds) *Handbook of clinical neurology*, Vol. II (Amsterdam: North Holland).

LURIA, A. R., 1973, *The working brain* (New York: Basic Books).

LURIA, A. R. and HOMSKYA, E. D., 1964, 'Disturbances in the regulative role of speech with frontal lobe lesions'. In J. M. Warren and K. A. Ahert (Eds) *The frontal granular cortex and behaviour* (New York: McGraw-Hill).

LURIA, A. R. and YUDOVICH, F., (Eds) 1972, *Speech and the development of mental processes in the child* (London: Penguin).

MACKWORTH, N. F., 1957, 'Some factors affecting vigilance', *Advances in Science*, **53**, 389–93.

MALEC, J., 1983, 'Training the brain injured client in behavioural self-management skills'. In R. Edelstein and E. C. Coutoure (Eds) *Behavioural assessment and treatment of the traumatically brain damaged* (New York: Plenum).

MEICHENBAUM, D., 1979, *Cognitive-behaviour modification: An integrative approach* (New York: Plenum).

MILLER, E., 1984, *Recovery and management of neuropsychological impairments* (Chichester: John Wiley and Sons).

MOSCOVITCH, M., 1979, 'Information processing and the cerebral hemispheres'. In M. S. Gazzaniga (Ed.) *Handbook of behavioural neurobiology. Vol II: Neuropsychology* (New York: Plenum).

NEISSER, U., 1967, *Cognitive psychology* (New York: Appleton).

PAVLOV, I. P., 1927, *Conditioned reflexes* (Oxford: Oxford University Press).

PIAGET, J., 1928, *Judgement and reasoning of the child* (New York: Harcourt, Brace, Jovanovich).

POSNER, M. I., 1980, 'Orienting of attention. The VII Sir Frederick Bartlett lecture', *Quarterly Journal of Experimental Psychology*, **32**, 3–5.

POSNER, N. and BOIES, S. J., 1971, 'Components of attention'. *Psychological Review*, **78**, 391–408.

POSNER, M. I. and RAFAL, R. D., 1987, 'Cognitive theories of attention and the rehabilitation of attentional deficits'. In M. J. Meier, A. L. Benton and L. Diller (Eds) *Neuropsychological rehabilitation* (New York: John Wiley).

PRIGATANO, G., 1986, *Neuropsychological rehabilitation after brain injury* (Baltimore: Johns Hopkins University Press).

REASON, J., 1984, 'Lapses of attention in everyday life'. In R. Parasurman (Ed.) *Varieties of attention* (London: Academic Press).

SCHACTER, D. L. and GLISKY, E. L., 1986, 'Memory remediation: Restoration, alleviation, and the acquisition of domain-specific knowledge'. In B. Uzzell and Y. Gross (Eds) *Clinical neuropsychology of intervention* (Boston: Martinus Nijhoff).

SHALLICE, T., 1982, 'Specific impairments in planning'. In D. Broadbent and L. Weiskrantz (Eds) *The Neuropsychology of Cognitive Functioning*, pp. 119–209 (London: The Royal Society).

SHALLICE, T., 1988, *From neuropsychology to mental structure* (New York: Cambridge University Press).

SHIFFRIN, R. M. and SCHNEIDER, W., 1977, 'Control in automatic human information processing. II. Perceptual learning, automatic attending and a general theory'. *Psychological Review*, **84**, 127–90.

SOHLBERG, M. M. and MATEER, C. A., 1987, 'Effectiveness of an attention training programme'. *Journal of Clinical and Experimental Neuropsychology*, **2**, 117–30.

SOHLBERG, M. M. and MATEER, C. A., 1989, *Introduction to cognitive rehabilitation, theory and practice* (New York: Guildford Press).

SOHLBERG, M. M., SPRUNK, H. and METZELAAR, K., 1988, 'Efficacy of an external cueing system in an individual with severe frontal lobe damage'. *Cognitive Rehabilitation*, **6**, 36–41.

STUSS, D. T. and BENSON, D. F., 1986, *The frontal lobes* (New York: Ravens Press).

STUSS, D. T., DELGARDO, M. and GUZMAN, D. A., 1987, 'Verbal regulation in the control of motor impersistence: A proposed rehabilitation procedure. *Journal of Neurologic Rehabilitation*, **1**, 1–6.

TEASDALE, G. and MENDELOW, D., 1984, 'Pathophysiology of head injuries'. In D. N. Brooks (Ed.) *Closed head injury: Psychological, social and family consequences* (Oxford: Oxford University Press).

VAN ZOMEREN, A. H., 1981, 'Reaction time and attention after closed head injury'. PhD Thesis, Rijksuniversiteit T Groningen.

VAN ZOMEREN, A. H. and BROUWER, F., 1987, 'Head injury and concepts of attention'. In H. S. Levin, J. Grafman and H. M. Eisenberg (Eds) *Neurobehavioural recovery from head injury* (New York: Oxford University Press).

VAN ZOMEREN, A. H., BROUWER, F. and DEELMAN, B. G., 1984, Attentional deficits: 'The riddles of selectivity, speed and alertness'. In D. N. Brooks (Ed.) *Closed head injury: psychological, social and family consequences* (Oxford: Oxford University Press).

VYGOTSKY, L. S., 1962, *Thought and language* (Boston: Harfmann and Baker, MIT Press).

VYGOTSKY, L. S. and LURIA, A. R., 1929, 'The function and fate of egocentric speech'. *Proc. Ninth Int. Psychol. Congress*, Newhaven, 1929, published in A. R. Luria and F. Yudovich (Eds) *Speech and the development of mental processes in the child*, 1971 (London: Penguin).

WEINSTEIN, E. A. and LYERLY, O. G., 1968, 'Confabulation following brain injury'. *Archives of General Psychology*, **18**, 348–54.

WILSON, B., 1982, 'Success and failure in memory training following a cerebral vascular accident'. *Cortex*, **18**, 581–94.

WILSON, B., 1987, *Rehabilitation of memory* (New York: Guildford Press).

WILSON, B., 1988, 'Models of cognitive rehabilitation'. In R. L. Wood and P. G. Eames (Eds) *Models of brain injury rehabilitation* (London: Chapman Hall).

WOOD, R. Ll., 1984, 'Management of attention disorders following brain injury'. In B. A. Wilson and N. Moffatt (Eds) *Clinical management of memory problems* (London: Croom Helm).

WOOD, R. Ll., 1987, *Brain injury rehabilitation: A neurobehavioural approach* (London: Croom Helm).

WOOD, R. Ll., 1988, 'Clinical constraints affecting human conditioning'. In G. Davey and C. Cullen (Eds) *Human operant conditioning and behaviour modification* (London: John Wiley and Sons).

WOOD, R. Ll., 1989, 'Salient factors in brain injury rehabilitation'. In R. Ll. Wood and P. G. Eames (Eds) *Models of brain injury rehabilitation*, (London: Chapman Hall).

WOOD, R. Ll., 1990a, 'The rehabilitation of attention disorders'. In B. A. Wilson and N. Moffatt (Eds) *Clinical management of memory problems*, Vol II, (London: Chapman Hall) in press.

WOOD, R. Ll., 1990b, 'A conditioning paradigm for brain injury rehabilitation'. In R. Ll. Wood (Ed.) *Neurobehavioural sequelae of traumatic brain injury* (London: Taylor and Francis) in press.

PART 2
REHABILITATION OF ATTENTION DISORDERS

Chapter 2

The Remediation of Attentional Disorders Following Brain Injury of Acute Onset

J. M. Gray

Introduction

Attentional difficulties are present in many forms of brain disease. This chapter discusses two of the most common patterns of deficit: general attention/concentration difficulties after diffuse brain injury and unilateral visual neglect, common after cerebrovascular accident (CVA). Both are important in their own right (Denes *et al.*, 1982; Brooks *et al.*, 1987), and both can compromise attempts at rehabilitation in other spheres.

Attention is not a well-defined term, and attentional processes overlap with frontal or executive processes. In the case of closed-head injury (CHI), generalized brain damage can coexist with focal lesions to frontal areas (Jennett and Teasedale, 1981), and both contribute to the general post-head injury picture. Patients with brain injury or disease may appear vague and unable to maintain focus on a particular object or problem, or they may be distractable, unable to resist the pull of irrelevant environmental stimuli. They may be unresponsive or have difficulty switching set according to the demands of the situation, and to perseverate on old responses long after they have ceased to be relevant. It is not clear which of these deficits should be considered attentional and which frontal. Executive deficits are, therefore, discussed here, but only as they relate to attentional dysfunction.

Theoretical rationale for attempts at cognitive rehabilitation have been organized into three broad categories (Robertson *et al.*, 1988). The mental exercise model assumes that practicing a mental function will improve that function. A behavioural shaping model uses the principles of learning theory to try to increase the probability of a given response. The functional reorganization model asserts that improvement occurs because the goal in question is now achieved by a different arrangement of spared mental functions. Proponents of this last model try to specify which alternative processes are mediating the improvement and attempt to foster these processes through specific training procedures (Luria, 1963). For either the behavioural shaping or the functional reorganization models, the first requirement is some description of the skills or behaviours to be taught.

Attention can be analysed at the level of overt behaviour. In this case the variables measured would include time on task, the time the eyes are actually oriented to the target, etc. The attempts to remedy left unilateral neglect, described later in this chapter, include components directed largely at 'looking behaviour'. This overt attending behaviour is, of course, a pre-requisite for attention, but, it is possible to produce increases in such behaviour without affecting the crucial information-processing aspects of attention (Wood, 1986).

Early information-processing models concentrated on the role of attention in perception; attention was seen as a mechanism for screening the vast amount of information that arrives at our senses and selecting out the important and relevant. Increasing evidence for the processing of unattended stimuli led to various reformulations including attenuation (Treisman, 1964) and late-selection theories (Deutsch and Deutsch, 1963). More recent models have embraced the role of attention in intellectual and mnestic processes (Baddeley, 1986) and in the control of action (Reason, 1984). In both cognition and action, most processing consists of running highly routinized schemata, which are activated more or less automatically by their internal and external context. Attention is involved when these routines are blocked for some reason or when different aspects of the context require different schemata and a choice is required. In this view, attention is a set of high-level processes concerned with the allocation of limited resources among various perceptual, sensori-motor and cognitive tasks. This set of processes includes components related to alertness, selectivity and capacity (Posner and Boies, 1971).

Alertness has been described in terms of two relatively distinct sets of mechanisms, tonic and phasic (Posner and Snyder, 1975; Posner and Rafal, 1987). Tonic alertness or arousal refers to a mechanism under internal, largely physiological control regulating global responsiveness to environmental stimulation, including the sleep-wakefulness cycle and maintenance of attention in vigilance tasks. Phasic alertness refers to more momentary changes in responsiveness, often under environmental or voluntary control, such as the processes occurring during the foreperiod in a reaction time task where alertness is developed very rapidly (i.e. over, say, 0.5 second).

Selectivity refers to the basic notion of attention, which is that some stimuli or tasks are processed at the expense of others. A high degree of selectivity is, of course, possible for unattended, or unconsciously attended, stimuli (Neisser, 1976). However, items selected for conscious attending have preferential access to memory (Nissen and Bullemer, 1987). In some cases, e.g. in simple reaction time tasks, attended stimuli may be processed more quickly and more efficiently. More often their processing is slow and laborious compared to unattended stimuli, but they have access to processes for creating novel responses to novel situations.

Limited capacity or effort applies to the intensive aspect of attention 'whereby the amount of attention devoted to a particular information source can be varied' (Davies, 1983, p. 10). This implies three things, 'voluntariness', effortfulness and the ability to allocate limited resources in different ways. The resources demanded by a particular task depend on the degree of automaticity with which the task is performed, with routine, automatic tasks requiring little resources and being perceived as involving little effort and novel tasks requiring more. Attention is now often defined as involving effortful, cognitive activity, with attentional, controlled, effortful processing contrasted with unconscious, automatic processing (Shiffrin and Schneider, 1977). Shallice (1982) has suggested a 'Supervisory Attentional System' for the selection of cognitive action and perceptual schemata where routine solutions are unavailable or fail, i.e. where controlled processing is necessary.

Generalized Attentional Deficit

Although the relationship between head injury and attentional problems has been recognized since the 19th century, there has been some difficulty about the precise description of the deficit, although most accounts will mention distractibility, slowed information processing and difficulties in coping with multiple or complex tasks, particularly under time pressure.

Certainly basic physiological arousal can be altered after CHI. Immediately post-trauma, patients are typically unconscious and recover through various degrees of unconsciousness as measured, for instance, by the Glasgow Coma Scale (Teasdale and Jennett, 1974). Klove (1987) has suggested that in many cases long-term behavioural disturbances may be largely attributable to chronic underarousal. As regards tonic alertness in extended information-processing tasks, Conkey (1938) concluded that CHI typically resulted in a reduction in the ability to sustain attention. However, van Zomeren and Brouwer (1988) have summarized the results of many studies on sustained attention: '. . . these subjects show poorer signal detection and longer reaction times to signals, but their performance over time is just as stable as the performance of control groups' (p. 407).

However, there is evidence, both at the electrophysiological (Rizzo *et al.*, 1978; Curry, 1981) and behavioural levels (van Zomeren *et al.*, 1986), that mechanisms underlying phasic alertness are damaged in CHI. Goldstein (1952) believed that CHI patients suffered from a failure of selectivity. However, Miller and Cruzat (1981), among others, have shown that these patients are not selectively disadvantaged at separating messages on the basis of simple stimulus characteristics, and in that sense basic selective mechanisms are intact. A series of experiments with the more complex

Stroop Colour Word Naming Test have consistently shown that head-injured patients have no specific difficulty over controls in inhibiting overlearned responses and focusing on the selected dimensions of familiar stimuli (Stuss *et al.*, 1985; van Zomeren *et al.*, 1986; van Zomeren and Brouwer, 1987).

It has been suggested that the crucial deficit in diffuse brain damage, and in traumatic head injury in particular, may be a Divided Attention Deficit, i.e. a specific impairment in controlled processing (Shiffrin and Schneider, 1977). Melamed *et al.* (1985) have lent credibility to this view by demonstrating that impairment on a divided attention task is related to the degree of difficulty in maintaining concentration, in participating in multi-party conversations and in reading, experienced by CHI patients. There is overwhelming evidence that diffuse brain injury leads to slowed information processing (Miller, 1970; van Zomeren *et al.*, 1986). Whether this is particularly so for controlled processing or whether all information processing is slowed is contentious. In either case, speed of information processing does place capacity limitations on controlled processing. Of course, not all difficulties with controlled processing need be due to capacity limitations. The sort of inability to exercise control by changing set, seen in the performance of some frontal patients on the Wisconsin Card Sort, is presumably due to an inability to engage in certain specific operations. Shallice (1982) has described how impairment of his one component of his Supervisory Attentional System would produce such a picture.

After traumatic brain damage, then, there is no evidence for specific impairment of basic selection processes or for a deficit in the ability to sustain heightened attention over time. Diffuse brain injury may result in rather gross impairment of basic level of arousal. More commonly, it results in impairment of the ability to produce momentary rises in readiness to respond and in resource allocation in multi-task situations, which may be due to speed/capacity limitations, impaired control processes or both.

Attentional difficulties after closed-head injury may be particularly evident in 'mental-control' tasks, such as serial sevens and backward digit span. These tasks involve not only storage in short-term memory (STM), which is largely unaffected, but the active manipulation of the material internally. The deficit here may reflect damage to control functions.

Most attention retraining packages have relied initially on reaction-time (RT) training with progress from simple to discrimination and choice RT paradigms and increasing stimulus–response incompatibility. Vigilance training and training in alternating and dividing attention are usually added (Ben-Yishay *et al.*, 1979; Rattock *et al.*, 1982; Scherzer, 1986). The underlying rationale for this type of training is given by Ben-Yishay *et al.* (1979) and involves reinforced practice of the basic operations involved. A hierarchy of processes is postulated from wakefulness through vigilance to attentional control in tasks with cognitive content. 'Saturation' training is given sequentially on tasks representing ascending levels of this hierarchy, and it is hypothesized that this will result in cumulative enhancement of the patients alertness-attention-concentration abilities.

Ben-Yishay's attention-training module has been embedded in a comprehensive cognitive rehabilitation program which includes components designed to address difficulties in other areas, such as visuo-spatial processing, memory, etc., and results are reported using simple pre/post design with plateaued patients (Ben-Yishay *et al.*, 1979; Rattock *et al.*, 1982). Of course, such studies can tell us nothing about the specific effects of the attentional component. Scherzer (1986) used Ben-Yishay's procedures in a quasi-experimental design and attempted to tease out the effects of the separate components by looking at the time course of the improvement in relation to the time course of the various treatment factors. He found improvements in psychomotor tests of attention and visual information processing, but the absence of adequate controls and the use of training measures as outcome measures vitiates the force of his conclusions.

Rattock *et al.* (1982) measured pre- and post-attentional function in a group of 40 consecutive CHI patients undergoing a specific attentional training module and found improvements in four tasks: visual reaction time, digit span, picture completion and describe a picture.

Other studies have attempted to evaluate attention-training modules in isolation (Gross *et al.*, 1982; Sohlberg and Mateer, 1987), although there have been no randomized group controlled trials. Gross *et al.* (1982) have used a set of procedures which seem designed to provide training in divided attention. A series of four, single-case studies produced some improvement, but limitations in the design make their results difficult to interpret with any confidence. Sohlberg and Mateer (1987) used more rigorous single-case experimental design with four patients having attention problems. The training procedures were computer-based vigilance tasks and more complex alternating and divided attention tasks, some with cognitive content such as arithmetical exercises. A multiple baseline by function design with a measure of attention as the target (Paced Auditory Serial Addition Task [PASAT]) and a measure of visuo-spatial functioning as the control measure showed that interventions could produce a change in measures of attentional function in the absence of global improvement in cognitive function.

In the studies described below, both information-processing speed/capacity and control processes are measured. The Wisconsin Card Sorting Test (WCST) (Nelson, 1976) is used to measure 'mindfulness', i.e. the integrity and efficiency of the control processes involved in the maintenance and switching of attention or set. The Controlled Word Association Test requires subjects to generate words to an arbitrary and unpracticed rule (words beginning with a particular letter) and to inhibit overlearned, semantic associations and is, therefore, a measure of controlled processing. The Paced Auditory Serial Addition Task, which is a paced task involving internal manipulation of numerical material, involves both mental control and paced information processing.

It is particularly sensitive to the effects of head injury (Gronwall and Wrightson, 1974; Gronwall, 1977) and has become the standard measure of attentional deficit post-head injury.

Study 1

Gray and Robertson (1989) treated three young men with attentional problems after severe head injury. The first patient was a 20-year-old, male road traffic accident (RTA) victim who suffered a diffuse brain injury with greater than eight weeks post traumatic amnesia (PTA). At entry to the trial he was oriented for person and place but not for time and was fully cooperative. His backward and forward digit span were five and four, respectively; he was unable to attempt PASAT even at the slower rate of one digit per four seconds. He had, therefore, severe attentional problems, including difficulties with mental control/working memory-type tasks.

An attempt was made over about two months to retrain his attention/concentration using two computerized tasks, Rapid Number Comparison (RNC) and Digit Symbol Transfer (Braun *et al.*, 1985) described below. A multiple baseline across function single-case experimental design was used. The target measure was a composite mental control score with contributions from forward and backward digit span and mental arithmetic. The control measure was a test of verbal long-term memory, which was not expected to change over training. There was a stable baseline for both control and target functions, followed by a gradual improvement during the intervention phase for the target function only.

Analysis of this patient's behaviour on the RNC task suggests verbal self-regulation strategies may be involved in his improvement. Initially he was required only to identify the identical numbers and speak them aloud. He rapidly became quite good at this. Then, when he was required also to enter the numbers into the computer, his performance plummeted. However, if he was required to speak the number out loud as he identified it, his performance was restored to its former level. One possibility must be that he was prone to interference effects in short-term memory and overt rehearsal prevented this.

Luria (1963) has suggested that brain-injured persons may be trained to compensate for their attentional impairment by increasing the functional importance of higher cortical mechanisms involved in the voluntary regulation of attention. One of these mechanisms is inner speech, which in Luria's system subserves a crucial role in the self-regulation, including the regulation of attention (see Wood, Chapter 1).

On the basis of this first patient, a new computer program was produced designed to provide training in control processes. The program, the Alternating Stroop task, is described below and formed part of the training package for the subsequent two patients. Verbal rehearsal of the instruction set was built in, as was 'correspondence training' between instruction set and action.

A commercial arcade-type game, 'Breakout', was also added to the package, since practice on this had previously been reported to produce gains in attentional function (Rivamonte and Redfield, 1987). As this was an exploratory study, different combinations of tasks were used with different subjects, making it impossible to attribute any effects to any specific component. A multiple baseline across function single-case experimental design showed gains on the target measure in the absence of generalized improvement for both patients.

Study 2

In a second study, microcomputer-delivered, attentional training tasks were selected on the basis that they provided the opportunity to train on self-modulation of arousal, on alternating attention or on dividing attention. Where possible, verbal self-regulation was built into the training procedure.

To be admitted to the trial, the subjects had to fulfil the following criteria: (1) either subjective reports of difficulty in concentrating in real-life situations, such as reading or following a conversation, or reports of lapses in concentration by relatives or care staff; and (2) either a score of one standard deviation below the mean or lower on PASAT (Gronwall, 1977) or more than five errors on the Modified WCST (Nelson, 1976).

Thirty-one patients with brain injury of acute onset and meeting these criteria were randomly allocated to an experimental attentional training group or a control group. The 17 subjects in the experimental group received between 13 and 18 hours computerized attentional retraining conducted in sessions of one to one-and-a-half hours over three to nine weeks. Retraining consisted of work on four types of program.

Reaction-time training

This involved practice with feedback and conjugate reinforcement on simple and discrimination reaction-time tasks. These tasks are intended to provide training in self-modulation of arousal.

Rapid Number Comparison (Braun *et al.*, 1985)

In this task, four equal-length strings of between one and six digits are displayed simultaneously at one of nine exposure durations from about 0.1 sec to 1 sec. One of the strings appears twice, and the task is to identify and enter this. Results are reported in terms of percentage correct and level (number of digits and exposure time). Subjects are encouraged to verbalize the numbers. This provides training in verbal rehearsal and, again, in the ability to 'ready' for perceptual input and information processing.

Digit Symbol Transfer (Braun *et al.*, 1985)

This is a computerized version of the traditional psychometric task where subjects are required to translate rows of symbols into digits according to a code displayed on the screen. Both this and the preceding task involve visual scanning and information processing under time pressure.

Alternating Stroop program

This is a computerized modification of the colour Stroop task (Dyer, 1973); responding is by pressing coloured and labelled keys. The initial set is, of course, to respond to the meaning of colour words. Subjects are trained to disregard meaning and respond to colour, then to switch from responding to meaning and then back again. The task is paced with variable rates of presentation of stimuli. There are three labels of cueing which are gradually faded until the subject is required to establish which rule is operating, maintain that rule and switch rule on error feedback. Verbal regulation is built into the training procedure. This program is intended to provide training in 'mindfulness', i.e. in monitoring current behaviour and of deliberately changing behaviour when appropriate.

Divided attentional tasks

These are numeric invaders, 'arcade' games which combine the sort of visuo-motor demands of 'space invaders' with mental arithmetic under time pressure.

The control group receive a mean of 12.7 hours recreational computing (sd = 3.8 hours) delivered in one to one-and-a-half hour sessions over three to nine weeks. The aim for the control group was to control, as far as possible, for any non-specific effects of the research or of using microcomputers. Thus, recreational computing was used as the control procedure, rather than, for example, no treatment or psychotherapy. The only restrictions were that they should not include any speed component, i.e. no externally paced tasks and no short or masked displays, nor should they include tasks with a large component of visual search. Most of the work was on anagram-type puzzles and on games like 'Reds and Greens', a simple problem-solving game similar to noughts-and-crosses. These computer programs provided a plausible and motivating session for the control subjects.

These procedures were expected to produce improvements in the experimental group on attentional function as measured by PASAT and WCST. However, subjects were also given a number of other psychometric tests which were thought to measure various aspects of attention or controlled processing. These were: Digit Span, Picture completion and Arithmetic subtests of the Wechsler Adult Intelligence Scale — Revised (WAIS-R) (Wechsler, 1981), letter cancellation (Diller *et al.*, 1974), time estimation (Benton *et al.*, 1964) and a measure of word fluency (Borkowski *et al.*, 1967). Other tests, such as the Wechsler Logical Memory (Wechsler, 1945), Rey-Osterreith (Rey, 1941), Neale Analysis of Reading (Neale, 1958) and the Block Design subtest of the WAIS-R (Wechsler, 1981), were also carried out.

At the end of training the scores achieved were analysed with initial values of the variables as covariates. There were only minor differences in attentional function. The experimental group did better on WAIS-R Picture completion ($F = 5.15$, $df = 1,28$; $p = 0.031$) and on PASAT Information Processing Rate ($F = 5.84$, $df = 1,26$; $p = 0.023$). However, when estimated premorbid IQ and weeks post-injury were added as covariates, there were no significant difference between groups. By the six month follow-up, the experimental group performed better on a variety of psychometric measures: Backward Digit Span ($F = 4.50$, $df = 1,27$; $p = 0.043$), Arithmetic ($F = 7.00$, $df = 1,24$; $p = 0.014$), PASAT Total Score ($F = 15.07$, $df = 1,26$; $p = 0.001$), PASAT Longest String ($F = 7.68$. $df = 1,26$; $p = 0.01$), Information Processing Rate ($F = 9.73$, $df = 1,26$; $p = 0.004$) and Block Design ($F = 8.11$, $df = 1,26$; $p = 0.008$).

When age, estimated premorbid IQ and weeks post-injury were entered as covariates, the experimental group scored higher for all variables derived from PASAT, i.e. total score at 4 sec ($F = 11.04$. $df = 1,24$; $p = 0.003$), longest string at 4 secs ($F = 4.75$, $df = 1,24$; $p = 0.039$) and IPR ($F = 5.90$, $df = 1,24$; $p = 0.023$), and for Arithmetic ($F = 4.85$, $df = 1,22$; $p = 0.038$).

The improvements were by no means trivial; the experimental group improved by an average of 2.14 points on Arithmetic versus 0.7 for the control group. Indeed, for Forward and Backward Digit Span, Picture Completion, Block Design and Arithmetic tests, performance in the experimental group was virtually normalized. Since it is unlikely that any remedial procedure would produce an improvement on pre-morbid status, the changes represent the maximum feasible change on these measures with the given levels of initial performance, and it may be that ceiling effects limited the differential improvement.

Discussion of Results

There are a number of possible explanations for such differences other than the specific effects of the attentional retraining procedures. Spontaneous recovery seems unlikely. Firstly, the groups were closely matched as regards demographic variables and initial values of the tests. There is no reason to suppose that one group was systematically more prone to spontaneous recovery. Also, the variable known to be most closely associated with extent of spontaneous recovery is time since injury. Allowing for the effects of this makes little difference to the results.

Perhaps some training or stimulating effect of using microcomputers produces an increase in test scores. In the context of differential sensitivity between the groups to these effects, this might have produced the observed greater improvement for the experimental group. The same considerations of matching and randomization apply as for spontaneous recovery.

Premorbid cognitive status (represented by National Adult Reading Test (NART) Estimated IQ), spared capacity (represented by the initial values for each test) and age are related, to extent of both spontaneous recovery and 'trainability'. Allowing for these made little difference to the results.

The results could be affected by different levels of motivation in the two groups. The general level of motivation in brain-injured patients to participate in any meaningful activity can be reduced in two quite different ways: by depression or other sorts of emotional disorder, existing independently of, as a reaction to, or as a consequence of the brain damage; and by the sort of apathy and lack of engagement characteristic of organic brain syndromes. Emotional distress is measured in this study using the 28 item version of the General Health Questionnaire (GHQ-28) (Goldberg, 1978) and the personality and motivational effects of organic syndromes by the Social Behaviour Assessment Schedule (SBAS) (Platt *et al.*, 1978). The groups were comparable on GHQ and SBAS.

One difficulty in this study was that most differences between the groups became apparent only at follow-up. In those tests for which significant differences emerged, the overall pattern was, for the experimental group, improvement starting in the training phase and continuing, sometimes less strongly, into the follow-up phase: for the control group, no real improvement occurred in either the training phase or the follow-up phase taken separately, but in some cases, there was improvement when both phases were taken together. The differential improvement, then, started during training but continued after formal training had stopped. This reflects the pattern obtained in Sohlberg and Mateer's earlier study on attentional retraining (Sohlberg and Mateer, 1987).

This pattern of results fits a skills-training model where one might expect some benefit as the skill is first learned and implemented but increasing benefit as it becomes more automated and integrated into a wider range of behaviours. There were age effects; in some cases, the age/dependent variable covariance was not homogeneous across the groups, implying a differential sensitivity to the treatment depending on age. This is what would be expected of any sort of training. Overall, taking account of age did attenuate (but did not destroy) the experimental effects.

Training may involve new, verbally mediated strategies. There is some reason to believe that verbal-mediated strategies for self-arousal and for combating interference effects in working memory are involved in the training tasks used here, and that this can produce improvement in non-trained tests of attentional function (Gray and Robertson, 1989). On the other hand, explicit training in the use of verbally mediated strategies failed to produce improvements in frontal function or 'mindfulness' as measured by the WCST. One possible reason for this might be found in Luria's observation that patients with lesions to the left frontal lobe were incapable of benefiting from self-instruction.

The training package was heavily weighted towards tasks involving the storage and manipulation of material working memory. A number of tests of these functions (PASAT, Arithmetic, and Backward Digit Span) seem to have improved as a result, indicating some possible specificity of effect. WAIS-R Block Design also showed greater improvement in the training condition. This task presumably involves the deployment of visual attention. Again, the training procedures for the experimental group included a number of tasks involving visual scanning. However, improvements were not seen in other tests involving visual attention, such as Letter cancellation. Also, block design involves frontal functions such as planning and sequencing. Frontal function was specifically targetted, yet no improvements were found on other frontal measures. It is difficult, then, to tie improvements in specific tests to specific training procedures.

Van Zomeren *et al.* (1986) have argued that the core deficit in diffuse brain injury is a 'Divided Attentional Deficit' (Shiffrin and Schneider, 1977), and that the core of this deficit is slowed (controlled) information processing. It seems inherently unlikely that such a relatively brief intervention could significantly affect such a basic parameter, however, phasic attention is disrupted in head injury. Phasic attention functions to provide short-lived increases in readiness to respond involving increased speed of information processing. The training effect may, at least in part, involve the learning of verbal habits for the regulation of arousal and the control of contents in working memory.

Unilateral Neglect

Unilateral visual neglect is a common result of CVA or other brain damage of acute onset (Denes *et al.*, 1982). It is more common after damage to the right hemisphere (Hècaen, 1962). The central feature is a relative lack of attention to, or response to, features on one side of space, usually the left. Although it is often found in association with visual field defects, it is not explained by them (Hècaen, 1962). There is good evidence that some data from the neglected portion of space is processed pre-attentively (Volpe, 1979) and that the amount of neglect varies with the information load (Pillon, 1981). Both phenomena locate neglect squarely within the attentional domain. It is a failure on the selectivity dimension of attention. However, it is certainly not a unitary phenomenon, and various features of the syndrome can be found in various combinations. It is important both in terms of its incidence (45% after CVA), and its rehabilitation significance, e.g. in activities of daily living (Denes *et al.*, 1982; Wade *et al.*, 1983).

Procedures for rehabilitating neglect have included training in systematic scanning, 'end-anchoring', line bisection, size estimation and spatial location and have generated some promising results (Diller *et al.*, 1974; Weinberg *et al.*, 1979, 1982; Gordon *et al.*, 1985; Gouvier *et al.*, 1987) suggesting that visual neglect is partially remediable.

Study 3

Robertson *et al.* (1988) studied the effects of computerized training procedures in three patients suffering from unilateral left visual neglect. One of the patients was head injured and two had suffered CVAs.

In the first two cases, training was based on a computer program (Gianutsos and Klitzner, 1981) which presented an array of shapes, all but one identical. The slightly different odd shape appeared an equal number of times on the left and on the right of the screen, and the subject's task was to press a key as soon as it was seen. The median search time for correct trials on left and right halves of the field provides an index of neglect. The aim of the training was to establish the habit for orienting leftwards, based on intact verbal processes and on intact abilities for cued eye, head and attentional shifts towards the left. A simple self-instructional procedure (Meichenbaum and Goodman, 1971) was employed. The command 'look left' being given loudly by the trainer just prior to the display. This was continued for a number of trials until the left-right discrepancy was reduced. The patient was then cued to give the command out loud, first softly, then without cueing, then sub-vocally. In the third case the procedure was more or less the same, but parts of it were automated in a custom-built program described later.

A multiple-baseline-by-function design showed selective improvements on tasks unrelated to the training procedures. These target functions included reading and other daily-living activities such as telephone dialling. In all cases, six or seven training sessions were given with sudden improvement on target functions generally appearing after one or two sessions.

Study 4

On the basis of this study, a controlled trial of the training was carried out. Thirty-six subjects were recruited to the trial. All showed significant unilateral, left visual field neglect according to the Behavioural Inattention Test (BIT) (Wilson *et al.*, 1987) and were aged 80 or under, oriented for time and place, not suffering from progressive or degenerative neurological conditions and were able to concentrate sufficiently to sit at a computer-based task for at least 15 minutes.

Subjects were randomly allocated to the experimental training and control procedures within blocks, the blocks comprising severe versus mild neglect on the one hand and stroke versus non-stroke cause of neglect on the other. Assessment was carried out blind at intake, end of training and six months follow-up. A wide range of psychological and neuropsychological tests were given.

The training procedure consisted of the three programs described below.

Search for the odd shape

A number of shapes are presented on the screen, all but one identical. The subject must identify the one which is different by touching the screen. The nature of the shapes can be varied and combined with different odd shapes, and the total number of shapes can be 4, 16 or 64. At the beginning of training, subjects were first given an assessment version of this program. They received intensive briefing about the nature of their problems as well as showing them computer-displayed bar charts illustrating the difference in left-right latencies.

Subjects were first trained in 'systematic clockwise scanning' (Weinberg *et al.*, 1982), using a 'scanning window' by touching each of the screen quadrants in a pre-determined order. The 'odd one out' task was presented with the 'scanning box' superimposed. In this task the person searches for the odd shape using the box as a viewfinder. A voice synthesizer and a flashing left-pointing arrow with the words 'Look Left' prominently displayed, cued the subject to look left, and subjects are encouraged to verbalize this. As the latencies decrease, cueing is gradually phased out.

Touch Left

This is a computerization of the 'end-anchoring' procedure used for reading training by Weinberg *et al.* (1979). A target is presented at the top of the screen and a series of matching targets and distractors below. The task is for the person to locate and touch the targets as quickly as possible. Accurate detection is signalled by auditory and visual reward related to the speed of response. Before each response, subjects must touch a red band at the far left of the screen which immediately turns green. Failure to do this results in the computer flashing a message 'Touch Left' across the screen, along with a flashing arrow, until the person touches the red band. The red band is gradually faded, until ultimately the person touches left without any visual cue.

Again after each cycle, the computer presents a bar chart showing left versus right latencies. As the latencies equalize, the difficulty is increased. This program allows an infinite number of tasks ranging from simple object matching tasks to ones requiring calculation (e.g. a target of 'numbers divisible by 9' and an array of numbers, some divisible by 9 and some not).

Block Design

Finally, a computerized visuo-spatial training program similar to Diller *et al.*'s (1974) block design training procedure was used. The mean number of training hours for the experimental group was 15.5 (s.d. 1.8). This time was close to the 20 hours of training which Weinberg *et al.* (1977) found to be effective in producing detectable improvements in neglect. Mean hours for the control group was 11.4 (s.d. 5.2), significantly less than the experimental group.

At end of training, only the Picture Completion test showed a statistically significant difference ($t = 2.5$; $df = 31$; $p = .018$). Analysis of covariance was performed with initial BIT as the covariate. Results remained essentially the same. Using the original selection criteria, there was no significant difference between the proportion of subjects in each group who continued to show neglect. When the subjects showing cognitive deterioration over the period of training were excluded, an analysis of covariance showed no treatment effect for this group of subjects. Twenty-seven subjects were followed up at six months. There were no significant differences between groups on any measure. If anything, the control group showed a greater proportion of improvers than the experimental.

Training had, therefore, no effect on the level or frequency of occurrence of neglect. Separate analysis of the more severe patients' data did not alter the initial findings. Similarly, exclusion of patients showing cognitive deterioration failed to yield any difference between groups. Less than a third of the subjects showed recovery of neglect during the training period, and significant further improvements were not observed over the next six months.

Discussion of Results

This finding is difficult to reconcile with the single-case studies published previously (Robertson *et al.*, 1988). One possibility is that the subjects in this trial were poor rehabilitation 'bets'. However, the analyses carried out above on the more severe and on the non-deteriorating patients do not support this. The three single-case studies lasted less than three weeks and a very rapid training effect was obtained. It may be that these training procedures induced insight learning in a number of patients in whom learning would have happened anyway, and that, in the longer term, these improvements were swamped by the natural recovery processes. Alternatively, the control procedure may have had some similar insight-producing effect.

There have been reports of lasting, widely generalized improvements in neglect, including improvements in practical activities ranging from physiotherapy to tasks such as serving tea, following training on computer-scanning tasks very similar to the ones described above with extensive training on a very large video screen, rather than on the standard computer screen. Certainly, the original studies of scanning training by Weinberg, Diller and Ben-Yishay (Diller *et al.*, 1974) used a scanning apparatus 2 metres across. Perhaps, where the effect depends on insight, the exact physical parameters of the training situation are not important and the amount of training need not be extensive. When the intention is to produce motor habits, on the other hand, training needs to be extensive, and the physical parameters should match as closely as possible the real-life situation.

Conclusions

Attention training seemed to produce improvements in attentional function in a mixed group of patients who suffered from the sort of generalized attentional problems common after closed-head injury, but not restricted to closed-head injury. In the single-case studies, in the group study, and in Sohlberg and Mateer's earlier study (Sohlberg and Mateer, 1987), the pattern of results fits a skills-training model. There was some reason from the single-case studies to believe that verbal-mediated strategies for self-arousal and for combating interference effects in working memory were involved in the improvement in non-trained tests of attentional function (Gray and Robertson, 1989). On the other hand, explicit training in the use of verbal strategies failed to produce improvements in maintaining and switching set (however, see Alderman and Burgess, Chapter 9). The results were compatible with those of the Ben-Yishay group (Rattock *et al.*, 1982), who report that their orientation-remediation programme improved scores of WAIS Picture Completion and Digit Span. How much these improvements on psychometric tests generalize to everyday function is an open question.

The results with patients suffering from unilateral neglect were disappointing. Initial success with the single-case studies was replaced by total failure in the group studies. Yet there is abundant evidence that neglect is remediable. The most likely explanation seems to be that while the single-case studies showed the effects of one sort of learning (insight learning), the group studies failed because the experimental procedures did not produce any useful form of incremental, motor habit learning. As no useful habit learning occurred due to the experimental procedures, this study also leaves open the role of verbal mediation in producing behaviour change.

It seems then that gains in certain aspects of attentional functioning can be produced by limited amounts of training. The precise mechanisms involved in producing changes in performance remain unclear, and, hence, the conditions for promoting useful learning generalized to everyday function also remain unknown.

References

BADDELEY, A., 1986, *Working Memory* (Oxford: OUP).

BENTON, A. L., VAN ALLEN, M. W. and FOGEL, M. L., 1964, 'Temporal orientation in cerebral disease'. *Journal of Nervous and Mental Disease*, **139**, 110–19.

BEN-YISHAY, Y., RATTOCK, J. and DILLER, L. A., 1979, 'A remedial "module" for the systematic amelioration of basic attentional disturbances in head trauma patients'. In *Working Approaches to Remediation of Cognitive Deficits in Brain Damaged Persons: Rehabilitation Monograph No. 61*, New York University Medical Center.

BORKOWSKI, J. G., BENTON, A. L. and SPREEN, O., 1967, 'Word fluency and brain damage'. *Neuropsychologia*, **5**, 135–40.

BRAUN, C., BARTOLINI, G. and BOUCHARD, A., 1985, *Cognitive Rehabilitation Software*. Université de Quebec à Montreal.

BROOKS, N., MCKINLAY, W., SYMINGTON, C., BEATTIE, A. and CAMPSIE, L., 1987, 'Return to work within the first seven years of severe head injury'. *Brain Injury*, **1**, 5–19.

CONKEY, R. C., 1938, 'Psychological changes associated with head injuries'. *Archives Psychology*, **33**, 1–62.

CURRY, S. H., 1981, 'Event-related potentials as indicants of structural and functional damage in closed head injury'. *Progress in Brain Research*, **54**, 507–15.

DAVIES, D. R., 1983, 'Attention, arousal and effort'. In *Physiological Correlates of Human Behaviour*, (London: Academic Press).

DENES, G., SEMENZA, C., STOPPA, E. and LIS, A., 1982, 'Unilateral spatial neglect and recovery from hemiplegia: a follow up study'. *Brain*, **105**, 543–52.

DEUTSCH, J. A. and DEUTSCH, D., 1963, 'Attention: some theoretical considerations'. *Psychological Review*, **80**, 80–90.

DILLER, L., BEN-YISHAY, Y., GERSTMAN, L., GOODKIN, R., GORDON, W. and WEINBERG, J., 1974, *Studies in Cognition and Rehabilitation in Hemiplegia. Rehabilitation Monograph No. 50*, New York University Medical Center.

DYER, F. N., 1973, The Stroop phenomenon and its use in the study of perceptual, cognitive and response processes'. *Memory and Cognition*, **1**, 106–20.

GIANUTSOS, R. and KLITZNER, C., 1981, *Computer P.ogrammes for Cognitive Rehabilitation, Volume 1* (New Jersey: Life Science Associates).

GOLDBERG, D., 1978, *General Health Questionnaire* (Windsor: NFER).

GOLDSTEIN, K., 1952, 'The effects of brain damage on personality'. *Psychiatry*, 15, 245–60.

GORDON, W., HIBBARD, M. R., EGELKO, S., DILLER, L., SHAVER, P., LIEBERMAN, A. and RAGNARSON, L., 1985, 'Perceptual remediation in patients with right brain damage: a comprehensive program'. *Archives of Physical Medicine and Rehabilitation*, **66**, 353–9.

GOUVIER, W., BUA, B., BLANTON, P. and UREY, J., 1987, 'Behavioural changes following visual scanning training: observation of five cases'. *International Journal of Clinical Neuropsychology*, **9**, 74–80.

GOUVIER, W., COTTAM, G., WEBSTER, J., BEISSEL, G. and WOFFORD, J., 1983, 'Behavioural interventions with stroke patients for improving wheelchair navigation'. *International Journal of Clinical Neuropsychology*, **1**, 186–90.

GRAY, J. M. and ROBERTSON, I., 1989, 'Remediation of attentional difficulties following brain-injury; 3 experimental single-case studies'. *Brain Injury*, **3**, 163–70.

GRONWALL, D. M. A. and WRIGHTSON, P., 1974, 'Delayed recovery of intellectual function after minor head injury'. *Lancet*, **ii**, 605–9.

GRONWALL, D. M. A., 1977, 'Paced Auditory Serial Addition Task: A measure of recovery from concussion'. *Perceptual and Motor Skills*, **44**, 367–73.

GROSS, Y., BEN-NAHUM, Z., MUNK, G., 1982, 'Techniques and applications of simultaneous information processing'. In L. E. Texler (Ed.) *Cognitive Rehabilitation: Conceptualisation and Intervention* (New York: Plenum).

HÈCAEN, H., 1962, 'Clinical symptomology in right and left hemispheric lesions'. In V. B. Montcastle (Ed.) *Interhemispheric Relations and Cerebral Dominance* (Baltimore: Johns Hopkins Press).

JENNETT, B. and TEASEDALE, G., 1981, *Management of Head Injuries* (Philadelphia: Davis).

KLOVE, H., 1987, 'Activation, arousal and neuropsychological rehabilitation'. *Journal of Clinical and Experimental Neuropsychology*, **9**, 297–309.

LURIA, A. R., 1963, *Restoration of Function after Brain Injury* (Oxford: Pergamon).

MEICHENBAUM, D., GOODMAN, J., 1971, 'Training impulsive children to talk to themselves: a means of developing self-control'. *Journal of Abnormal Psychology*, **77**, 115–26.

MELAMED, S., STERN, M., RAHMANI, L., GROSSWASSER, Z. and NAJENSON, T., 1985, 'Attention capacity limitation, psychiatric parameters and their impact on work involvement following brain injury'. *Scandinavian Joiurnal of Rehabilitation Medicine Supplement*, **12**, 21–6.

MILLER, E., 1970, 'Simple and choice reaction time following severe head injury'. *Cortex*, **6**, 121–7.

MILLER, E. and CRUZAT, A., 1981, 'A note on the effect of irrelevant information on task performance after mild and severe head injury'. *British Journal of Social and Clinical Psychology*, **20**, 69–70.

NEALE, M., 1958, *Neale Analysis of Reading Ability* (London: Macmillan).

NEISSER, U., 1976, *Cognition and Reality* (San Francisco: Freeman).

NELSON, H. E., 1976, 'A modified card sorting test sensitive to frontal lobe deficit'. *Cortex*, **12**, 313–24.

NISSEN, M. J. and BULLEMER, P., 1987, 'Attentional requirements of learning: evidence from performance measures'. *Cognitive Psychology*, **19**, 1–32.

PILLON, B., 1981, 'Negligence de l'hemi-espace gauche dans des spreuves visuo-constructive. (Influence de la complexite spatiale et de la methode de compensation)'. *Neuropsychologia*, **19**, 317–20.

PLATT, S., HIRSCH, S., WEYMAN, A., 1978, *Social Behaviour Assessment Schedule (3rd Edition)*, (Windsor: NFER).

POSNER, M. I. and BOIES, S. J., 1971, 'Components of attention'. *Psychological Review*, **78**, 391–408.

POSNER, M. I. and SNYDER, C. R. R., 1975, 'Attention and cognitive control'. In R. L. Solso (Ed.) *Information Processing and Cognition: The Loyola Symposium* (New Jersey: Erlbaum).

POSNER, M. I. and RAFAL, R. D., 1987, 'Cognitive theories of attention and the rehabilitation of attentional deficits'. In M. J. Meier, L. Diller and A. L. Benton (Eds) *Neuropsychological Rehabilitation* (London: Churchill Livingston).

RATTOCK, J., BEN-YISHAY, Y., ROSS, B., LAKIN, P., SILVER, S., THOMAS, L. and DILLER, L. A., 1982, 'Diagnostic-remedial system for basic attentional disorders in head trauma patients undergoing rehabilitation: A preliminary report'. In *Working Approaches to Remediation of Cognitive Deficits in Brain Damaged Persons: Rehabilitation Monograph No. 64*, New York University Medical Center.

REASON, J., 1984, 'Lapses of attention in everyday life'. In R. Parasuraman and D. R. Davies (Eds) *Varieties of Attention* (Orlando, Florida: Academic Press).

REY, A., 1941, 'L'examen psychologique dans le cas d'encephalopathie traumatique'. *Archives de Psychologie*, **28**, 286–340.

RIVAMONTE, V. and REDFIELD, J., 1987, 'Differential effects of video game training and psychotherapy in rehabilitation of right CVA patients'. Presented at *15th Annual Meeting of the International Neuropsychological Society*, Washington DC.

RIZZO, P. A., AMABILE, G., CAPORALI, M., SPADARO, M., ZANASI, M. and MOROCUTTI, C., 1978, 'A CNV study in a group of patients with traumatic head injuries'. *Electroencephalography and Clinical Neurophysiology*, **45**, 281–5.

ROBERTSON, I., GRAY, J. and MCKENZIE, S., 1988, 'Microcomputer-based cognitive rehabilitation of visual neglect: three multiple baseline single-case studies'. *Brain Injury*, **2**, 151–63.

SCHERZER, B. P., 1986, 'Rehabilitation following severe head trauma: Results of a three year program'. *Archives of Physical Medicine Rehabilitation*, **67**, 366–74.

SHALLICE, T., 1982, Specific impairments of planning. *Philosophical Transactions of the Royal Society of London*, **298**, 199–209.

SHIFFRIN, R. and SCHNEIDER, W., 1977, 'Controlled and automatic human information-processing: Perceptual learning, automatic attending, and a general theory'. *Psychological Review*, **84**, 127–90.

SOHLBERG, M. and MATEER, M., 1987, 'Effectiveness of an attention-training programme'. *Journal of Clinical and Experimental Neuropsychology*, **9**, 117–30.

STUSS, D. T., ELY, P., HUGENHOLTZ, H., RICHARDS, M. T., LA ROCHELLE, S., POIRIER, C. A. and BELL, I., 1985, Subtle neuropsychological deficits in patients with good recovery after closed head injury'. *Neurosurgery*, **17**, 41–7.

TEASDALE, G., JENNETT, B., 1974, 'Assessment of coma and impaired consciousness: A practical scale'. *Lancet*, **2**, 81–6.

TREISMAN, A., 1964, 'Monitoring and storage of irrelevant messages in selective attention'. *Journal of Verbal Learning and Verbal Behaviour*, **3**, 449–559.

VAN ZOMEREN, A. H. and BROUWER, F., 1987, 'Head injury and concepts of attention'. In H. S. Levin, J. Grafman and H. M. Eisenberg (Eds) *Neurobehavioural Recovery from Head Injury* (New York: Oxford University Press).

VAN ZOMEREN, A. H., BROUWER, F. and DEELMAN, B. G., 1986, 'Attentional deficits: The riddles of selectivity, speed and alertness'. In D. N. Brooks (Ed.) *Closed Head Injury: Psychological, Social and Family Consequences* (Oxford: OUP).

VOLPE, B. T., LEDOUX, J. E. and GAZZANIGA, M. S., 1979, 'Information processing of visual stimuli in the extinguished field'. *Nature*, **282**, 722–44.

WADE, D., SKILBECK, C. and LANGTON-HEWER, R., 1983, 'Predicting Barthel ADL score at 6 months after an acute stroke'. *Archives of Physical Medicine and Rehabilitation*, **64**, 24–8.

WECHSLER, D., 1945, 'A standardized memory scale for clinical use'. *Journal of Psychology*, **19**, 87–95.

WECHSLER, D., 1981, *The Wechsler Adult Intelligence Scale-Revised* (Ohio: The Psychological Corporation).

WEINBERG, J., PIASETSKY, E., DILLER, L. and GORDON, W., 1982, 'Treating perceptual organisation deficits in non-neglecting RBD stroke patients'. *Journal of Clinical Neuropsychology*, **4**, 59–75.

WEINBERG, J., DILLER, L., GORDON, W., GERSTMAN, L., LIEBERMAN, A., LAKIN, P., HODGES, G. and EZRACHI, O., 1977, *Archives of Physical Medicine Rehabilitation*, **58**, 479–86.

WEINBERG, J., DILLER, L., GORDON, W., GERSTMAN, L., LIEBERMAN, A., LAKIN, P., HODGES, G. and EZRACHI, O., 1979, 'Training sensory awareness and spatial organisation in people with right brain damage'. *Archives of Physical Medicine Rehabilitation*, **60**, 491–6.

WILSON, B., COCKBURN, J. and HALLIGAN, P., 1987, 'Development of a behavioural test of visuospatial neglect'. *Archives of Physical Medicine Rehabilitation*, **68**, 98–102.

WOOD, R. Ll., 1986, 'Rehabilitation of patients with disorders of attention'. *Journal of Head Trauma Research*, **1**, 45–53.

Chapter 3

The Use of Computers in the Rehabilitation of Attention Disorders

J. Ponsford

Introduction

In recent years there has been increasing recognition of the implications of the cognitive and behavioural changes which result from brain injury. In many cases these represent the greatest impediments to successful rehabilitation. This has led to the birth of a new discipline — 'cognitive rehabilitation' (Gianutsos, 1980; Ben-Yishay and Diller, 1981; Diller and Gordon, 1981; Powell, 1981; Trexler, 1982; Miller, 1984; Uzzell and Gross, 1986; Meier *et al.*, 1987). At its foundation lies the assumption that disorders of attention, memory, concept formation and thought organization can be improved by remediation.

The use of computers in the rehabilitation of cognitive deficits has increased so rapidly in recent years that it has become almost synonymous with the term 'cognitive rehabilitation'. The computer certainly offers a number of advantages as a medium of therapy. A large amount of software is now available for the treatment of specific cognitive deficits. However, as with many approaches to cognitive rehabilitation, its development and use has not always been clearly based on a careful analysis of brain-behaviour relationships and scientific evaluation of its effectiveness. The aim of this chapter is to explore the use of computers within the context of the evolving discipline of cognitive rehabilitation.

Approaches to the Remediation of Cognitive Deficits

A review of the literature reveals that there are well over 100 studies in which cognitive rehabilitation techniques have been described or evaluated in recent years. These studies have been classified by several authors in terms of their conceptual approach to remediation (Powell, 1981; Miller, 1984), and these will be outlined briefly. Pharmacological treatments will not be discussed within the confines of this chapter.

Non-directed stimulation or practice

This method, described by Powell (1981), is probably the most commonly used in rehabilitation settings, perhaps because it is the way skills are most commonly acquired in our lives. The patient is asked to practice on tasks he/she finds difficult. Its use is based on the assumption that cognitive functions, such as memory, respond like 'mental muscles', and that exercising them on one task will strengthen them for use on other tasks. However, there is no experimental evidence to support this 'mental muscle' view (Schacter and Glisky, 1986). Powell (1981) has expressed the view that the use of repeated practice may take patients more quickly to their plateau level, but there is no reason to suppose that it carries them beyond this plateau of spontaneous recovery, because it does not teach any extra skills.

Directed or specific stimulation

In the practice or non-directed stimulation paradigm, the brain is stimulated by the tasks imposed on the patient, but little regard is paid to the precise functional relationship between brain and task and the manner in which they interact (Powell, 1981). The second paradigm, directed or specific stimulation, necessitates a careful analysis of such relationships. A pre-requisite to such an approach is, of course, a detailed neuropsychological assessment, which offers a description in terms of lost functions or skills, and their neuroanatomical correlates. The next step is to find a task which adequately and directly reflects this skill. Repeated, but highly structured practice is given on this task, gradually changing parameters, such as complexity, quantity, speed of presentation or the amount of cuing given, depending on the goal of therapy.

Much of the work of Diller, Ben-Yishay, Gordon, and their colleagues fits into this category, most notably what Diller and Gordon (1981) refer to as the 'psychometrist' and 'biologist' models of cognitive rehabilitation. Their work is impressive, not only in terms of the careful way in which the training programmes were devised and implemented, but also because they were evaluated in terms of their generalization to certain everyday tasks.

However, based on recent reviews of the literature on recovery of function by authors such as Laurence and Stein (1978), one must seriously question the apparent assumption underlying this approach, that our understanding of brain-behaviour relationships is such that one can be sure that specific abilities or parts of the brain are being stimulated by a given task. Indeed, many of the tasks used in this approach, including those which are computer-mediated, are multi-factorial in nature, so that it becomes difficult to separate such therapy from the non-specific stimulation or practice paradigm. Unfortunately, whilst there are many papers describing therapy according to the non-directed and directed stimulation paradigms, there is a marked dearth of proper evaluative studies which control adequately for spontaneous recovery, practice effects and non-specific treatment effects to assess the degree to which training generalizes to aspects of everyday life and whether gains are maintained over time.

Behaviourist approach

This third form of therapy involves the use of feedback and reinforcement to maximize the speed, extent and level of learning or recovery on the part of the patient. Whilst there is a paucity of group studies, there is now quite a body of evidence from single-case studies supporting the efficacy of the use of behaviour modification techniques to treat not only disturbed behaviour, but also speech behaviour (Horton, 1979), memory problems (Dolan and Norton, 1977; Wilson, 1984, 1987) and activities of daily living (Godfrey and Knight, 1988) following brain injury.

Compensation

The aim of this approach is to facilitate functional reorganization or adaptation to disability, rather than to restore lost function. It is thus linked conceptually with the theory that recovery of function occurs by such processes. The emphasis is shifted from the patient's weaknesses to his/her strengths, since it is intact abilities which must be utilized to overcome difficulties or learn to manage despite them. Clearly, the extent to which simple, functional substitution is possible depends on the extent to which the function is amenable to alternative modes of processing (Powell, 1981).

Compensatory approaches which have been advocated for the treatment of memory problems have included the use of visual imagery mnemonics to compensate for verbal memory deficits (Patten, 1972; Cermak, 1975; Crovitz, 1979, Gasparrini and Satz, 1979; Binder and Schreiber, 1980) and the use of verbal mediation to overcome visual or non-verbal problems (Glasgow *et al.*, 1977). An important question, however, is whether the use of such techniques, whilst helpful in a laboratory situation, can be effective for patients in their everyday lives. It would appear that many of the techniques are either quite impractical or too complex for everyday use.

Environmental manipulation

This may involve designing environments to benefit brain-injured people, such as job situations which are not noisy or stressful, where duties have been broken down for those who think concretely and which place minimal demands on memory. It may also involve training relatives and friends or using other external means to control or shape the brain-injured person's behaviour or provide necessary prompting and structure in order to achieve therapeutic goals, especially in cases where the brain-injured client lacks the capacity to learn (Wood, 1984). There has been relatively little emphasis on such approaches in the cognitive rehabilitation literature to date.

The Use of Computers in Cognitive Rehabilitation

Computers have most commonly been applied to the remediation of cognitive deficits according to the non-directed and directed stimulation paradigms. Workers such as Bracy (1982, 1983), Gianutsos (1980), Gianutsos and Klitzner (1981), Lynch (1983), and Sbordone (1983) have designed and used computer programs to assess and stimulate specific functions such as reaction time, visual scanning, attention, speed of information processing, recent memory and problem solving. These programs have subsequently been marketed and used widely in rehabilitation settings. As already pointed out, they offer a number of advantages over traditional methods of presenting therapy tasks. They allow the therapist to systematically alter task parameters and monitor and record patients' responses objectively. They save time for therapists, both occupying patients therapeutically and recording their performances, thereby cutting costs. They provide immediate feedback to patients, thereby potentially increasing their awareness of their limitations. They are also intrinsically motivating. It is not clear, however, that their development and use has been the result of such a careful process as that used by Ben-Yishay, Diller and their colleagues.

There have been relatively few published studies examining the effects of computer-assisted cognitive retraining according to the non-directed or directed stimulation paradigms. Early studies examined the effects of playing video games. Okoye and Hollander (unpublished study, 1980) found, in a small sample of 'perceptually handicapped' children, that playing video games, in lieu of more standard perceptual motor skills training, resulted in greater improvement on measures of visual-motor coordination in comparison with controls. Jones *et al.* (1981) and Kennedy *et al.* (1981), both cited by Lynch (1984), described the use of commercial video games substituted for conventional methods of training visual tracking in naval trainees. They found that video game training was generally equivalent to standard training.

Sivak and others (1983) evaluated the effects of training on computer-based cognitive retraining programs upon driving-related perceptual deficits. Right cerebrovascular accident (CVA) subjects showed improvement on several measures, whilst the two head-injured subjects improved only on selected measures. No control group was included, and, as this was a pilot study, the results must be evaluated with extreme caution.

Malec *et al.* (1984) used a randomized double cross-over design to evaluate the effectiveness of a video game, 'Target Fun', on sustained attention in 10 head-injured subjects who were less than six months post-injury. No significant differences were found between the games and no games conditions, although as a group the subjects showed improvement in sustained attention, as measured on a range of psychometric measures.

Wood and Fussey (1987) reported the results of a study in which a group of seven severely head-injured subjects were trained on a number of computer-mediated tasks with the aim of improving attentional skills (reaction time, selective attention, speed of processing). Results showed some positive effects on a couple of psychomotor tasks, but overall there was little evidence that the programme had a significant effect on performance on dependent psychometric measures. There was, however, a significant improvement in attentional behaviour, as measured in the therapy situation.

Sohlberg and Mateer (1987) employed a single-case, multiple baseline across behaviours design to assess the impact of training on a hierarchy of five sets of treatment tasks aimed at different aspects of attention and labelled 'Attention Process Training' (APT). Training was conducted over a period of four to eight weeks in four brain-injured subjects who were more than twelve months post-injury. All subjects showed improvement in their scores on the Paced Auditory Serial Addition Test (PASAT) (Gronwall and Sampson, 1974) during the attention training phase, and improvements remained above baseline levels throughout the period of post-attention training measurement. Training of and improvement in attentional skills was not routinely associated with improvements in visual processing abilities, and training of visual processing did not generally impact upon PASAT performance. The authors reported other functional gains made by their subjects, noting that these gains correlated in time with improvements in cognitive peformance. However, this study has some limitations. The baseline phase was significantly shorter than the intervention phases in most cases, placing limitations on the interpretation of trends seen in the data points. Furthermore, no attempt was made to control for the effects of the concurrent intervention subjects were receiving in activities of daily living, prevocational and psychosocial skills. In the absence of such controls, it is not valid to attribute the functional gains made by the subjects to the attentional training alone.

Finally, Robertson, Gray and McKenzie (1988) reported the results of three, single-case studies, again using a multiple baseline across behaviours design, in which attentional problems were treated through computer training on various combinations of a range of information-processing tasks. In each case, significant gains were made on target measures of attention (digit span and arithmetic) during the intervention phase, whilst no gains were made on the control measures (discrimination reaction time, Buschke Selective Reminding Test). However, given that the control measures also measured aspects of attention which were involved in the training tasks, one is first led to question why they were selected as control measures in the first place and second, why the training had no impact on these measures. One is able to glean nothing from these studies regarding which specific aspects of attention were being trained and how the target measures were related to these.

There have also been a number of descriptive reports of uncontrolled case studies by Bracy (1982), Gianutsos (1980), Lynch (1983) and Molloy and Garner (1988) which have shown positive results.

Thus, studies evaluating the impact on cognitive deficits of stimulation using computer-mediated tasks have shown mixed results. However, all of these studies showed certain limitations. In particular, there were no reported attempts to analyse the nature of the cognitive deficit in the patients being studied in order to establish a clear relationship between the deficit, the training tasks used and the dependent measures of effectiveness of training. With the exception of the study by Wood and Fussey (1987), all of the studies used performance on neuropsychological tests as the sole measure of the effectiveness of the remedial intervention. In recent years, however, a number of authors have demonstrated that neuropsychological test data do not necessarily reflect everyday functioning of the patient, that is, they lack ecological validity (Hart and Hayden, 1986). The majority of the studies thus failed to demonstrate objectively the impact of training on the everyday lives of the patients.

It is also important to control for therapist attention, other forms of therapy given concurrently or practice effects. Wood and Fussey (1987) suggested that a possible reason for their failure to find significant effects was the fact that their subjects were one to two years post-injury. The findings of Black *et al.* (1975) support the view that early remedial intervention may be more beneficial than such late intervention, although this raises the methodological problem of separating response to treatment from spontaneous recovery. The studies by Malec *et al.* (1984), Sohlberg and Mateer (1987) and Gray and Robertson (1989) were the only ones in which a single-case design was utilized, thus enabling the examination of the individual responses of each subject to the intervention. This would seem to be particularly important in the case of closed-head injury, where injuries are heterogeneous.

Evaluation of a Remedial Programme for Attentional Deficits Resulting from Closed-Head Injury

In view of the limitations of these studies, Ponsford (1989) and Ponsford and Kinsella (1988) designed a study to evaluate the effectiveness of a remedial programme for attentional deficits resulting from closed-head injury.

The aims

In order to achieve this, the first aim of the study was to assess the nature of the attentional deficit in the severely head-injured population being studied and find which measures best reflected the deficit. The second aim was to design and validate a scale for measuring the patients' everyday attentional behaviours, to examine their correlation with the neuropsychological measures being used and their intra- and inter-rater reliability. The third aim was to design the treatment programme itself, based on the analysis of the attentional deficit, comparing the effectiveness of directed stimulation with computer-mediated attentional tasks alone with that of directed stimulation accompanied by therapist feedback and reinforcement. The final aim was to examine the individual responses of each subject with a view to establishing which head-injured patients were most likely to respond to such a programme and at what point in their recovery.

In order to fulfil the first aim of the study, Ponsford (1989) studied several aspects of attention in a group of 54 severely head-injured subjects. Those aspects of attention studied included selective attention [specifically, the presence of focused and divided attention deficits, as defined by Schneider and Shiffrin (1977)], sustained attention or vigilance as defined by Parasuraman (1984) and the Supervisory Attentional System, as defined by Shallice (1982). Consistent with the findings of previous studies, such as those of Miller (1970), Gronwall and Sampson (1974), van Zomeren (1981), van Zomeren and Brouwer (1987), Brouwer and van Wolffelaar (1985) and Stuss *et al.* (1985), Ponsford (1989) found no evidence for the presence of deficits in focused attention, sustained attention or Supervisory Attentional Control in the severely head-injured subjects studied. There was, however, ample evidence of the presence of divided attention deficits. These appeared to result from reduced speed of information processing, which, in turn, reduced the information processing capacity of the subjects. The neuropsychological measures of this deficit which best discriminated the head-injured subjects from controls included the Symbol Digit Modalities Test (Smith, 1973), simple and choice reaction time tasks (van Zomeren, 1981), colour naming and word reading scores on the Stroop (Stroop, 1935), a Letter Cancellation Task and the Paced Auditory Serial Addition Test (Gronwall and Sampson, 1974). In the light of these findings, speed of information processing was selected as the focus of treatment.

The next step was to develop and validate a rating scale of attentional behaviour, as it was manifested in functional performance in everyday settings, to be used by therapists as a measure of the effectiveness of the remedial intervention on the patients' attentional behaviour in therapy settings. The rating scale covered a number of components of attention, including alertness, aspects of selective attention, such as speed of thinking, distractibility, the capacity to pay attention to more than one thing at once and attention to detail, and the ability to sustain attention, as they were most likely to be manifested in a behavioural sense. Each of the 14 items selected was to be rated by the therapist on a scale from 0 to 4, representing the frequency with which the problem was apparent at the time the rating was made (0 = Not at all; 1 = Occasionally; 2 = Sometimes; 3 = Almost Always; 4 = Always).

The results of the study, in which 50 patients with severe closed-head injury of traumatic origin were rated on the scale by their Occupational Therapist at intervals of three days, showed that the scale had a very high level of internal consistency, and the intra-rater reliability was above 0.9. The scale showed correlations of 0.4 or above with a number of the neuropsychological measures of speed of information processing used in the previous study. It was concluded that the scale could be successfully used by one therapist over time as a measure of the impact of therapeutic interventions on attentional behaviour in the therapy setting.

The Remedial Programme

Ponsford and Kinsella (1988) went on to design a remedial programme which focused on deficits in speed of information processing following closed-head injury. In view of the findings of Black *et al.* (1975), which supported the view that early remedial intervention may be more beneficial than late intervention, the programme was implemented during the first 12 months after injury.

Participants in the study were 10 severely traumatically head-injured subjects (four males), ranging in age from 17 to 38 years, who were admitted to Bethesda Hospital, Melbourne, for rehabilitation. The average interval between injury and entry into the study was 13.8 weeks, the range being six to 34 weeks. The subjects' length of post-traumatic amnesia (PTA) ranged from 10 days to 12 weeks (mean = 5.5 weeks; sd = 4.8 weeks), indicating that the group fell into the very severely head-injured category. The subjects had an average of 11 years of education. On neuropsychological assessment, all subjects exhibited slow information processing and poor selective attention. Some also showed difficulties in sustaining attention and/or distractibility. On the rating scale of attentional behaviour, they were all judged clinically, by their Occupational Therapist, as exhibiting impaired attentional behaviour.

A single-case multiple baseline across subjects' design was employed, in which the treatment is applied in sequence across subjects. This design accommodated the potential heterogeneity of the subjects, the possibilities of an improving baseline due to practice effect or spontaneous recovery and an irreversible intervention effect. Staggering the onset of treatment served to separate out improvements due to factors unrelated to the specific remedial programme, such as practice, other forms of therapy or recovery. Baseline phases of just two lengths (three weeks and six weeks) were selected.

During the first three weeks of the programme, all subjects were given baseline procedures. During the baseline phase (A) and indeed all phases, neuropsychological measures of speed of information processing were taken three times per week. Subjects were otherwise engaged in their normal rehabilitation programme, which involved daily sessions of Occupational Therapy, Speech Therapy and Physiotherapy. During the next three weeks, five subjects continued in baseline and the other five commenced training in phase (B). During phase (B), which lasted three weeks, each subject underwent half-hour daily training sessions (totalling 15) on computer-mediated tasks designed to assess and train speed of visual reaction time, visual search and selective attention. Two of the training tasks (REACT and SEARCH) were designed by Gianutsos and Klitzner (1981), and the other three selective attention tasks were designed by the present author. Speed and accuracy scores were recorded. The therapist gave no feedback or reinforcement to the subject regarding his/her performance.

Phase (BC) was added on the basis that many head-injured patients lack insight, motivation and the capacity for carry-over from one therapy session to the next. It was felt that therapist feedback and reinforcement might maximize these factors. In this phase (BC), the same training tasks were given for a further three weeks, but the therapist took a reinforcing role by giving contingent verbal reinforcement consisting of (1) telling the patients they were doing well, (2) telling them their score for each task and recording it in a graph and (3) showing the patients by how much they had improved their performance when they had performed the task faster. When they performed more slowly than their former best time, they were simply told to move on to the next task. The final three-week phase involved a return to baseline, in order to see whether the gains, as measured by performance on the dependent measures of speed of information processing, were lost, maintained or consolidated once training had ceased.

Three forms of dependent measures were selected. The first three were neuropsychological measures of speed of information processing, selected from the first study on the basis that they discriminated significantly between head-injured and control subjects and were subject to minimal practice effect if alternate forms were used. They included (1) a four-choice reaction time task (as used by van Zomeren, 1981); (2) the Symbol Digit Modalities Test (Smith, 1973), of which five alternate forms were generated; and (3) a two-letter cancellation task, of which six alternate forms were generated. A further cognitive measure, not involving speed, was added as a control measure. This was the WAIS Similarities subtest, a measure of verbal conceptual ability. The fifth measure was the rating scale of attentional behaviour, which was rated by the patients' Occupational Therapist. The final measure of the impact of the remedial programme on the attentional behaviour of the patient in the therapy setting consisted of a half-hour video of the patient performing a clerical task in the Occupational Therapy Department. This was rated according to the percentage of the period which the patient spent directed to the task (defined by his/her eyes being focused on it). The Similarities subtest, rating scale of attentional behaviour and video were administered at the beginning and the end of each phase.

Findings

Results were analysed at both a group and a single-subject level. Group means for each

Figure 3.1 Mean results for each group on the choice reaction time task.

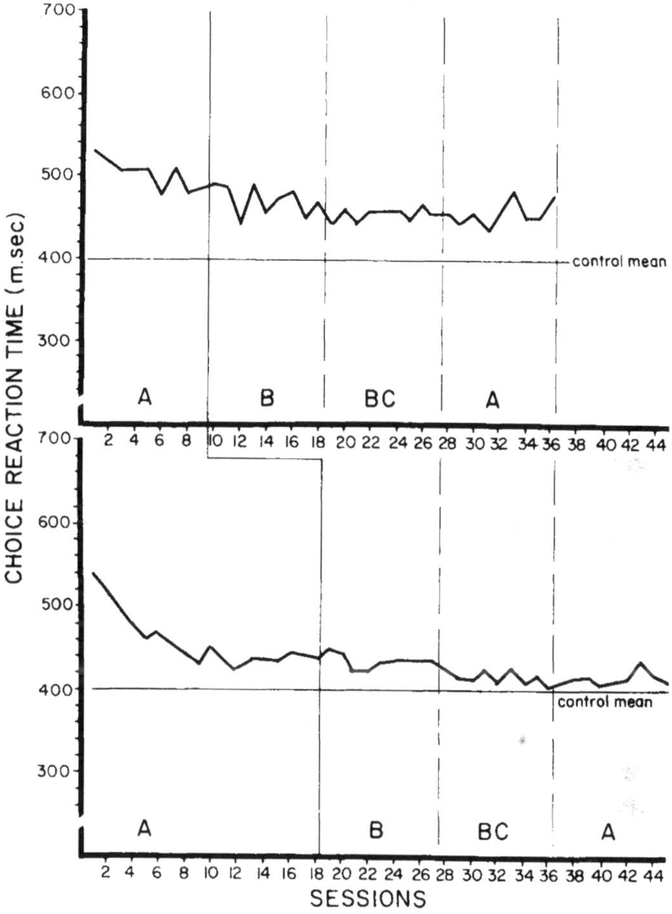

dependent measure, depicted in Figures 3.1 to 3.6, indicate that the subjects, divided into two groups according to length of baseline phase, showed a gradual improvement across all phases. Clearly spontaneous recovery was occurring. In order to examine the effectiveness of the interventions, it was necessary to determine whether the rate of that improvement increased during the intervention phases. A linear function was fitted to these data in order to obtain the slope of the measures within each phase. Slope was then used as the dependent variable in a two-way repeated measures analysis of variance in order to examine whether there were significant changes in slope across phases. There were no significant intervention effects on any of these measures or on the rating scale, the Similarities subtest or the video, although there was clearly a ceiling effect on the video measure.

Figure 3.2 Mean scores for each group on the Symbol Digit Modalities Test — written and oral versions.

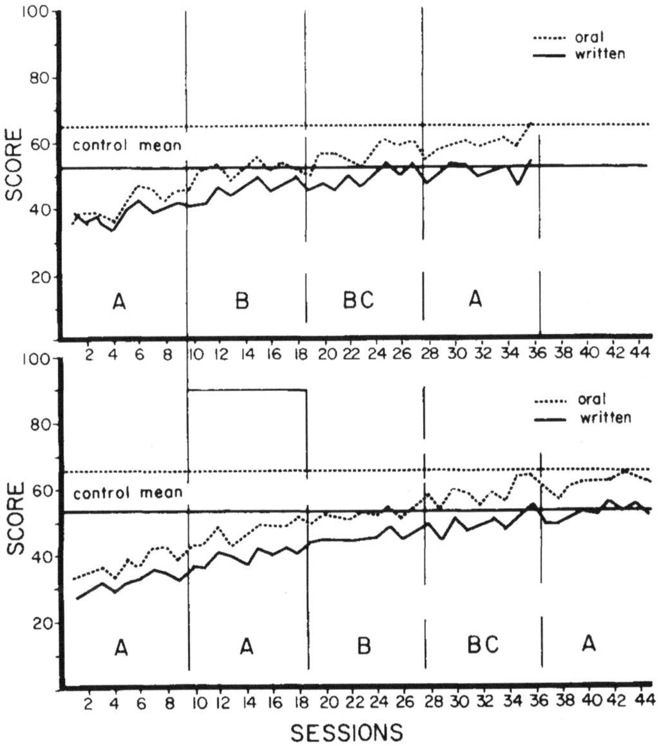

Each subject's results on the neuropsychological measures were also analysed individually, using Gottman's Interrupted Time-Series Experiment (ITSE) (Williams and Gottman, 1982). Comparisons across all phases confirmed the presence of a gradual improvement in each subject. Comparisons between adjacent phases revealed few significant changes, and the majority of the significant results failed to indicate positive effects of the intervention. There were, however, a number of instances of significant responses to feedback and reinforcement, when this was added to computer training in phase (BC), for three of the subjects. It was not possible to differentiate these subjects

Figure 3.3 Mean scores for each group on the Letter Cancellation task — time taken and per cent correct.

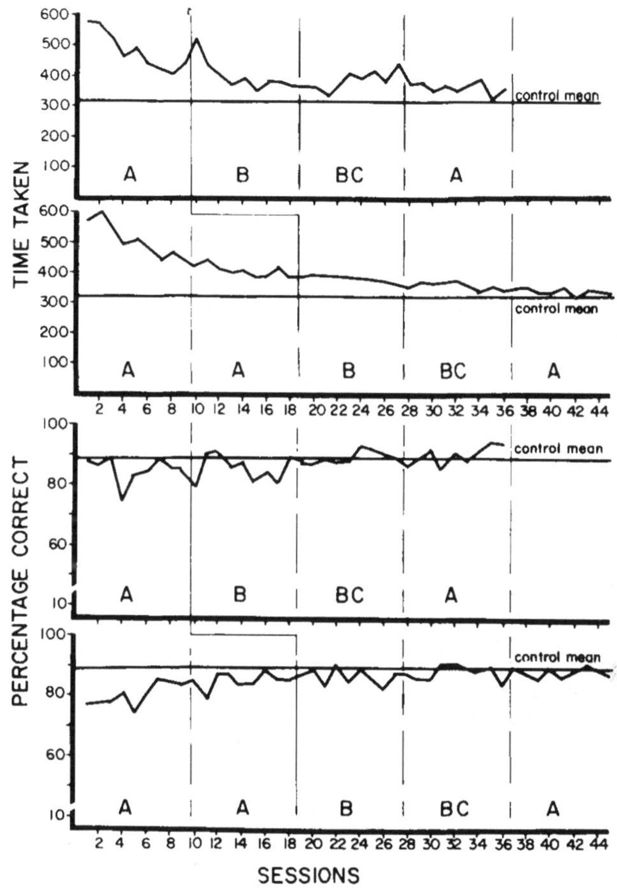

from the others on the basis of age, sex, educational background, length of PTA, time since injury, the nature of their neuropsychological deficits or the severity of attentional deficit, and thereby to identify factors which may have contributed to their positive response to feedback and reinforcement.

Figure 3.4 *Mean scores for each group on the Similarities subtest.*

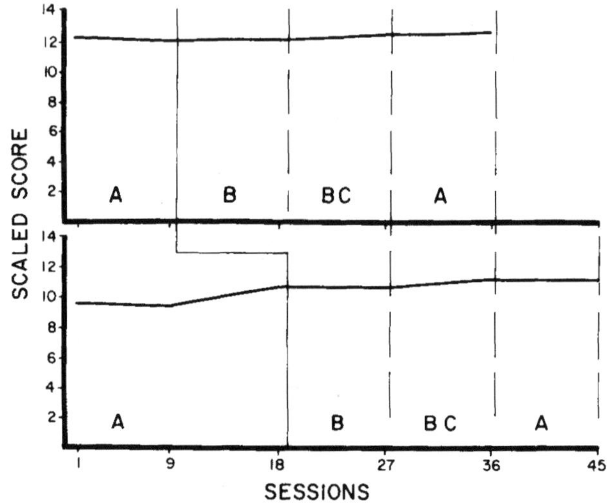

Figures 3.5 *Mean scores for each group on the Rating Scale of Attentional Behaviours.*

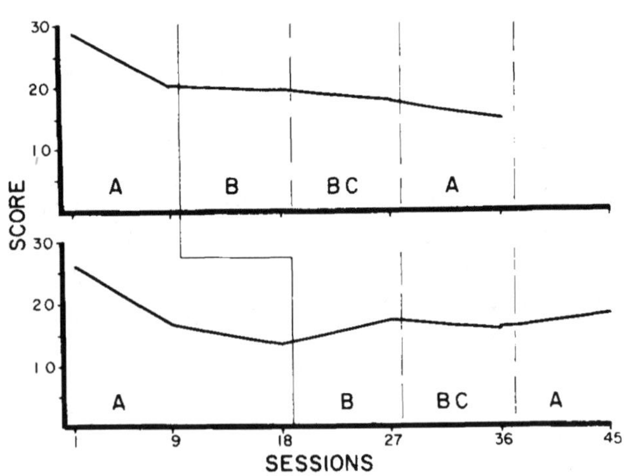

Figure 3.6 Mean results obtained for each group from the video in terms of the percentage of time spent directed to the task.

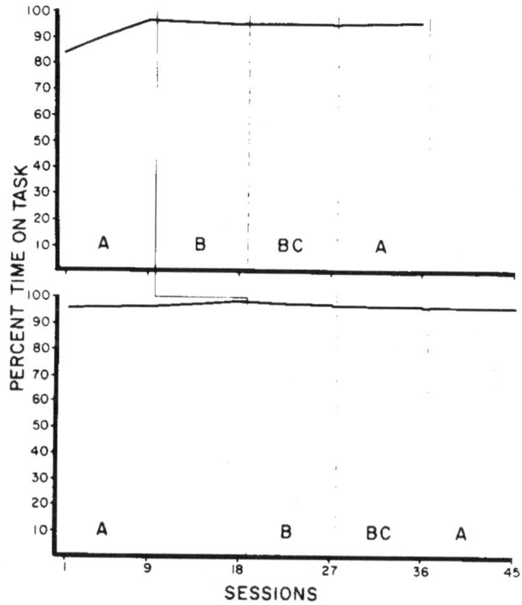

Summary

The results of the study by Ponsford and Kinsella (1988) indicated that the head-injured subjects improved significantly over the course of the remedial programme, both on neuropsychological measures of speed of information processing and on the rating scale of attentional behaviour. This would be expected on the basis of natural recovery of cognitive ability during the first twelve months following head injury. There was, however, no conclusive evidence that, when such recovery, as well as the effects of practice, therapist attention and other forms of therapy, was controlled for, the subjects showed a significant response to remedial intervention, which involved repeated practice on computer-mediated tasks designed to improve speed of information processing. This was the case whether such practice was or was not accompanied by therapist feedback and reinforcement, although there was a tendency for some subjects to respond to the feedback and reinforcement given. This result suggested the need to explore the responses of individual subjects over time, whilst examining the influence of such factors as mood and motivation. (However, for an alternative view, see Mateer, Sohlberg and Youngman, Chapter 4).

These findings were generally consistent with those of Malec *et al.* (1984) and Wood and Fussey (1987), both of whom utilized computer-mediated training tasks in attempting to rehabilitate attentional deficits in head-injured subjects but failed to document significant treatment effects. The studies by Sohlberg and Mateer (1987) and Gray and Robertson (1989) did show more positive results from training subjects very intensively in several different aspects of attention simultaneously. However, the methodological problems of these studies, already discussed, place limitations on the interpretation of their success.

No studies published to date have conclusively demonstrated that training on computer-mediated tasks, whether they be video games, as used by Malec *et al.* (1984), or tasks focusing on specific aspects of attention, as used in the study by Ponsford and Kinsella (1988) and others, has an impact on the everyday attentional problems of head-injured subjects suffering from attentional deficits. This has been so whether the intervention has been made during the early phase of recovery, less than 12 months post-injury or after recovery has plateaued.

There is no doubt that it is difficult to demonstrate the efficacy of any remedial intervention in a conclusive fashion. One could argue that training more intensively or over a longer period might bring more positive results. Certainly, computers have many advantages in rehabilitation settings, in monitoring patients' responses objectively and systematically, saving time for therapists and providing useful feedback to patients. The motivational aspects of using the computer should not be underestimated. Patients are almost invariably much more willing and interested in engaging in tasks on the computer than they are in other aspects of therapy, particularly those involving paper and pencil tasks. Moreover, for some patients at least, engaging in computer-mediated tasks may give them a feeling of tackling their problems constructively, thereby leading to an increase in self-esteem and motivation, which may lead to other improvements. At the very least, this may take patients more rapidly to their plateau level.

However, the results of studies conducted to date, applied to a range of cognitive deficits, certainly lead one to question the assumption underlying the directed stimulation approach to cognitive retraining, that repeated practice on tasks exercising a given cognitive function, no matter how specifically directed they are, necessarily leads to the restoration of that function following brain injury. It would seem that it is time to explore alternative approaches, which do not necessarily preclude the use of the computer.

A very important issue in terms of exploring approaches to cognitive rehabilitation is that of how 'recovery' should be defined, and, following from this, how remedial interventions should be designed and their success or otherwise be assessed. Should recovery mean restoration of the impaired function? Studies using the so-called directed stimulation approach to therapy and neuropsychological measures as means of evaluating the effectiveness of interventions or monitoring recovery presumably make this assumption. Or perhaps, as Schacter and Glisky (1986), O'Connor and Cermak (1987) and others have recently suggested, should recovery be defined in terms of the alleviation of the disability or handicap which results from the impairment? According to this paradigm, recovery is assessed in terms of goals achieved rather than the means used to attain those goals. Some agreement on these issues might lead to more constructive advances in the development and evaluation of remedial techniques. At the very least, clinicians and researchers working in this area need to define their goals in terms of recovery clearly from the outset.

There have been a few studies conducted to date, using computers, which have taken a compensatory approach to therapy. Early studies, such as that of Gianutsos and Gianutsos (1979), demonstrated the effectiveness of compensatory strategies, such as mnemonic elaboration, in improving the ability of brain-injured patients with significant memory difficulty to recall word lists. As these authors acknowledged, however, no attempt was made to examine the functional significance of the gains. More recently, Robertson *et al.* (1988) reported success in training three brain-injured subjects, suffering from unilateral spatial neglect, to use verbal cuing to overcome their visual scanning difficulties on a range of computer-mediated tasks. These authors were able to demonstrate some evidence of generalization of gains to functionally relevant tasks, such as reading and telephone number dialling. This finding, which is comparable to that of Weinberg *et al.* (1977), suggests that computers may be used successfully to provide training in the use of compensatory strategies to overcome cognitive deficits, such as visual scanning.

Studies which have focused more directly on the alleviation of specific difficulties the patient is experiencing in his/her daily life, by utilizing remaining intact functions or manipulating the environment, seem to have demonstrated a greater and a longer lasting impact on the patient's quality of life. One outstanding example of this, involving the use of a computer, is the recent study by Glisky and Schacter (cited in Schacter *et al.*, in press) who devised a training programme to teach a severely amnesic woman the knowledge and skills needed for a data entry job. The aim of the therapy was not to decrease the extent of this woman's amnesia, and indeed this remained very severe, but rather to teach her functional skills using her intact abilities, which enabled her to continue to lead a productive life style. These results suggest that computers might be used more productively, not to restore impaired functions through directed stimulation, but rather as a medium through which patients may be taught new skills or practice the use of compensatory strategies.

Others, such as Kirsch (1984) and Kreutzer (1987), have demonstrated that a computer may be programmed to provide necessary instruction, structure and prompting for brain-injured subjects to perform activities in the home, ranging from the daily routine of getting up, dressed and off to work, to the performance of more complex tasks, such as cooking a recipe. Such programmes must, however, be simple and practical enough for the brain-injured patient to use on a daily basis.

Nevertheless, it is clear that no single approach to treating cognitive deficits will provide the answer to all problems. It is probable that all or most of the approaches to therapy outlined earlier may be used successfully in various permutations and combinations to assist different patients to overcome their difficulties at various stages of their recovery.

Computers are now widely used in rehabilitation settings, and they have many potential uses. However, the absence of support for the use of repeated practice on computer-mediated tasks in remediating cognitive deficits seen in a number of studies conducted to date, suggests that therapists should be cautious in assuming the effectiveness of such programmes. The computer is no more than a tool, and its usefulness depends on the creativity of the therapist in helping patients to overcome or adapt to the specific difficulties they experience in their daily lives as a result of their cognitive deficits. Above all, since the effectiveness of any approach to cognitive rehabilitation is far from established, it is vital that therapists be prepared to assess objectively the impact of their interventions on the lives of their patients, both in the short and the longer term.

References

BEN-YISHAY, Y. and DILLER, L., 1981, 'Rehabilitation of cognitive and perceptual defects in people with traumatic brain injury'. *International Journal of Rehabilitation Research*, **4**, 208–20.

BINDER, L. M. and SCHREIBER, V., 1980, 'Visual imagery and verbal mediation as memory aids in recovering alcoholics'. *Journal of Clinical Neuropsychology*, **2**, 71–4.

BLACK, P., MARKOWITZ, R. S. and CIANCI, S., 1975, 'Recovery of motor function after lesions in motor cortex of monkey'. In Ciba Foundation Symposium No. 34, *Outcome of severe damage to the central nervous system* (Amsterdam: Elsevier), pp. 65–84.

BRACY, O. L., 1982, *Cognitive rehabilitation programmes for brain-injured and stroke patients* (Computer Programs) (Indianapolis, In: Psychological Software Services, Inc.).

BRACY, O. L., 1983, Computer based cognitive rehabilitation. *Cognitive Rehabilitation*, **1** (1), 7–8.

BROUWER, W. H. and VAN WOLFFELAAR, P. C., 1985, 'Sustained attention and sustained effort after closed head injury: detection and 0.10 Hz heart rate variability in a low event rate vigilance task'. *Cortex*, **21**, 111–9.

CERMAK, L. S., 1975, 'Imagery as an aid to retrieval for Korsakoff patients'. *Cortex*, **11**, 163–9.

CROVITZ, H. F., 1979, 'Memory retraining in brain damaged patients: the airplane list'. *Cortex*, **15**, 131–4.

DILLER, L. and GORDON, W. A., 1981, 'Rehabilitation and clinical neuropsychology'. In S. B. Filskov and T. J. Boll (Eds) *Handbook of clinical neuropsychology* (New York: John Wiley & Sons), pp. 702–733.

DOLAN, M. P. and NORTON, J. C., 1977, 'A programmed training technique that uses reinforcement to facilitate acquisition and retention in brain damaged patients'. *Journal of Clinical Psychology*, **33**, 496–501.

GASPARRINI, B. and SATZ, P., 1979, 'A treatment for memory problems in left hemisphere CVA patients'. *Journal of Clinical Neuropsychology*, **1**, 137–50.

GIANUTSOS, R., 1980, July-September, 'What is cognitive rehabilitation?' *Journal of Rehabilitation*, 36–40.

GIANUTSOS, R. and GIANUTSOS, J., 1979, 'Rehabilitating the verbal recall of brain injured patients by mnemonic training: an experimental demonstration using single-case methodology'. *Journal of Clinical Neuropsychology*, **1**(2), 117–35.

GIANUTSOS, R. and KLITZNER, C., 1981, *Computer programs for cognitive rehabilitation* (Computer programs) (Bayport, New York: Life Science Associates).

GLASGOW, R. E., ZEISS, R. A., BARRERA, M. and LEWINSOHN, P. M., 1977, 'Case studies on remediating memory deficits in brain damaged individuals'. *Journal of Clinical Psychology*, **33**, 1049–54.

GODFREY, H. P. D. and KNIGHT, R. G., 1988, June, 'Memory training and behavioural rehabilitation of a severely head-injured adult'. *Archives of Physical Medicine and Rehabilitation*, **69**, 458–60.

GOODKIN, R., 1969, 'Changes in word production, sentence production and relevance in an aphasic through verbal conditioning'. *Behaviour Research and Therapy*, **7**, 93–9.

GRAY, J. M. and ROBERTSON, I., 1989, 'Remediation of attentional difficulties following brain injury: 3 experimental single case studies'. *Brain Injury*, **3**(2), 163–70.

GRONWALL, D. M. A. and SAMPSON, H., 1974, *The psychological effects of concussion* (Auckland: Auckland University Press).

HARRIS, J., 1984, 'Methods of improving memory'. In B. A. Wilson and N. Moffat (Eds) *Clinical management of memory problems* (London: Croom Helm), pp. 46–62.

HART, T. and HAYDEN, M. E., 1986, 'The ecological validity of neuropsychological assessment and remediation'. In B. P. Uzzell and Y. Gross (Eds) *Clinical neuropsychology of intervention* (Boston: Martinus Nijhoff Publishing), pp. 21–50.

HORTON, A. M., 1979, 'Behavioural neuropsychology: rationale and research'. *Clinical Neuropsychology*, **1**(2), 20–3.

JONES, M., KENNEDY, R. S. and BITTNER, A. C., 1981, 'A video game for performance testing'. *American Journal of Psychology*, **94**, 143–52.

KENNEDY, R., 1981, 'Video game and conventional tracking'. *Perceptual and Motor Skills*, **53**, 310.

KIRSCH, N., 1984, March, 'A compensatory microcomputer intervention for patients with cognitive limitations'. Paper presented at the symposium: *Models and Techniques of Cognitive Rehabilitation — IV*, Indianapolis, Indiana.

KREUTZER, J. S., 1987, June, 'Acquisition of daily living skills through computer-assisted cognitive rehabilitation'. Paper presented at the *Postgraduate Course on Rehabilitation of the Brain-Injured Adult and Child*, Williamsburg, Virginia.

LAURENCE, S. and STEIN, D. G., 1978, 'Recovery after brain damage and the concept of localisation of function'. In S. Finger (Ed.) *Recovery from brain damage* (New York: Plenum Press), pp. 369–407.

LEZAK, M. D., 1987, 'Assessment for rehabilitation planning'. In M. J. Meier, A. L. Benton and L. Diller (Eds) *Neuropsychological rehabilitation* (New York: Churchill Livingston), pp. 41–58.

LYNCH, W. J., 1983, 'Cognitive retraining using microcomputer games and commercially available software'. *Cognitive Rehabilitation*, **1**, 19–22.

LYNCH, W. J., 1984, January, Computer-assisted cognitive retraining. Paper presented at the conference *Controversies in rehabilitation for neurological trauma and disease*, Miami, Florida.

MALEC, J., JONES, R., RAO, N. and STUBBS, K., 1984, 'Video-game practice effects on sustained attention in patients with cranio-cerebral trauma'. *Cognitive Rehabilitation*, **2**(4), 18–23.

MEIER, M. J., BENTON, A. L. and DILLER, L. (Eds) 1987, *Neuropsychological rehabilitation* (New York: Churchill Livingston).

MILLER, E., 1970, 'Simple and choice reaction time following severe head injury'. *Cortex*, **6**, 121–7.

MILLER, E., 1984, *Recovery and management of neuropsychological impairments* (London: John Wiley & Sons).

MOLLOY, M. and GARNER, J. A., 1988, *Neuropsychological rehabilitation — recovery from head injury* (Melbourne: Spectrum Publications).

O'CONNOR, M. and CERMAK, L., 1987, 'Rehabilitation of organic memory disorders'. In M. J. Meier, A. L. Benton and L. Diller (Eds) *Neuropsychological rehabilitation* (New York: Churchill Livingston), pp. 260–279.

OKOYE, R. and HOLLANDER, A., 1980, October, 'Multisensory video games: an adjunctive tool for treatment of learning disabilities'. Paper presented at the *Annual Meeting of the New York State Occupational Therapy Association*, New York.

PARASURAMAN, R., 1984, 'The psychobiology of sustained attention'. In J. S. Warm (Ed.) *Sustained attention in human performance* (New York: John Wiley & Sons), pp. 66–84.

PATTEN, B. M., 1972, 'The ancient art of memory: usefulness in treatment'. *Archives of Neurology*, **26**, 25–31.

PONSFORD, J. L., 1989, *Assessment and rehabilitation of attentional deficits following closed head injury*. Unpublished PhD Thesis, La Trobe University, Melbourne.

PONSFORD, J. L. and KINSELLA, G., 1988, 'Evaluation of a remedial programme for attentional deficits following closed head injury'. *Journal of Clinical and Experimental Neuropsychology*, **10**(b), 693–708.

POWELL, G. E., 1981, *Brain function therapy* (London: Gower).

ROBERTSON, I., GRAY, J. M. and MCKENZIE, S., 1988, 'Microcomputer-based cognitive rehabilitation of visual neglect: three multiple-baseline single-case studies'. *Brain Injury*, **2**(2), 151–63.

SBORDONE, R. J., 1983, July, *A computerised approach to cognitive rehabilitation for individuals with severe traumatic head injury*. Paper presented at the *International Conference on The Management of Traumatic Brain Injury*, London.

SCHACTER, D. L. and GLISKY, E. L., 1986, 'Memory remediation: Restoration, alleviation, and the acquisition of domain-specific knowledge'. In B. Uzzell and Y. Gross (Eds) *Clinical neuropsychology of intervention* (Boston: Martinus Nijhoff Publishing), pp. 257–282.

SCHACTER, D. L., GLISKY, E. L. and MCGLYNN, S. M. (in press). 'Impact of memory disorder in everyday life: awareness of deficits and return to work'. In D. Tupper and K. Cicerone (Eds) *The neuropsychology of everyday life. Volume 1. Theories and basic competencies* (Boston: Martinus Nijhoff).

SCHNEIDER, W. and SHIFFRIN, R. M., 1977, 'Controlled and automatic human information processing: I. Detection, search and attention'. *Psychological Review*, **84**(1), 1–66.

SHALLICE, T., 1982, 'Specific impairments to planning'. In D. E. Broadbent and L. Weiskrantz (Eds) *The neuropsychology of cognitive function* (London: The Royal Society), pp. 199–209.

SIVAK, M., HILL, C. S. and OLSON, P. L., 1983, *Computerised video task as training techniques for driving-related perceptual deficits of persons with brain damage: A pilot evaluation*. Unpublished manuscript, University of Michigan Transportation Research Institute, Rehabilitation Engineering Centre, Ann Arbor, Michigan.

SMITH, A., 1973, *Symbol Digit Modalities Test*. Los Angeles: Western Psychological Services.

SOHLBERG, M. M. and MATEER, C. A., 1987, 'Effectiveness of an attention-training program'. *Journal of Clinical and Experimental Neuropsychology*, **9**(2), 117–30.

SPARKS, R., HELM, N. and ALBERT, M., 1974, 'Aphasia rehabilitation resulting from Melodic Intonation Therapy'. *Cortex*, **10**, 303–16.

STROOP, J. R., 1935, 'Studies of interference in serial verbal reactions'. *Journal of Experimental Psychology*, **18**, 643–62.

STUSS, D. T., ELY, P., HUGENHOLTZ, H., RICHARDS, M. T., LA ROCHELLE, S., POIRIER, C. A. and BELL, I., 1985, 'Subtle neuropsychological deficits in patients with good recovery after closed head injury'. *Neurosurgery*, **17**(1), 41–7.

TREXLER, L. E. (Ed.) 1982, *Cognitive rehabilitation* (New York: Plenum Press).

UZZELL, B. P. and GROSS, Y. (Eds) 1986, *Clinical neuropsychology of intervention* (Boston: Martinus Nijhoff Publishing).

VAN ZOMEREN, A. H., 1981, *Reaction time and attention after closed head injury* (Lisse: Swets and Zeitlinger B.V.).

VAN ZOMEREN, A. H. and BROUWER, W. H., 1987, 'Head injury and concepts of attention'. In H. S. Levin, J. Grafman and H. M. Eisenberg (Eds) *Neurobehavioural recovery from head injury* (New York: Oxford University Press), pp. 398–415.

WEINBERG, J., DILLER, L., HODGES, W. A., GERSTMAN, L. J., LIEBERMAN, A., LAKIN, P., HODGES, G. and EZRACHI, O., 1977, 'Visual scanning training effect on reading-related tasks in acquired right brain damage'. *Archives of Physical Medicine and Rehabilitation*, **58**, 479–86.

WILLIAMS, E. A. and GOTTMAN, J. M., 1982, *A user's guide to the Gottman-Williams time-series analysis computer programs for social scientists* (Cambridge: Cambridge University Press).

WILSON, B. A., 1984, 'Memory therapy in practice'. In B. A. Wilson and N. Moffat (Eds) *Clinical management of memory problems* (London: Croom Helm), pp. 89–111.

WILSON, B. A., 1987, *Rehabilitation of memory* (New York: Guilford Press).

WOOD, R. L., 1984, 'Behaviour disorders following severe brain injury: their presentation and psychological management'. In Neil Brooks (Ed.) *Closed head injury: Psychological, social and family consequences* (Oxford: Oxford University Press), pp. 195–219.

WOOD, R. L. and FUSSEY, I., 1987, 'Computer-based cognitive retraining: a controlled study'. *International Disability Studies*, **9**(4), 149–54.

Chapter 4

The Management of Acquired Attention and Memory Deficits

C. A. Mateer, M. M. Sohlberg and P. K. Youngman

Introduction

The distribution of kinetic energy which occurs in closed-head injury results in diffuse microscopic changes to the cerebral structures. This reduces attentional capacity (van Zomeren, *et al.*, 1984) and causes many individuals to experience stress from the feeling of 'information overload' and the continual mental effort and concentration necessary to perform tasks that were once relatively easy. As well as diffuse damage, head-trauma patients also sustain damage to frontal structures, causing deficits in the ability to control, direct, organize and monitor their activity, both motor and mental. Such a control deficit diminishes the ability to utilize attentional capacity. Patients may be able to attend fairly well if someone else gets them started on a particular task and reminds them to stay on the task until it is completed. When left to their own initiative, however, they easily lose track of what they are doing, saying or thinking, and become distracted. They also have difficulty moving their focus of attention from one task to another in a controlled but flexible way. Attention thus underlies many daily activities and mental capacities, including memory, communication and problem solving.

This chapter will focus on the treatment of attentional deficits in individuals who experience cognitive changes as a result of minor head injury. These persistent, post-concussional symptoms often affect everyday living and work, yet this class of injury, whilst frequent among the divisions of traumatic brain injury, has been least studied in terms of intervention strategies and approaches. Historically, physicians and other medical practitioners have tended to view the minor brain-injury syndrome as a psychiatric, emotionally based or psychosomatic disorder. More recent evidence has confirmed its biological basis. In this paper, results of cognitive rehabilitation in a set of patients from this population will be described. As attention and memory deficits are among the most frequently diagnosed following minor brain injury, the paper will focus on these two areas of cognitive processing.

Treatment of Attentional Disorders

The majority of studies on attention have focused on attempts to retrain underlying attentional skills. The assumption behind attention training is that it is more efficient to focus on cognitive functions underlying daily activities than it is to focus on the training of such activities directly — i.e. to focus on causes rather than symptoms. Used in this way, cognitive rehabilitation differs from a purely functional approach to treatment, but since the ultimate goal of rehabilitation is to improve skills which allow individuals to regain independence or employment, improvement in cognitive function (based on training activities) must therefore be shown to generalize and improve the performance on functional skills as well.

To date, 14 studies addressing the treatment of attentional disorders have appeared in the literature. Eight of these utilized exposure to and repetition of specific laboratory-based activities or tasks which provided opportunity to exercise attentional skills. The remaining studies looked at the effectiveness of a behavioral token economy, EEG Biofeedback and pharmacologic intervention.

In a series of monographs Ben-Yishay and Diller (1978–1983) developed five training tasks (one auditory, four visual) which were hierarchically ordered in terms of the number of subfunctions involved and the relative difficulty level. The five tasks were only loosely related to existing cognitive models of attention but included references to Posner's (1975) model of effortful processing. Goals included improved self-monitoring and efficient utilization of feedback about performance. Eleven head-injured subjects were evaluated in a multiple baseline design to determine improvement on training tasks and generalization to independent untrained tests. Task-specific training effects were reported as well as improvements in reaction time, attention to visual details and visuo-motor speed.

Sturm *et al.* (1983) evaluated the effect of attention training on two groups of 15 patients (each in a full-time in-patient rehabilitation setting) and two groups of normal controls. Patient and control subjects in the experimental group received seven hours of training on tasks involving visual and auditory stimuli which were manipulated for complexity and speed. Improvement in the experimental groups was seen on a number of independent measures taken from common German intelligence and vocational tests. Results of the study are somewhat confounded, however, by the relatively early stage of recovery (10 months mean chronicity) and the high percentage of cerebro-vascular as opposed to head-trauma patients.

Kewman *et al.* (1985) evaluated the efficacy of attention training in a group of head-injured subjects (N = 13, average chronicity 3.7 years) and a head-injured and normal control group. The experimental training required the subjects to manoeuvre a modified battery-powered wheelchair along courses of increasing difficulty while they responded to auditory and visual stimuli. The head-injured control group attended a classroom driving course but had no exposure to the attention tasks. Normal control subjects participated in advanced parts of the experimental training. All groups underwent on-the-road evaluation prior to and after training. Both experimental groups improved significantly on the training tasks as well as in on-the-road driving skills as compared to the head-injured control group. The study demonstrated effects of cognitive training on a functional skill.

Wood (1986), using visual and auditory training tasks, reported increases in attentive behavior during therapy sessions in some severely head-injured patients using a token reinforcement procedure. Some generalization was noted on certain memory tasks as well as on attentive behavior in other therapeutic environments. A different approach was employed by Klove (1987) who described beneficial effects of stimulant medication in three of four patients with chronic arousal deficits.

In 1987, Sohlberg and Mateer reported on the effectiveness of a cognitive rehabilitation program specifically designed to address a broad range of attentional deficits (Attention Process Training) combined with selective work book or computer-based programs. We based the administration of hierarchically organized treatment tasks on a five-level model of attention including focused, sustained, selective, alternating and divided attention. Over 60 exercises were given, each corresponding to specific components of attention. This provided repeated exercise of attention in a gradual and progressively more demanding sequence. Treatment was individualized and varied from four to eight weeks with each subject receiving seven to nine sessions per week. Attention training and visual process training were used in a multiple baseline design replicated across four subjects. Gains in attention, as measured by performance on the Paced Auditory, Addition Task serial were seen during and following attention training, and gains on a visual task were seen during and after visual-process training. Results were interpreted to indicate domain-specific cognitive improvement. We went on to report positive effects on memory performance following attention training in a series of five additional subjects (Mateer and Sohlberg, 1988). In this way attention training was demonstrated to have a beneficial effect on another cognitive process which was dependent on attention.

Niemann (1989) evaluated the effects of attention training versus memory training in two groups of head-injured subjects. Attention-training tasks were similar to those described by Sohlberg and Mateer (1987). Memory training consisted of training on a variety of mnemonic strategies. Results indicated gains on specific measures of attention and of memory function in the group receiving attention training. Similar gains were not seen in the group receiving memory training. Neither group, however, demonstrated gains on an independent set of neuropsychological measures administered pre- and post-treatment.

Ruff *et al.* (1989), using two groups of head-injured patients, conducted a controlled study which compared the efficacy of neuropsychological treatment with a non-structured treatment providing equivalent professional attention and psychological support. Subjects received eight weeks of treatment with a total of 160 hours of treatment per patient. Although analysis of pre- and post-treatment data on neuropsychological functioning demonstrated significant improvements for both groups, the group receiving targeted treatment of cognitive deficits achieved relatively greater gains on measures of memory and error reduction tasks for selective attention.

Weber (1990) describes an approach to the treatment of two patients, one with an attentional capacity deficit and one with an attentional control deficit. Although the same basic tasks were used to treat both sorts of deficits, the way in which they were used was varied according to the relative proportions of capacity and control difficulties. Weber argued that an individual whose main problem is limited capacity will primarily make errors of omission on monitoring tasks, whereas the person with control problems makes frequent commission (or false positive) errors in addition to omissions. The patient with limited-capacity benefits from repetition of the task, increasing familiarity and knowing where the 'danger spots' are so that he/she can increase attentional effort at these particular places. The patient also benefits from learning relaxation and self-pacing techniques to reduce/prevent 'overload'. The patient with a control-deficit may respond to repetition and feedback about errors by becoming more entrenched in an error pattern, and the retraining procedure needs to include ways of preventing or disrupting such inappropriate response sets and teaching the person how to do this independently through role-reversal strategies, goal-setting and task-structuring techniques.

In contrast to these studies, several negative reports regarding the efficacy of attention training have appeared (Malec *et al.*, 1984; Wood and Fussey, 1987; Ponsford and Kinsella, 1988). Wood and Fussey (1987) did not report significant improvement on psychomotor or vigilance tasks in head-injured patients who were at least one year post-injury. Training, however, may have been too limited or narrow in that only one computerized visual attention task was utilized in treatment.

Using ten patients with severe head injury, Malec *et al.* (1984) evaluated the effects of a two-week, visual attention training program within six months after the trauma. Improvements were found but were independent of training. Problems may have emerged here due to the interaction with spontaneous recovery, the short training period and the use of a single visual attention task. In addition, the authors used a withdrawal treatment design. Subjects were assigned to an ABAB or a BABA condition where a week of training (A) was altered with a week of non-training (B). It may be that treatment effects on a cognitive function cannot be withdrawn as can intervention for more behaviorally controlled variables.

Ponsford and Kinsella (1988) trained 10 patients with an average chronicity of nine months or less on five visual tasks (e.g. simple and choice reaction time, visual search) in a staggered, baseline design. Total time on treatment tasks was 15 hours. One of two treatment phases was associated with reinforcement and feedback, while the other was not. Attention tests, an attention-rating scale and a video evaluation of attentive behaviors were used as independent measures. None of the measures revealed treatment-related effects though three of the ten patients were reported to respond favorably to feedback and reinforcement. The nature and amount of feedback given to patients about their training task performance may well be a significant factor in determining outcome of treatment and in explaining some of the discrepant findings between studies.

Despite these somewhat conflicting studies on the efficacy of attention training, reasons for optimism remain and further investigation is clearly warranted. Several factors emerge from these investigations which may be critical to treatment success. All three of the attention-training studies with negative effects used only visually based training tasks, and two studies provided a very limited number of relatively unmodifiable tasks. Studies reporting greater success tended to use a much broader range and number of training tasks. Retraining of underlying cognitive skills is likely to require not only sufficient repetitive practice but exposure to tasks of a sufficiently broad and demanding attentional load.

Issues of what training tasks are beneficial, for what patients, at what time post-injury and with what effects have only just begun to be critically addressed. Just as the direction in neuropsychological assessment has been toward development of task measures which more adequately reveal the way in which a cognitive process is disrupted, process-oriented cognitive rehabilitation must increasingly move toward applying specific treatments to specific patients based on the individual nature of their deficits. Sohlberg and Mateer's (1987) model of treatment provides for the application of specific attentional training exercises (i.e. sustained, selective, alternating and divided attention) based on the particular profile of deficits a patient demonstrates. In a similar vein, Weber's (in press) approach argues for matching the attention treatment plan to the individual's specific attentional deficits (capacity and control).

In summary, the targeted treatment of attention appears to be an appropriate and promising focus for rehabilitation efforts. In order for the field to progress, clinicians will need to incorporate current models of attentional functioning into treatment efforts. Training tasks must not only emerge from such models but must reflect and incorporate everyday aspects of attentional functioning.

Rehabilitation of Memory Functions

Disturbances of memory are among the most frequently voiced complaints and demonstrated impairments of individuals with head trauma. Damage to many areas of the brain can impact different aspects of memory functioning (see Sohlberg and Mateer, 1989a, for review). Specific approaches to the rehabilitation of memory include methods which attempt to restore or improve memory function per se and approaches which might help the individual with a memory deficit cope with the effects of memory impairment. Restorative approaches would include pharmacological therapies (Goldberg *et al.*, 1982; McLean *et al.*, 1987), surgical interventions or the use of behavioral exercises or drills which would restore memory to a level closer to pre-morbid function. Compensation approaches would include the development and training of internal or external strategies which might help the individual access information more efficiently.

Restorative approaches of a behavioral nature have focused on repetitive practice or drill of recall tasks. Commonly included in this approach and exemplified by many work-book activity and computer programs for memory, are list-learning or paragraph-recall tasks. Published studies have, however, quite consistently documented the failure of such approaches to substantially improve scores on untrained memory tasks or to impact functional memory outside the clinic (Prigatano *et al.*, 1984; Godfrey and Knight, 1985; Schacter *et al.*, 1985).

As discussed in the previous section, several authors (Mateer and Sohlberg, 1988; Niemann, 1989) have reported gains in memory function following targeted training of attentional skills. Since attention is critical to the receipt and registration of information, it is reasonable that improvement in this first stage of the information-processing system for memory would have positive effects on memory for those individuals whose memory deficits are secondary to attentional deficits.

An alternative approach to memory restoration proposed by Sohlberg and Mateer (1989a) is the development of 'prospective memory' capacity. Prospective memory refers to the capacity to carry out future intended actions — in a sense, to remember to remember! This kind of memory, which involves such common everyday activities as remembering to take medications, remembering to return a phone call or remembering to pick items up at the store, has been proposed to be an ecologically important component of memory. We have reported preliminary findings which suggest that the length of prospective memory (the duration of time over which actions can be recalled and independently carried out) can be increased and that such increases are related to improved scores on independent measures of memory function.

Compensatory approaches typically involve environmental modifications or the training of internal or external memory strategies. Internally based compensatory memory techniques are strategies which the individual applies from within to enhance the ability to encode, store or retrieve information to be recalled. These techniques focus on increasing organization of information to be recalled, rehearsing information to be remembered or training of specific mnemonic devices, such as peg words or visual imagery (Wilson and Moffat, 1984). Although several studies have suggested that recall performance in memory-disordered patients can be improved through training of such internal, mnemonic learning schemes (Cermak, 1975; Lewinsohn *et al.*, 1977; Gasparrini and Satz, 1979; Gianutsos and Gianutsos, 1979; Wilson, 1981, 1982; Parente and Anderson, 1983), none of these studies have clearly demonstrated the degree to which these strategies are maintained or that they generalize to naturalistic settings. There is some indication that use of such internally generated strategies may be beneficial in patients with mild head injuries who have considerable residual memory ability (Wilson, 1987). Patients with moderate to severe memory deficits have been found to have difficulty generating and applying mnemonic strategies spontaneously (Crovitz *et al.*, 1979). Since these techniques place heavy demands on already jeopardized cognitive systems, they are generally inappropriate for persons with severely compromised intellectual or memory functions.

Similar criticisms, in terms of a need for high-level abstraction skills, can be levelled against verbal mediation techniques, such as chaining or linking, alphabetical cuing and semantic or phonetic elaboration. Overall results of these studies suggest that for the majority of head-injury patients, gains are likely to be short-lived and positive results may not relate to everyday tasks. In addition, only a limited number of everyday situations lend themselves to imagery or to other restricted mnemonic associations and are thus not easily generalized.

A second strategy for development of compensatory approaches in individuals with memory impairment involves training in the use of external memory aids. External memory aids consist of organizational devices, prospective memory devices and environmental modification. Organizational devices include such tools as electronic memories, memory notebook systems and computers that allow an individual to organize, store and retrieve significant amounts of information. Prospective memory devices include tools to remind a memory-impaired person to perform a particular action at a specific future time. These would encompass alarms, calendars, buzzers and watches. Environmental modifications involve restructuring or alteration of the environment to decrease the impact of memory deficits on everyday functions, including posted checklists, labelled shelves, alphabetized cupboards and specially structured work environments.

Effective use of such systems often involves a fairly complex set of activities. Given the inherent problems patients have with new learning as well as with initiation, planning and insight into, appropriate training in how to use these devices has not routinely been provided. Sohlberg and Mateer (1989b) describe a three-stage behavioral approach for the training of memory devices which is based on learning theory and identification of needs for memory-system usage in the patients' daily life. Phases involve the acquisition of knowledge about the memory system, the application of the memory system through role-play activities and the adaptation of the memory system (i.e. notebook use) in a naturalistic setting via community retraining.

Cognitive Outcomes from a Post-Acute Rehabilitation Program

In the previous sections we have discussed the theory and principles behind approaches to the training of attentional process, as well as the use of this and other techniques in working with individuals who demonstrate memory impairments. In the following section we will present cognitive and vocational outcome data on five individuals who had sustained brain injury and who were seen in a post-acute rehabilitation program.

Three years ago we developed, in the Center for Cognitive Rehabilitation at Good Samaritan Hospital, an outpatient program specifically tailored to the needs of individuals with so-called mild head injury (CCR II). Participants included individuals who may have initially sustained what appeared to be mild blows to the head, concussions or whiplash injuries. Some had sustained more severe injuries from which they appeared to have relatively good recovery. Despite recovering independence in self-care and basic communication, these individuals continued to experience physical limitations, problems with cognitive functioning, altered social-emotional functioning and difficulty with effective return to work. Physical problems often included pain-related complaints (headache and back and/or neck pain), dizziness with postural changes, blurred vision and fatigue. Cognitive complaints most frequently included problems with memory, difficulty dealing with more than one thing at a time and specific word-retrieval problems. Social-emotional changes included irritability, loss of self-esteem, worry and reactive depression. At work, concerns most commonly centered around loss of efficiency, increased frequency of errors, increased need for vigilance, sensitivity to noise and difficulty learning new information or tasks.

Participants were entered into an individually tailored program which took place three days per week. Each person received approximately four, individual, cognitive therapy hours per week, two individual psychosocial sessions and two sessions with a vocational rehabilitation counsellor. Weekly cognitive, pragmatic, psychosocial and vocational groups were also held. Neuropsychological testing yielded a very high incidence of deficits on attention tests, particularly those involving higher levels of selective, alternating and divided attention. Corresponding deficits on immediate recall tasks and on measures of new learning were judged to be, in large part, due to attentional deficits. For this reason, each participant received extensive training and practice in the use and application of attentional skills using Attention Process Training (Sohlberg and Mateer, 1987) and related materials. Participants received an average of 64 instruction hours over an eight-month period. Aside from attention training, no formal restorative memory education was undertaken. Participants were, however, given extensive and systematic training in the development and use of compensatory memory aids and personal organization systems. The overall goals of this program were to restore or assist the individual in compensating for reduced cognitive function, to increase insight into understanding and acceptance of cognitive and behavioral change, to increase self-regulatory function and to enhance vocational outcomes through work stations and job placement.

A brief description of five recent graduates from this program follows, summarized in Table 4.1.

Case 1

JM, a 46-year-old male electrician, sustained a head injury when a cable he was replacing came free and he fell down nine stairs. No loss of consciousness or post-traumatic amnesia were noted, but a subsequent EEG showed left hemisphere slowing. After the injury, he attempted to return to work but was unable to maintain regular employment. He stated that this was due to an inability to follow directions and read blueprints and that his speed of performing tasks had significantly decreased.

Case 2

AK, a 32-year-old man, was struck by an oncoming vehicle while driving. He apparently hit his head on the steering wheel or windshield. His wife reported he lost consciousness momentarily and appeared dazed. No medical attention was sought until the following day, when he saw his family physician because of a severe headache. Several months later, he was referred for a neuropsychological evaluation, upon his own insistence that something was wrong. He had worked as a correctional officer prior to the injury and attempted to return to that job one week after the accident. However, he experienced difficulties and, after six months, was placed on medical leave.

Case 3

AC, a 40-year-old woman who worked as a sales clerk for a large department store, sustained an injury at work after she slipped on perfume from a broken bottle and fell to the floor, striking her head. Loss of consciousness was between 5 and 15 minutes. At a local hospital emergency room, she was found to have a contused scalp and non-depressed skull fracture of the left occiput. She was placed on medical leave of absence. Twenty-two months after the head injury, she continued to report significant pain, in addition to the more typical cognitive and psychosocial difficulties.

Case 4

LM is a 46-year-old woman who was injured when the car she was driving was struck from the rear. No loss of consciousness or post-traumatic amnesia were reported. Following her injury, she attempted to return to work but experienced memory, concentration and word-finding problems, as well as head, neck, shoulder and back pain, dizziness and fatigue.

Case 5

AJ is a 42-year-old woman who underwent five weeks of immediate hospitalization following a head-on motor vehicle accident in which she sustained significant internal injuries and multiple fractures. She experienced only a brief loss of consciousness but had traumatic amnesia for approximately two weeks. The impact of the head injury was not recognized for four years, although she reports attempting to explain her problems to a series of medical practitioners. An attempt to work following a recovery period was successful largely due to the support of her employer. Initially at half days, she was gradually able to work back into a full-time position as a Technical Clerk for the phone company, with a reduced work load. She described many problems upon return to work, including decreased attention/concentration, fatigue, difficulty with memory and an increased rate of errors.

Table 4.1 Subject characteristics.

Case	Sex	Age	Injury	LOC	PTA	Neurological exam	Pre-injury employment
1–JM	M	46	Fall	No	No	(L) EEG Slowing	Electrician
2–AK	M	32	MVA	Brief	No	WNL	Correctional Officer
3–AC	F	40	Fall	5–15 min	No	Occipital skull fracture	Sales Clerk
4–LM	F	46	MVA	No	No	WNL	Technical Editor
5–AJ	F	42	MVA	Brief	Two weeks	WNL	Technical Clerk

Attention Process Training: The Model and Methods

The clinical model of attention and its treatment used with these patients was based on the experimental attention literature, clinical observation and patients' subjective complaints (Sohlberg and Mateer, 1987). It considers attention as a multi-dimensional cognitive capacity critical to memory, new learning and all other aspects of cognition. There are five levels of attention addressed in the treatment model: focused attention, sustained attention, selective attention, alternating attention and divided attention. Given this five-component model of attention, a set of specific exercises was developed or selected. In the following sections, definitions and sample treatment tasks are presented. Many of those that were specifically developed in the context of this model are included in the commercially available set of materials entitled *Attention Process*

Training or APT (Sohlberg and Mateer, 1987). Clinicians are, of course, encouraged to use existing tasks or to develop new ones based on their relevance to the clinical model described.

Focused Attention

This is the ability to respond discreetly to specific visual, auditory or tactile stimuli. Although almost all patients recover this level of attention, it is often disrupted in the early stages of emergence from coma. The patient may initially be responsive only to internal stimuli (pain, temperature, etc.) and only gradually start responding to specific external events or stimuli. None of the subjects discussed in this report has difficulty at this basic level.

Sustained Attention

This refers to the ability to maintain a consistent behavioral response during continuous and repetitive activity. It incorporates the notion of vigilance. Disruption of this level of attention is implied in the patient who can only focus on a task or maintain responses for a brief period (i.e., seconds to minutes) or who fluctuates dramatically in performance over even brief periods (i.e., variable attention or attentional lapses). It also incorporates the notion of mental control or working memory on tasks that involve manipulating information and holding it in mind.

Sustained attention treatment tasks require consistent responding to either aurally or visually presented information. Visually based exercises include a variety of cancellation tasks in which the patient scans an array of targets and crosses some out. Simple levels of the task might include crossing out one or two target letters or numbers. Auditory stimulation is often preferred; the transient nature of auditory stimuli puts greater demands on the attentional system. The APT materials include a set of 16 audio cassette tapes; patients respond to targets by pushing a buzzer. At higher levels of sustained attention training, there are greater and greater demands on mental control and information processing. Subjects might be asked to respond to sequences of ascending or descending numbers or letters, days of the week or months of the year.

Other APT tasks include the Serial Numbers, Mental Number Control and Alphabetical Sequences. Serial Numbers are exercises in counting backwards by 2s, 3s, 4s or 5s. The complexity of serial-number counting can be increased by adding additional mathematical operations, for example, adding 2, then subtracting 1 or subtracting 4, then adding 2, consecutively, as numbers go up or down. Mental Number Control requires ordering four numbers presented auditorally in ascending or descending sequence. For example, after hearing the numbers 27, 13, 9, 18, the correct response for a descending trial would be 27, 18, 13, 9. Difficulty level is dependent on using single- or double-digit numbers and on using strings of four or five numbers. Criterion is set at 90% correct on two or three sets of ten stimuli with a 20% reduction from baseline performance time. Alphabetical Sequences exercises require that the person repeat words from 4- to 6-word sentences in alphabetical order. For example, after hearing 'Seattle is an original city', the person would respond 'A city is original Seattle'. These mental exercises appear to tap, and thus exercise, attentional capacities.

An example of performance charting on a sustained attention activity is given in Figure 4.1. This data was generated by Subject AK, the 32-year-old, male Corrections Officer. The task was to give back, in alphabetical order, five words presented in a sentence. Initial performance in trial 1 indicates a total time of 370 seconds with three errors on a set of ten sentences. On this basis, a target time goal of 295 seconds, repre-

Figure 4.1 Five Word Alphabetized Sentences (10 Sentence Sets). Criterion: 295 seconds (20% decline from baseline); no more than 1 error in 10 sentences (10% error rate).

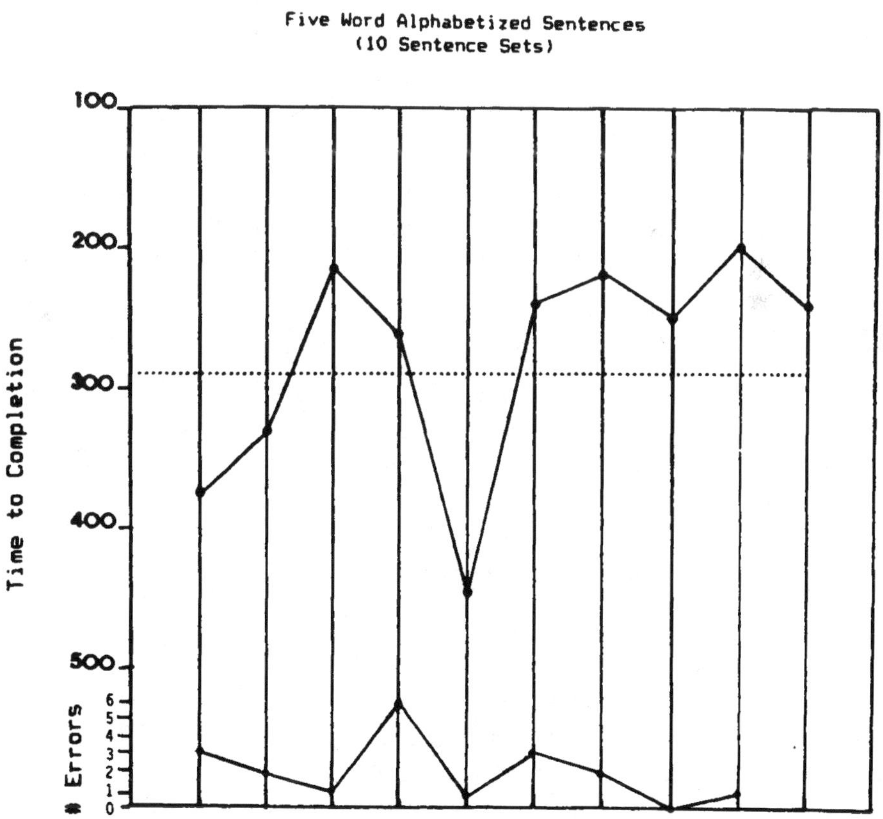

senting a 20% decrease in response time, was set. An accuracy goal was set at 90%, that is no more than one incorrect response in a set of ten sentences. These goals were met once in trial 3, but the criterion for task mastery required meeting the time and accuracy goals on two of three consecutive sets of ten sentences. This was achieved on February 27 after ten total trials (seven sessions) utilizing the task.

Of particular note in the data is AK's strikingly poor performance on trials 4 and 5, both administered on one day. When speed was acceptable, the error rate was extremely high (60%); when he slowed substantially, error rate met criterion (10%). Review of the file revealed that both psychosocial and vocational counselling sessions that day dealt with difficult, though important, issues. Under that additional stress, cognitive performance demonstrated clear and characteristic decline. Charting of data in this way is critical to an understanding and appreciation of a patient's response patterns and cognitive/behavioral course. It is what allows the clinician to make critical treatment decisions regarding stopping, changing or modifying treatment tasks.

Selective Attention

This level of attention refers to the ability to maintain a behavioral or cognitive set in the face of distracting or competing stimuli. It thus incorporates the notion of 'freedom from distractibility'. Individuals with deficits at this level are easily drawn off task by extraneous, irrelevant stimuli. These can include both external sights, sounds or activities (the 'cocktail party effect') and internal distractions (worry, rumination or focus on personally important thoughts). Examples of problems at this level include an inability to perform therapy tasks in a stimulating environment (e.g. an open-treatment area) or to prepare a meal with the children playing in the background.

Training at this level involves the incorporation of distracting or irrelevant information during task performance. For visual cancellation tasks, plastic overlays with distracting designs have been found to be useful. In the auditory modality, the same attention tape stimuli are used but the targets are now embedded in a background of distracting noise. This may be in the form of a news broadcast, a sports commentary, cafeteria noise or conversation. Although the APT tapes used for selective attention training have pre-recorded background stimuli, use of novel or individually adapted distraction is encouraged. The patient with social interests might be most distracted by a tape of lunchtime conversation between staff members; another may be most distracted by a football game; yet another may be vulnerable to music or to the sound of children playing. Tapes can easily be made and used in conjunction with these tasks. Making such tapes is preferable to just turning on a TV or radio because the stimuli are better controlled, and repeated data trials will be more comparable. Some patients are more disrupted by internal than external distraction, that is, worry, rumination or pre-occupation with personal concerns or agendas. With these patients, focusing on reducing these distractions may be primary. Techniques, such as writing things down and then setting the paper aside before beginning a task, may be helpful.

There is a wide variety of other exercises, including computer programs, that appear to fit within this clinical model. In particular, the Visual Reaction Stimulus Discrimination 1 and Auditory Reaction Stimulus Discrimination, published by Psychological Software Services, provide tasks that require inhibition of responses during target-reaction tasks. Clinicians can incorporate the notion of distraction into many different kinds of exercises. Consider, for example, utilizing a simple computer task at the same time a noise tape is played. A humorous Groucho Marx audio tape has proved very distracting to many of our clients.

Alternating Attention

This level of attention refers to the capacity for mental flexibility that allows individuals to shift their focus of attention and move between tasks having different cognitive requirements thus controlling which information will be selectively attended to. Problems at this level are evident in the patient who has difficulty changing treatment tasks once a 'set' has been established and who needs extra cueing to pick up and initiate new task requirements. Real-life demands for this level of attentional control are frequent. Consider the student who must shift between listening to a lecture and taking notes, or the secretary who must continuously move between answering the phone, typing and responding to inquiries.

Training of attentional deficits at this level requires flexible redirection and reallocation of attention. Effective tasks have requirements of repeated changes in task demands. The patient might, for example, be called to respond first to ascending numbers and then on cue to descending numbers or to add and then, on cue, subtract number sets. Training tasks often involve material that can be treated, or responded to, in different ways. Requirements are for frequent and repeated changes in cognitive or response set.

Divided Attention

This stage involves the ability to respond simultaneously to multiple task demands. Two or more behavioral responses may be required or two or more kinds of stimuli may need to be monitored. This level of attentional capacity is required whenever multiple, simultaneous demands must be managed. Performance under such conditions (i.e. driving a car while listening to the radio or holding a conversation during meal preparation) may actually reflect either rapid and continuous alternating attention or dependence on more unconscious automatic processing for at least one of the tasks. Modelling this level as a separate component of attention emphasizes its importance in the rehabilitation context and provides a foundation for retraining.

Training in this area involves the use of tasks in which multiple kinds of information must be attended to simultaneously, or it involves the simultaneous use of two or more tasks. It would be common, for example, to combine two simple vigilance tasks, one auditory and one visual, in a divided attention activity. The person might, for example, be asked to listen to a news report while simultaneously completing a letter-cancellation task and then be asked to recount important details of the news report. Another example of a divided attention activity is the APT Card Sorting task in which the patient sorts cards by suit but also must pay attention to and turn over any card with a target letter in its name (e.g. turning over twos, threes, eights, tens, if the target letter is 't').

Task Selection

The most critical characteristic in selecting attention training activities is that they be addressed to a specific component of attention as defined by the model. At any one time, three to four attention tasks are typically being utilized, but these all fall in one or perhaps two areas of attention. A combination of auditory and visual tasks is usually selected. Data is kept on all tasks and an individual patient's performance on any one task is what determines whether the exercise is repeated or modified in some way. In this way, a patient is gradually introduced to and masters more and more challenging attention tasks.

Training Use of Compensatory Memory Devices

In the mild head-injury program, memory deficits are dealt with in two primary ways. For many individuals, memory deficits are secondary to attentional limitations, and training of attentional processing is used to boost memory function. The second approach is to train individuals in the systematic use of compensatory memory aids. Some individuals come in with systems they have developed on their own (see Deelman *et al.*, Chapter 6). These are reviewed for organizational effectiveness. If workable, they are further developed and their systematic use ascertained through treatment exercises. For individuals with no current system, one is selected and developed. Usually, this takes the form of a notebook system [as, for example, the use of a 'process diary' (Finset and Andresen, Chapter 5)]. The approach described in this chapter is of a 'Daytimer System' which we have found particularly flexible and adaptable.

The first stage of training with a compensatory memory device is to ascertain whether the person is knowledgeable about the name and purpose of each notebook section. Sections typically include basic information (personal information, phone numbers, etc.), a calendar, a daily log of activities and a planning or 'things to do' section. A set of ten questions about the notebook structure, contents and purpose is developed, and the person is asked to answer these questions accurately (i.e. 'Where are appointments recorded?'). When the person is able to answer these questions with 100% accuracy on two consecutive days, the next training phase is normally begun.

In the second phase, role-play activities or exercises involving notebook use are introduced. These exercises or assignments require that the person use their book to record and then carry out some action. They may involve bringing something to the clinic, making a phone call, or remembering to follow-up a plan of action. Data is kept on the assigned and due dates, the assignment or task, who assigned it, when the action was carried out and the accuracy of task completion. Criteria are set individually, but usually target 80–100% accuracy over at least five consecutive assignments (Sohlberg and Mateer, 1989b).

Results

Case 1: JM

During the initial, cognitive, baseline assessment, this individual's test scores did not appear to reflect the difficulties he was reporting. Most of his test results were well within a normal range. Cognitive therapy was designed to assess the point at which he was unable to maintain the high level of efficiency he exhibited on the testing measures. A mild attentional deficit clearly did show up early in the first sessions of cognitive therapy, without the structure and noise restrictions of the assessment period. When put on a 'work station' to assess cognitive and psychosocial ability, his memory and executive function deficits became more apparent. The memory difficulties showed up as missed appointments and forgotten tools left at work site, for example. Executive function skills were not reliable when he needed to plan ahead on the job, to know what tools to take or how to organize the day to complete all his work. When engaged in conversation, he exhibited mild, word-finding difficulties and, on occasion if questioned, it became apparent that he had missed parts of the conversation.

In the area of attention/concentration, extensive work on mental control and mental flexibility was initiated during individual cognitive therapy when baseline testing was completed. The tasks included Serial Number Computations and Mental

Number Control (ordering random, non-sequential digits from highest to lowest order and vice versa), as well as Add/Subtract, Odd/Even, and Progressive Letter Cancellation (tasks involving rapid switches between cognitive sets, using numbers and letters). Independently, he was working two hours a week on commercial computer programs which exercised the targeted attention skills. A compensatory memory strategy was introduced in the first week of therapy. This particular individual found the organizational and memory notebook to be convenient and beneficial. He habitually carried it in his shirt pocket and, after ten weeks he proved sufficiently reliable, allowing external clinical monitoring to be stopped.

Just prior to meeting his goal in the area of compensatory memory strategies, executive function tasks were introduced in individual therapy. Work-book exercises arranged hierarchically by degree of difficulty were used throughout the remaining months of cognitive therapy. Over time, he progressed to very high-level and difficult organization and planning tasks, demonstrating increased competency. Carry-over was observed on the work station when the supervisor and co-workers noticed more efficiency and thoroughness on the job. As he was making these changes in executive abilities, his attentional capacity also demonstrated improved efficiency, and therapy was refocused onto attention levels which were more challenging. Weekly group sessions, some designed specifically to address communication problems, provided a structured place for verbal and auditory processing skills to develop. Although he continued to report mild word-finding problems, these were not apparent to those around him.

Overall, this was an individual whose intellectual abilities challenged the clinicians to find increasingly difficult tasks at a very high-skill level. As demonstrated by pre- and post-treatment test scores, he made gains in areas targeted during cognitive treatment. The carry-over onto the work stations was apparent not only to the vocational counsellor, but to his supervisor and coworkers. His success was particularly noteworthy in light of the difficulty he had in accepting and responding to the structure and accountability of the CCR program.

Following eight months of treatment, which began one year after his injury, he returned to work as an electrician, in a higher paying position than his previous job. His new employer was willing to adapt the position to a non-climbing one, as he continued to exhibit balance problems. Discharge testing indicated a 14-point increase in Performance IQ, improved speed on Trails A and B and substantial gains on a verbal learning test.

Case 2: AK

AK exhibited mild deficits across a range of cognitive abilities, including attention/concentration, memory/new learning, executive functions and communication. Only a minimal amount of work was needed to develop a compensatory memory system, as he had developed an independent system which was quite functional. It was apparent that he valued the organizational notebook system, and that he relied upon regular use of it. Therefore, the first three months of cognitive therapy focused only on establishing a strong foundation in sustained and selective attention. Tasks of alternating attention, or mental flexibility, were then introduced, as well as executive function exercises. This man set extremely high standards of performance for himself; because of this, the clinicians gave him constant feedback about his levels of expectation for scores on therapy tasks. The performance issue was an important focus of psychosocial treatment during the same time period, and the cognitive sessions provided opportunities to reinforce the work being done with the psychosocial counsellor.

Performance expectations also became apparent to the participating group members during AK's interaction in weekly groups. During communication sessions, he was given feedback about his manner of presentation to others. Most noticeably, his 'hard-driving' personality was reflected in his communication style by speech that was too rapid, a tendency not to listen to the content of what others presented (affecting his ability to adjust to changes in communication) and a general inability to express his feelings verbally. These pragmatic issues were targeted in groups throughout his seven months at CCR. Excellent changes were noted in his communications skills, as well as in overall intellectual testing (30 point gain on Full Scale IQ), on higher level attention tasks (Trails B and PASAT) and in acquisition of new information (Randt).

Throughout treatment, AK demonstrated a strong determination to maximize his recovery. Pacing was an issue confronted regularly, as his tendency was to take on more than the recommended number of activities, whether it be work, treatment or daily living activities. His aggressive perserverance was at times deemed detrimental by the clinical staff, but ultimately, he made gains that resulted in an excellent vocational outcome. The CCR-II vocational placement specialist negotiated with the correctional institution, and this individual was placed part-time in his previous position as a corrections officer, on a trial basis, while still in treatment at CCR. At program completion, he returned full-time to his previous position with no job modifications. The institution reports complete satisfaction with his current job performance. He was a valued employee prior to the injury, which assisted in the ultimate vocational outcome.

Case 3: AC

Initial baseline testing of cognitive processes indicated overall depressed cognitive functioning. Scores on individual tests reflected a severe memory deficit, moderate to severe difficulties with attention/concentration and communication abilities, a moderate impairment of reasoning/problem, and a mild executive function deficit. In addition, she exhibited a fear of driving to new places and had stopped cooking all but the most basic meals for her family. She was no longer participating in social activities, including entertaining at home.

In cognitive therapy, work was initiated in sustained attention and compensatory memory strategy training. Two months of cognitive treatment time were spent at this more basic level of attention in order for this women to meet goals and establish a strong attentional skills base. In three subsequent months of treatment, the areas of selective, alternating and divided attention were targeted and mastered. Upon entrance to the program, this woman reported consistent use of her own organizational system which also served memory requirements. Early in treatment she was given assignments to test how well the system met her needs. She completed the work assigned at only 77% accuracy, and it became apparent that she was not consistently using the system, nor was her use of it broad enough to cover all areas of her life. Her future requirements for memory assistance on the job were taken into consideration, and a series of questions based on functional usefulness were designed and trained. When she was able to respond accurately (100% of the time) to the questions for two consecutive days, criterion was met. During that training time, more extensive assignments were introduced which incorporated use of the new memory/organization system. When her scores reflected consistency and accuracy in its use, random assignments were given during the remaining three months of treatment.

While scores in attention and compensatory strategies were improving, a third cognitive process area was introduced. Executive functions were targeted in a task involving categorizing wooden objects while considering three principles: size, colour and shape. Reasoning tasks and a series of hierarchically ordered problem-solving worksheets were also introduced. Communication difficulties included word-finding and auditory processing problems. These were largely targeted in group sessions, with all program staff attending to her individual communication needs during the one-to-one treatment sessions. For example, in a vocational counselling session, she was questioned regarding the information just presented to her and reminded to take notes on verbal instruction. At a work station, the supervisor was advised that the participant needed to take written notes when new information was given and then was asked to provide documentation to the treatment team as to whether or not this was occurring.

In cognitive therapy, more direct targeting of communication abilities was completed with exercises using comprehension of information presented and generation of appropriate words and phrases for a specific instance. In the final months of treatment, she proved ready to target her fear of driving to new places. Gradually, assignments of increasing complexity were introduced, and she completed each of them successfully. For the first assignment only, a member of the clinical staff drove with her to the designated place. Likewise, assignments were provided for her cooking difficulties. She participated in independent food preparation for all of the seven discharge parties which occurred during her eight months of treatment. Over time, her preparations became more elaborate. Several home-cooking assignments were also completed successfully. Discharge testing revealed 10-point gains in Verbal and Performance IQ and marked improvement on all measures of attention and memory.

AC participated in two 'work stations' during her program. The success that she experienced on the hospital-based work station provided her with the confidence she needed to try a community placement. This final work station was at a county medical bureau and involved general office clerical tasks. Upon discharge from the CCR program, a comparable permanent full-time position was created for this individual by a local distributing company. The manager of the company sits on the CCR business advisory council and had heard of this woman during one of the council meetings and had asked to meet her. He was so impressed with her resumé and presentation, that he developed a place in the company to use her skills.

Case 4: LM

Goals for cognitive therapy with LM initially focused on sustained, as well as alternating attention and the development of compensatory memory strategies. Eventually, her program targeted each of the other areas in which deficits were demonstrated on baseline testing. These included selective and divided attention, reasoning/problem solving, executive functions, communication, visuo-motor speed and coordination and memory/new learning.

Over time, LM met goals on the first levels of sustained attention training, and within three months she was working at the most difficult alternating attention exercises and on selective attention tasks. She quickly adapted to the use of an organization and compensatory memory system, grateful to have one place to record and locate the information she needed. Visuo-motor skills were then targeted, in addition to the ongoing work in attention and the memory-book assignments. A variety of exercises for problem solving and executive functions were done concurrently during the final weeks of therapy. Worksheets which taxed both visual processing and reasoning abilities proved beneficial. LM participated in communication groups using the opportunity to develop a better awareness of pragmatics and to practice new skills. All staff members and most of the group members assisted in providing feedback to LM regarding her accuracy and timeliness of response to auditorily received information. At the end of her eight-month program, her auditory-processing skills had improved, although she continued to note that it often 'felt like' it took a long time for her to develop her responses in conversation.

Use of learned cognitive and psychosocial skills was measured through her participation on one communication-based work station and through selected work samples administered at CCR. Excellent carry-over was documented. Discharge testing indicated an 18-point gain in Full Scale IQ and significant gains on one or more portions of all attentional and memory measures administered. When LM entered the program, her goals for discharge did not include return to work. Upon discharge, she was able to carry through on her plans to take an extended vacation and to relocate to the east coast. A significant reduction in physical pain was reported at the end of her program.

Case 5: AJ

This woman came to CCR for rehabilitation five-and-a-half years after incurring a head injury. During those years, she had undergone numerous operations for other injuries resulting from the same motor-vehicle accident. She continued to suffer significant chronic pain in her head, neck, jaw and knees. When she arrived at CCR, her cognitive testing indicated deficits in attention/concentration, memory/new learning, executive functions and communication. Initial therapy focused on sustained and selective attention and assessment of her own compensatory memory system.

AJ arrived with a very elaborate memory and organization system, which she had developed out of need over the years since the accident. Little modification of the system resulted from the trial assignments given to assess it's usefulness. Additional compensatory strategies were suggested for times when AJ was unable to record information immediately, and she reported success with some of the new strategies. AJ worked at various levels of attention training (sustained through divided) during her eight months of treatment, with executive functions formally added at the fifth month. Work-book exercises in this area were supplemented by several computer programs which effectively train the ability to plan ahead, to look at a 'bigger picture', to gather information, and to develop suitable strategies. The computer games are structured to provide opportunities for correction and repair. Communication abilities were targeted in groups and individual sessions, with growth demonstrated in auditory processing and pragmatics. Discharge testing revealed a 19-point increase in Verbal IQ and gains in complex attention, memory and new learning.

Carry-over of cognitive skills and psychosocial gains was noted initially by AJ and then by others at her work stations and in her social-support system. AJ attended treatment and struggled to work 32 hours a week throughout her eight months at CCR. A work station, at her place of employment, allowed direct intervention by the therapists for the problems which arose on the job. For six years prior to injury, AJ had successfully held this position. However, the difficulties she now experienced led her to request a lower level position, three months prior to discharge. Her decision to make this change resulted from a desire to reduce the stress and fatigue she was experiencing and to allow herself the energy to participate in non-work activities she enjoyed. AJ reported success in learning the requirements of her new position, and the company indicated satisfaction with her work. Gains were made despite having started the program 65 months post-injury.

Summary

These case scenarios have been included to illustrate the need for individualized programming and to reinforce a focus on functional outcomes. Objective and quantifiable outcomes based on neuropsychological assessment are provided in Table 4.2. Following statistics on the sex, age and time post-injury commencement of treatment for the five participants, the pre- and post-treatment scores are provided for a measure of general intelligence, the *Wechsler Adult Intelligence Scale-Revised* (*WAIS-R*), (Wechsler, 1981). Bold scores indicate significant improvements at post-treatment testing (> 1 SD or 20% change). Following this are pre- and post-treatment results for two measures of attention: *Trial Making A and B* (Reitan, 1985) in seconds to completion, and total correct responses on the first three (slowest) trials of the *Paced Auditory Serial Addition Test* (PASAT), (Gronwall, 1977). The last four columns include pre- and post-treatment scores on two memory measures. These include total correct words recalled on Trials I–V and delayed recall on the *Auditory Verbal Learning Test* (Rey, 1964) and scores on the *Randt Memory Test* (Acquisition score, Recall score and Overall Memory Index) (Randt and Brown, 1983).

Inspection of Table 4.2 reveals a total of 65 separate scores. Of these, 39 were significantly improved following treatment, 2 declined and 24 remained unchanged. All of the participants made gains on one or more measures of general intellectual function. All subjects showed gains on one or both of the measures of attention and on one or both of the measures of memory. Average group gains were seen on all of the measures except the PASAT on which scores were more variable within and across individuals.

The results suggest that statistically significant gains, sometimes to even above-average level performance, could be seen on independent, untrained and unpracticed measures of general intellectual function, sustained, selective and alternating attention and on measures of acquisition and new learning following a period of cognitive rehabilitation as described. Attention training appeared to have benefits for both attentional and memory functioning in much the same way that we and others had previously described (Mateer and Sohlberg, 1988; Niemann, 1989). Attention training also appeared to support gains in general speed of information processing and in both verbal and non-verbal reasoning and problem solving. We recognize that training in the use of external memory aids and executive functions, psychosocial counselling and/or participation in vocational work stations may have contributed to the measured gains on psychometric tests. It is unlikely that spontaneous recovery played a role as all participants were at least 12 months post-injury with one seen over five years post-injury. Gains in cognitive functioning are believed to contribute substantially to the improved vocational functioning of these individuals, although employability and job efficiency are clearly related to many pre- and post-injury variables.

Table 4.2 *Cognitive outcomes following attention training in a mild head-injury population.*

Subject variables	Intelligence		Attention				Memory			
Subject # Sex/Age Months Post-Injury	*WAIS-R* VIQ PIQ FSIQ		*Trails* A B		*PASAT* Trial 1 Trial 2 Trial 3		*AVLT* Total T1–T5 Delayed Recall		*Randt* Forms A–E Acquisition Recall Memory Index	
	Pre	Post	Pre	Post	Pre	Post	Pre	Post	Pre	Post
1	127	123	37	**19**	53	45	48	**68**	125	127
M–46 yrs	124	**138**	56	**43**	48	39	11	**14**	104	111
12 months	129	134			42	35			116	121
2	88	**124**	23	56	47	48	52	53	94	**113**
M–32 yrs	98	**110**	65	**41**	38	43	13	14	116	104
18 months	91	**121**			20	**31**			106	109
3	78	**88**	72	**32**	36	**44**	52	**63**	64	**108**
F–40 yrs	85	**95**	168	**76**	32	**45**	10	**13**	72	**99**
22 months	81	**90**			30	**37**			63	**104**
4	99	**113**	31	**23**	31	**44**	42	50	111	116
F–46 yrs	99	**121**	76	**50**	33	**39**	8	**10**	71	**83**
24 months	99	**117**			39	33			89	**99**
5	101	**120**	22	20	40	**48**	44	**61**	93	101
F–42 yrs	118	121	43	42	34	**40**	5	**12**	78	**95**
65 months	109	**124**			37	33			83	**97**
Means	98.6	**113.6**	37.0	**30.0**	41.4	45.8	47.6	**59.0**	97.4	**113.0**
40.8 yrs	104.8	**117.6**	81.6	**50.4**	37.0	41.2	9.4	**12.6**	88.2	**98.4**
28.2 months	101.8	**117.2**			33.6	33.8			91.4	**106.0**

Conclusion

Overall, this research and our experience with many other individuals seen in our post-acute programs have led us to believe that targeted training of attentional skills and compensatory memory strategies can have substantial benefits in a package of rehabilitation services (see Chapters 5 and 6, this volume). This is true, not only for the moderately to severely head-injured patient, but also for the patient with apparently milder injuries. Reduction in high-level linguistic, reasoning or problem-solving skills is less likely to occur than is reduced efficiency for basic underlying capacities, such as attention. The delivery of theoretically based, systematic treatment which focuses on a hierarchy of attentional processes appears to be an important and effective restorative facet of cognitive rehabilitation. This should be combined with structured training in and facilitation of compensatory systems and strategies. All treatment activities must incorporate functional activities and settings. Generalization should never be expected; it should be planned for, trained for, and evaluated.

References

BEN-YISHAY, Y. and DILLER, L., 1983, 'Cognitive deficits'. In M. Rosenthal (Ed.) *Rehabilitation of the head injured adult* (Philadelphia: F. A. Davis), pp. 162–81.

BEN-YISHAY, Y. and DILLER, L., 1978–1983, 'Working approaches to remediation of cognitive deficits in brain damaged persons'. New York University Medical Center, *Rehabilitation Monographs Nos. 59–62, 64, 66.*

BEN-YISHAY, Y., PIASETSKY, E. B. and RATTOCK, J., 1987a, 'A systematic method for ameliorating disorders in basic attention'. In M. J. Meier, A. L. Benton and L. Diller (Eds) *Neuropsychological Rehabilitation* (New York: Guilford Press), pp. 165–81.

BEN-YISHAY, Y., SILVER, S. and PIASETSKY, E., 1987b, 'Relationship between employability and vocational outcome after intensive holistic cognitive rehabilitation'. *Journal of Head Trauma Rehabilitation*, **2**, 35–48.

BIRBAUMER, N., ELBERT, T., ROCKSTROH, B. and LUTZENBERGER, W., 1986, 'Biofeedback of slow cortical potentials in attentional disorders'. In W. C. McCallum, R. Zapolli and F. Denoth (Eds) Cerebral psychophysiology: Studies in event-related potentials. *Electroencephalography and Clinical Neurophysiology* (Suppl.), **38**, 42–9, 440–2.

CERMAK, L. S., 1975, 'Imagery as an aid to retrieval for Korsakoff patients', *Cortex*, **11**, 163–9.

CROVITZ, H. F., 1979, 'Memory retraining in brain-damaged patients: The airplane list'. *Cortex*, **15**, 131–4.

CROVITZ, H. F., HARVEY, M. T. and HORN, R. W., 1979, 'Problems in the acquisition of imagery mnemonics: Three brain-damaged cases'. *Cortex*, **15**, 225–34.

DILLER, L. and WEINBERG, J., 1977, 'Hemi-inattention in rehabilitation: The evolution of a rational remediation program'. In E. A. Weinstein and R. P. Friedland (Eds) *Advances in Neurology*, **18**, 63–82.

FRAZIER, L. M., 1980, 'Biofeedback in coma rehabilitation: Case study'. *American Journal of Clinical Biofeedback*. **3**, 148–54.

GASPARRINI, B. and SATZ, P., 1979, 'A treatment for memory problems in left hemisphere CVA patients'. *Journal of Clinical Neuropsychology*, **91**, 66–73.

GESCHWIND, N., 1982, 'Disorders of attention: A frontier in psychology'. *Philosophical Transactions of the Royal Society of London*, **B298**, 173–85.

GIANUTSOS, R. and GIANUTSOS, J., 1979, 'Rehabilitating the verbal recall of brain-injured patients by mnemonic training: An experimental demonstration using single-case methodology'. *Journal of Clinical Neuropsychology*, **2**, 117–35.

GLASGOW, R. E., ZEISS, R. A. and BARRERA, M. Jr., 1977, 'Case study on remediating memory deficits in brain-damaged individuals'. *Journal of Clinical Psychology*, **33**, 1049–54.

GLISKY, E., SCHACTER, D. and TULVING, E., 1985, 'Acquisition and retention of new knowledge in amnesic patients: Method of vanishing cues'. Paper presented at the *13th Annual Meeting of the International Neuropsychological Society*, San Diego, CA.

GODFREY, H. and KNIGHT, R., 1985, 'Cognitive rehabilitation of memory functioning in amnesiac alcoholics'. *Journal of Consulting Clinical Psychology*, **43**, 555–7.

GOLDBERG, K., GERSTMAN, L. J. and MATHIS, S., 1982, 'Selective effects of cholinergic treatment on verbal memory in post-traumatic amnesia. *Journal of Clinical Neuropsychology*, **4**, 219–34.

GOLDSTEIN, G. and RUTHVEN, L., 1983, *Rehabilitation of the brain-damaged adult* (New York: Plenum).

GRONWALL, D., 1977, 'Paced auditory serial addition task: A measure of recovery from concussion'. *Perceptual Motor Skills*, **44**, 367–73.

JACOBS, H., 1988, 'The Los Angeles head injury survey: Procedures and initial findings'. *Archives of Physical Medicine and Rehabilitation*, **69**, 425–31.

JOHNS, D. F., 1978, *Clinical Management of Neurogenic Communication Disorders* (Boston: Little Brown & Company).

KEWMAN, D. G., SEIGERMAN, C., KINTNER, H., CHU, S., HENSON, D. and REEDER, C., 1985, 'Simulation training of psychomotor skills: Teaching the brain-injured to drive'. *Rehabilitation Psychology*, **9**, 297–309.

KLOVE, H., 1987, 'Activation, arousal and neuropsychological rehabilitation'. *Journal of Clinical and Experimental Neuropsychology*, **9**, 297–309.

KREUTZER, J., WEHMAN, P. and MORTON, M., 1988, 'Supported employment and compensatory strategies for enhancing vocational outcome following traumatic brain injury'. *Brain Injury*, **2**, 205–23.

LEWINN, E. B. and DIMANCESCU, M. D., 1978, 'Environmental deprivation and enrichment in coma'. *The Lancet*, **2**, 156–7.

LEWINSOHN, P. M., DANAHER, B. G. and KIKEL, D., 1977, 'Visual imagery as a mnemonic aid for brain-injured persons'. *Journal of Consulting and Clinical Psychology*, **45**, 717–23.

LEZAK, M. D., 1978, 'Living with the characterologically altered brain-injured patient'. *Journal of Clinical Psychiatry*, **39**, 592–8.

LEZAK, M. D., 1983, *Neuropsychological Assessment* (New York: Oxford University Press).

LEZAK, M. D., 1987, 'Relationships between personality disorders, social disturbances, and physical disability following traumatic brain injury'. *Journal of Head Trauma Rehabilitation*, **2**, 57–9.

LYNCH, J. J., 1978, 'The simple act of touching'. *Nursing*, **8**, 32.

MALEC, J., JONES, R. and RAO, N., 1984, 'Video game practice effects on sustained attention in patients with craniocerebral trauma'. *Cognitive Rehabilitation*, **2(4)**, 18–23.

MATEER, C. A. and SOHLBERG, M. M., 1988, 'A paradigm shift in memory rehabilitation'. In H. Whitaker (Ed.) *Neuropsychological studies of nonfocal brain damage: Dementia and trauma* (New York: Springer Verlag), pp. 204–19.

MATEER, C. A. and SOHLBERG, M. M., 1989, 'Vocational outcomes following post-acute rehabilitation'. *Bulletin of the Center for Cognitive Rehabilitation*, Puyallup, Washington: Good Samaritan Hospital.

MCLEAN, A. Jr., STANTON, K. M. and CARDENAS, D. D., 1987, 'Memory training combined with the use of physostigmine'. *Brain Injury*, **1**, 145–59.

NIEMANN, H., 1989, 'Retraining of attention in head injured individuals'. Doctoral dissertation, University of Victoria, British Columbia, Canada.

PARENTE, R. and ANDERSON, J. K., 1983, 'Techniques for improving cognitive rehabilitation: Teaching organizational and encoding skills'. *Cognitive Rehabilitation*, **1**, 20–2.

PONSFORD, J. L. and KINSELLA, G., 1988, *Journal of Clinical and Experimental Neuropsychology*, **10**, 693–708.

POSNER, M. I., 1975, 'Psychobiology of attention'. In M. S. Gazzeniga and C. Blakemore (Eds) *Handbook of Psychology* (New York, London: Academic Press), pp. 441–80.

PRIGATANO, G., 1986, *Neuropsychological rehabilitation after brain injury* (Baltimore, Johns Hopkins University Press).

PRIGATANO, G., FORDYCE, D., ZEINER, H., ROUECHE, J., PEPPING, M. and WOOD, B., 1984, 'Neuropsychological rehabilitation after closed head injury in young adults'. *Journal of Neurology, Neurosurgery, and Neuropsychiatry*, **47**, 505–13.

RANDT, C T. and BROWN, E. R., 1983, *Randt Memory Test*, Bayport, New York: Life Science Associates.

RAPPAPORT, M., HALL, K. M., HOPKINS, K. and BELLEZA, T., 1982, 'Disability rating scale for severe head trauma: Coma to community'. *Archives of Physical Medicine and Rehabilitation*, **63**, 118–23.

REEDER, C., 1985, 'Simulation training of psychomotor skills: Teaching the brain-injured to drive'. *Rehabilitation Psychology*, **30**, 11–27.

REITAN, R. M., 1958, 'Validity of the trail making test as an indication of organic brain damage', *Perceptual Motor Skills*, **8**, 271–276.

REY, A. L., 1964, *L'Examen Clinique en Psychologie*, Paris, Presses Universitaires de France.

RUFF, R. M., BASER, C. A., JOHNSON, J. W., MARSHALL, L. F., KLAUBER, S. K., KLAUBER, M. R. and MINTEER, M., 1989, 'Neuropsychological rehabilitation: an experimental study with head-injured patients'. *Journal of Head Trauma Rehabilitation*, **4**, (3), 20–36.

SCHACTER, D., RICH, S. and STAMPP, A., 1985, 'Remediation of memory disorders: Experimental evaluation of the spaced-retrieval technique'. *Journal of Clinical and Experimental Neuropsychology*, **7**, 79–96.

SOHLBERG, M. M. and BROCK, M., 1985, 'Taking the final step: The importance of post-medical cognitive rehabilitation'. *Cognitive Rehabilitation*, **3**, 10–4.

SOHLBERG, M. M. and MATEER, C. A., 1987, 'Effectiveness of an attention-training program'. *Journal of Clinical and Experimental Neuropsychology*, **9**, 117–30.

SOHLBERG, M. M. and MATEER, C. A., 1989a, *Introduction to cognitive rehabilitation: Theory and practice* (New York: Guilford Press).

SOHLBERG, M. M. and MATEER, C. A., 1989b, 'Training use of compensatory memory books: A three stage behavioral approach'. *Journal of Clinical and Experimental Neuropsychology*, **11**, 871–91.

SOHLBERG, M. M. and MATEER, C. A. (1990), 'Evaluation and treatment of communications skills'. In J. S. Kreutzer and P. Lehman (Eds) *Community integration following traumatic brain injury* (Baltimore, MD: Paul H. Brookes Publishing Company), pp. 67–83.

SOHLBERG, M. M., SPRUNK, H. and METZELAAR, K., 1988, 'Efficacy of an external cuing system in an individual with severe frontal lobe damage'. *Cognitive Rehabilitation*, **6**, 36–41.

STURM, W., DAHMEN, W., HARTJE, W. and WILLMES, K., 1983, 'Ergebnisse eines Trainingsprogramms zur Verbesserung der visuellen Auffassungsschnelligkeit und Konzentrationsfahigkeit bei Hirngeschadigten'. (Results of a progam for the training of perceptual speed and attention in brain damaged patients). *Archiv fur Psychiatrie und Nervenkrankheiten* (Archives of Psychiatry and Neurological Sciences), **233**, 9–22.

STUSS, D. T. and BENSON, D. F., 1986, *The frontal lobes* (New York: Raven Press).

VAN ZOMEREN, A. H., BROUWER, W. H. and DEELMAN, B. G., 1984, 'Attentional deficits: The riddles of selectivity, speed, and alertness'. In N. Brooks (Ed.) *Closed head injury. Psychological, social, and family consequences* (New York: Oxford University Press), pp. 74–107.

WEBER (1990), 'A practical clinical approach to understanding and treating attentional problems'. *Journal of Head Trauma Rehabilitation*, **5**, 73–85.

WEINBERG, J., DILLER, L., GORDON, W. A., GERSTMAN, L. J., LIEBERMANN, A., LAKIN, P., HODGES, G. and EZRACHI, O., 1977, 'Visual scanning training effect on reading-related tasks in acquired right-brain damage'. *Archives of Physical Medicine and Rehabilitation*, **58**, 479–86.

WEINBERG, J., DILLER, L., GORDON, W. A., GERSTMAN, L. J., LIEBERMANN, A., LAKIN, P., HODGES, G. and EZRACHI, O., 1979, 'Training sensory awareness and spatial organization in people with right brain damage'. *Archives of Physical Medicine and Rehabilitation*, **60**, 491–6.

WILSON, B., 1981, 'Teaching a patient to remember people's names after removal of a left temporal tumor'. *Behavioral Psychotherapy*, **9**, 338–44.

WILSON, B., 1982, 'Success and failure in memory training following a cerebral vascular accident'. *Cortex*, **18**, 581–94.

WILSON, B., 1987, *Rehabilitation of Memory* (London: Guilford Press).

WILSON, B. and MOFFAT, N. (Eds) 1984, *Clinical management of memory problems* (Rockville, Maryland: Aspen).

WOOD, R. L., 1986, 'Rehabilitation of patients with disorders of attention'. *Journal of Head Trauma Rehabilitation*, **1**, 43–53.

WOOD, R. L., 1987, *Brain injury rehabilitation: A neurobehavioral approach* (Rockville, Maryland: Aspen).

WOOD, R. L., 1989, 'Clinical model for sensory stimulation for patients in coma and PVS'. Paper presented at the *Santa Clara Valley Medical Center Twelfth Annual Conference*, San Jose, CA.

WOOD, R. L. and FUSSEY, I., 1987, 'Computer-based cognitive retraining: A controlled study'. *International Disability Studies*, **9**, 149–53.

PART 3
REHABILITATION OF MEMORY DISORDERS

Chapter 5

The Process Diary Concept: An Approach in Training Orientation, Memory and Behaviour Control

A. Finset and S. Andresen

Introduction

Problems of orientation, memory and behaviour control are rather common after traumatic head injury (Griffith, 1983; Prigatano, 1986). They represent typical challenges to the rehabilitation team as the patient may often have problems of behaviour control which prohibits the use of many memory training techniques. On the other hand, memory problems may seriously complicate the effectiveness of the team in treating behavioural problems. Any awareness or insight arrived at during a therapy session may all too easily be forgotten, and the therapist may have to start the counselling process all over again.

The characteristic combinations of the neuropsychological deficits after traumatic head injury reflects the complexity of pathophysiology in brain trauma — and the multiple ways in which brain injury affects cognition. In any individual patient referred for rehabilitation, the team may find examples both of limited functional losses due to focal damage (contusions, haematomas), such as a specific memory problem or language disturbance, and of a more generalized reduction in the basic level of cognitive functioning, for instance due to diffuse axonal damage (Miller, 1983).

The nature of the focal damage may be different in the head-injured patient than in many other categories of brain disease. For instance, after a stroke, the focal neuropsychological symptoms may be limited to one or a few functional systems, such as visuo-spatial or verbal functions based on posterior cortical processing. The posterior cortex, containing primary sensory projection fields and providing higher order integration of these, specializes in what may be called 'representative' functions as they provide perceptual representations of the environment. In the head-injured patient, however, the focal damage tends to involve anterior temporal or frontal structures (Stuss and Benson, 1986), which often leads to a breakdown of processes such as initiating behaviour, adequate shifting from one action sequence to another, inhibition of inadequate impulses and the general planning and structuring of behaviour. Tucker (1988) denotes these processes as 'regulatory' as opposed to representative functions. This dichotomy parallels Pribram's (1981) distinction between epicritic and protocritic processing. Whereas representative (epicritic) processing involves perceptual analysis and integration, regulatory (protocritic) functions are responsible for a broad range of behavioural control processes.

Basic to the concept of regulatory processing is the notion of cerebral interaction. In his discussion of representative and regulatory functions, Tucker (1988) pointed to the research on the reciprocal connections between each major cortical region and frontal cortex (Nauta, 1971). Recent studies indicate that each of the cognitive operations of the posterior cortex is paralleled by activity in specific pre-frontal areas not directly involved in motor processing (Roland, 1984). Thus, the regulatory processing involves the influence of frontal structures over processing in other areas of the brain.

In this view, the brain is functioning as a system of interconnected subsystems. Let us take language as an example. Verbal behaviour involves what we call representative functioning. But there are centres in the frontal lobes that exert regulatory influence on language behaviour: initiating talking, regulating the shift of subject, verbally perseverating, planning what to do next. Thus, pre-frontal damage may function to inhibit or excite the functioning of the language centres located elsewhere in the brain.

The breakdown of regulatory functions are among the most problematic kinds of sequelae after traumatic head trauma. It seems to be less complicated to work with a single skill or concrete task than to cope with aspects of complex deregulation of behaviour. In patients with deficits in regulatory processing, the challenge to the treatment team may be described as to further the release of function in intact areas of the brain that may not be available and useful to the patient without special intervention.

Treatment Strategies in Training Orientation, Memory and Behaviour Control

Methods described in the rehabilitation literature

Many approaches have been adopted to treat orientation, memory and behaviour control in head-injury patients. Problems in general orientation have been addressed in various forms of reality-orientation therapy programmes, individually or in group therapy (Cerny and McNeny, 1983). Orientation therapy is very basic to all head-injury rehabilitation, and some approach to this category of training should be included in all head-injury programmes, at least in early stages of treatment. Patients should be provided with clocks, calendars, name tags, signs, etc. to promote orientation in the environment.

Memory training has been described many times in the last few years with a wide variety of techniques and procedures being used; little explicit attention has been given to memory-training techniques in the context of behaviour-control problems.

In recent years, some approaches have also been described, specifically designed for treatment of the deficits in regulatory functions and behaviour control. One obvious approach is behaviour therapy. As early as the late 1960s a few references were available on the application of behaviour therapy in the treatment of brain-damaged patients (Goodkin, 1966; Walls, 1969), but only recently has behaviour therapy been described as a comprehensive treatment approach in head-trauma rehabilitation (Muir *et al.*, 1983; Eames and Wood, 1985). Over the last few years, therapy approaches have been described in very different treatment settings, ranging from acute care, head-injury units (Howard, 1988) to community reintegration programmes (Hogan, 1988).

Some authors have described different problem-solving techniques applied in retraining of regulatory functions (Craine, 1982). Both laboratory tasks, computer games and puzzles of different kinds may be of value in a training programme, but nonetheless the question of transfer of training or generalizing will arise as far as these methods are concerned. It is reasonable to believe that problem-solving techniques will be more useful when the regulatory deficits comprise problems in cognitive flexibility and executive functions rather than, for instance, impulsivity or deficient behaviour initiation.

Different types of psychotherapeutic approaches have been described (Prigatano, 1986). Obviously, the memory problems of the patient will interfere with treatment, and Prigatano gives several suggestions on how to cope with this, such as applying short sessions, providing frequent repetitions of main points in therapy, etc.

Requirements of a treatment method for problems of behavioural control

We have indicated a need for a programme that specifically addresses both the orientation and memory problems of the patient and the problems associated with aspects of behaviour control (i.e. regulatory functions). Our emphasis will be on the latter and, for our purposes, what we need is a treatment approach that includes the following:

1 Even if behaviour control is the main objective of the treatment programme, it must be specifically oriented to the memory problem of the patient. Whatever intervention is chosen, it must be stored in a way that is available to the amnesic patient. If the interventions are kept on record, on tape, in a book or wherever, they must be used actively and repeated frequently if they are to be remembered by the patient.

2 A basic problem of the frontal lobe-injured patient is the lack of structure. The very nature of regulatory functions is to provide structure to the environment for the individual. When this in-built structure is deficient, the treatment method must be able to provide structure to the patient, explicit enough for the patient to recognize.

3 Also, the patient with deficient regulatory functions has a reduced ability to use feedback provided by others in the environment (Craine, 1982). Therefore, we must find an approach that very explicitly provides the patient with feedback. Giving feedback, of course, is the very essence of behaviour therapy, but the reinforcement of behaviour therapy is very much a here-and-now phenomenon. Reinforcements work to make the patient learn — by constant repetitions over a long time or by the application of learning principles to a limited set of behaviours. However, behaviour therapy is not specifically directed towards increasing deficit awareness, which is shown to be positively related to treatment performance among head-injury patients (Lam *et al.*, 1988). We need a feedback procedure that — possibly in addition to functioning as positive reinforcement — may relate to cognitive content in order to increase deficit awareness.

4 The method should also give the patient an opportunity to take an active part in the assessment process, applying the method of self-monitoring, which has been shown to be a useful therapeutic technique in cognitive psychotherapy (Kendall and Norton–Ford, 1982) and is also discussed in the management of emotional disorders by Alderman and Burgess, Chapter 10.

5 The method should be related, as directly as possible, to the everyday tasks the patient needs to learn to cope with and master, in order to assist with the transfer of training. The more relevant the tasks are, the easier is the process of teaching the patient to apply the method outside the clinical programme.

6 The method should be available to the whole rehabilitation team. Often, the team members do not know what goes on in other therapy sessions, therefore the methods used for training should be recorded so that all members of the team understand the content of training. Self-explanatory training procedures may be useful simply to inform other team members of what goes on in treatment.

The Process-Diary Concept

The notebook or diary — a common tool in cognitive rehabilitation

In our search for a method that would meet the above requirements, we chose a diary as a basic tool for treatment. This is certainly not a new idea, the notebook or diary is one of the most common and obvious external aids applied in memory training (Harris, 1978, 1984). The way we apply the diary, however, is specifically designed for use with patients with problems of behaviour control.

The applicability of a diary or notebook for this purpose is not obvious. As indicated, most often the diary is used for purposes of memory training. Very often, when such a book is to serve several purposes, the structure is lost; frequently we find diaries with many categories of entries, but not organized in a way that makes them available for patients with difficulties initiating and structuring behaviour. Most often a therapist will apply a notebook or diary with the emphasis on the content. Our approach is concerned with emphasizing process as well, thus the name 'process diary'.

The setting for treatment

Before describing the treatment approach in more detail, it may seem appropriate to briefly describe the setting in which the process-diary concept has been developed. Sunnaas Rehabilitation Hospital, Nesodden, Norway, is the largest and most highly specialized rehabilitation hospital in Norway, with programmes for head-injury rehabilitation, spinal cord rehabilitation, stroke rehabilitation and a special programme for patients with other disabilities. The hospital serves basically the two southeastern regions of Norway, covering about half the Norwegian population of some 4 million people, but patients from western and northern Norway may also be admitted for treatment. The head-injury programme consists of a 17-bed unit, with most of the patients admitted a few weeks post-injury. The unit is divided into three subsections, each located in a separate wing in the head-injury ward (Finset, 1989).

The North Wing Programme (four beds) is specialized for evaluation and treatment of patients with very severe sequelae after head injury, including patients in or close to vegetative states. Most of these patients are admitted for an evaluation of their rehabilitation potential. They are usually returned to their local hospitals after evaluation. The East Wing Programme (six beds) is designed for patients with severe head injuries but with at least some capacity to communicate and cooperate in treatment. Most patients will have both physical and psychological sequelae and stay for treatment for three to five months. The South Wing Programme (seven beds) offers evaluation and treatment for patients who walk and talk but who suffer from deficits in cognitive, regulative and emotional areas. The programme is to a large extent based on group treatment.

The Format of the Process Diary

The process diary is a notebook of a loose-leaf letter-file type in standard A4 format. The treatment consists of individual sessions, where the patient works with a therapist (psychologist, occupational therapist, special education teacher or nurse trained in cognitive rehabilitation). A series of standard work sheets has been developed, a couple of examples are given in Figures 5.1 and 5.2. The sheets are produced on the hospital word-processing system and may easily be changed to meet individual needs. All the sheets are available in the head-injury ward and may be easily used by nurses or other trained personnel. Treatment starts with assessment in the area of cognitive functions in question and of behaviour in general. Assessment is done by the clinical neuropsychologist as well as by other team members.

The first step in treatment should be to formulate treatment goals, but as the very formulation of treatment goals is a basic part of the treatment process, we may start by simply stating to the patient that this book is used during therapy sessions without giving him or her an explanation. Very often cognitive training begins with orientation and memory tasks, and the book is introduced as a tool to be used in memory training.

As the work with the process diary progresses, the diary is divided into sections, separated with divider sheets. Most often, each of the category of work sheets mentioned below will constitute one section. Some examples of standard work sheets in the different categories or sections include:

Orientation

One work sheet states the name of the weekday, date, month and year. One such sheet is filled in every day, most often in the morning, and is supervized by one of the nurses on the ward. Another work sheet contains a series of questions such as: What is the name of the hospital? When were you admitted? Why are you staying here? What was the date of your injury? Where did you go first after injury? The diary will also often include a calendar in the orientation section of the book.

Another standard orientation and memory aid is the daily schedule. To aid amnesic patients, we have produced small passport-size pictures of team members that may be attached to schedules, etc. as stickers.

Planning

Several work sheets are concerned with different aspects of planning, both of the treatment sessions and of planning activities in the hospital or during weekend visits in the home. One sheet lists the goals for treatment, another one a plan for assignments during the week, etc.

Memory

Many patients have a smaller datebook, developed within the programme, with the daily schedule presented and space to record how each session went. The process diary itself may be used in many different ways as a memory-training tool, just as other diaries are described in the memory-training literature (Harris, 1984).

Diary

One section of the book may simply contain a diary, written every day, if necessary with a special work sheet for each day, to remind the patient of this assignment.

Self-evaluation

A series of work sheets is concerned with self-evaluation. The strong-points-and-weak-points sheet (Fig. 5.1) is commented on in more detail in the brief case example (Case A) in the following section. The diary may be used in many different ways to promote self-evaluation.

Special assignments

The patient may be given assignments to be carried out between therapy sessions, such as watching TV and telling, in a subsequent therapy session, what the news programme was about, etc.

Feedback on behaviour

In some patients with impulsivity and disinhibition problems, we use the diary to give feedback on behaviour in a more systematic way. With one patient for instance, we designed two special feedback sheets. On one page, all violations of agreed upon rules concerning certain target behaviours were recorded, primarily by the nursing staff and preferably immediately after the rule was violated. On another page, examples of tasks the patient actually did master were recorded in the same way. The method seemed to make the patient more aware of his actions and to some extent shape his behaviour in the desired direction.

Training initiative

Training patients to take more initiative will be briefly mentioned in the two case examples. In working with passive patients, the psychologist may, for instance, write assignments in the notebook. The assignment may concern some sort of activity that the patient is supposed to perform toward one of the nurses: ask a specific question, discuss a topic, give a message, etc. The assignment should be available in the book for the nurse to see, but she should not remind the patient about the assignment. The assignment may also be a more general reminder to read the papers, take a walk, etc. or include a structured schedule for the patient's spare time. The patient should remember the assignment and be supposed to take the initiative to perform the task. The intervention may help the patient to a better awareness of his problems in taking initiative and eventually overcoming them.

Evaluation of treatment

After each brief period of treatment, usually one week, a specific sheet evaluating treatment is filled in (Fig. 5.2). The therapist and the patient go back to the planning sheet for the week and evaluate to what extent the plans have been carried out and which goals have been attained.

As the work with the diary progresses, the patient gradually should become more responsible for what occurs. In the beginning, everything in the book is initiated by the therapist. As time goes on, the patient may learn to work with the book more independently, and the structure of the book will usually become more complicated, with more sections and dividing sheets. The assignments may become more difficult, and the range of activities may be broader. Only imagination will limit the application of the process diary.

Case example A: John F. — Training in Structure, Initiative and Awareness of Own Behaviour

John F. — a 32-years-old, married bus driver — sustained a severe head injury in a traffic accident. He was in a coma for over a week, and CT-scans showed signs of a right frontal contusion. As he emerged from coma in the second week post-injury, he was found to have a left hemiplegia. He was admitted to the head-injury unit of a major rehabilitation hospital a little less than two months post-injury. By this time he had recovered fairly well from his pareses but still suffered from disorientation in time and space, to the point of delusions; he also had considerable memory problems. He confabulated, showed little or no initiative, suffered from marked irritability and showed no ability to plan and structure his own behaviour. He had little or no insight into his own situation and had no clear understanding of what had actually happened

Figure 5.1 Worksheet used for the patient's self-evaluation of weak and strong points in his/her own functioning.

THE PROCESS DIARY

NAME:............................ Date:......... Sign.:......

STRONG POINTS AND WEAK POINTS IN MY FUNCTIONING

THESE THINGS I TACKLE FAIRLY WELL:

1.

2.

3.

THESE THINGS ARE TROUBLESOME FOR ME:

1.

2.

3.

to him. Neuropsychological tests did not reflect the severity of this problem. Perceptual and certain other cognitive functions were operating close to the normal range of scores for his age group.

During the first two weeks of treatment in the rehabilitation hospital, John F. was extremely disoriented. After a few more days, his orientation gradually progressed. He had occasional episodes of disorientation with a complete confusion as to where he was. It was hard to discriminate between confabulation and outright delusions. He could, for instance, insist that a specific friend of his was on the ward, but every time he said it, the friend was absent. As his orientation improved, we decided to start the process diary. John's intellectual capacities were well preserved and his orientation had recovered to the point where it was basically intact, making it possible to quit the orientation and memory preludes and go straight to a more complex variant of the process diary.

The neuropsychological assessment, as well as team observations, revealed that in spite of his relatively preserved posterior hemisphere functions, John had massive problems in the structure of behaviour. He was physically able to perform all daily life activities but was not able to carry them out properly without prompting. He showed very little initiative and did not commit himself to anything during the days on the ward. He would typically be found passive in a chair, possibly watching TV, or roaming aimlessly around the corridor. He showed little insight into his own problems.

We decided to work with three interrelated sets of problems in the process-diary programme: (1) structure, (2) initiative and (3) insight. A diary with five sections separated with dividing sheets was designed. The first section of John's book was a 'planning and scheduling' section. Here we had the daily schedule and a planning sheet for every week of treatment. The second section was the actual diary section. Here he wrote a little story for each day. Third came the 'strong-points/weak-points' section. This work sheet contained three items under the heading 'strong points' and three items with 'weak points' (Fig. 5.1).

The fourth section was allotted for different assignments. Here we worked with homework-type assignments, such as reading newspapers and telling the contents, etc. Finally, the fifth section in John's book was the evaluation section. One evaluation sheet (Fig. 5.2) was filled in every week of the treatment.

In working with John, we first emphasized planning and structuring of the treatment and of the day in general. In the treatment sessions with the psychologist, we repeated his daily schedule over and over again. We set up a plan for treatment sessions and started the session with references to the plan. We asked John to write a diary and informed the afternoon nurses so that they could supervize his writing. Some days he actually wrote a little, but with very short and somewhat laconic entries.

Early in treatment we started to fill in the strong-points/weak-points sheet (Fig. 5.1). He had little awareness of his deficits, and under the heading 'These things are troublesome for me', he wrote down some variations of the theme 'I'm bored in the hospital'. We responded to his 'I'm bored' talk by giving him assignments such as reading interesting stories in the newspaper (c.f. the fourth section for assignments in his process diary). He complied to his assignments but without enthusiasm.

After some time, John actually began to show more interest in the strong-points/weak-points sheet. We discussed the sheet in several therapy sessions; we advized him to talk to his wife about it, and gradually he became more realistic and to the point in his self-evaluations. He became aware of his passivity, and showed more effort and interest in treatment. Gradually the sessions, that at one time were daily,

Figure 5.2 Evaluation sheet used towards the end of each week of treatment.

THE PROCESS DIARY

NAME:.......................... Date:......... Sign........

HOW WELL HAVE WE BEEN WORKING THIS WEEK ?

Time period: ....

WHAT WE PLANNED	HOW IT WORKED OUT
1.	
2.	
3.	
4.	

became less frequent, and John started to work with some of the sheets on his own. By the time of his discharge, after some three months in the unit, he clearly showed more initiative, was better able to structure his day and had a better awareness of his assets and deficits.

Case Example B: Assessment of Treatment Efficacy

Assessment of treatment efficacy of a method designed to treat behavioural control is not easy. The variables involved, such as initiation of behaviour, perseverations, distractibility, impulsivity, disinhibition, ability to plan and structure behaviour and even day-to-day memory, are far more difficult to measure than such cognitive tasks as memory span, verbal acquisition, spatial perception, etc.

In our head-injury unit, we are presently engaged in developing assessment procedures, designed to evaluate treatment methods such as the process-diary concept. The procedures include lists of target behaviour relevant for each of the aspects of behaviour regulation mentioned above. For each individual patient, we select ten items on the relevant list, observe the patient over a number of baseline observations then during treatment and finally over a short period of post-training assessments, basically following a conventional single-case study approach (Kazdin, 1982).

One case example illustrating both the treatment approach described in this paper and our developing methods of assessing treatment efficacy will be presented. Patient B is a 40-years-old, married, male carpenter who sustained a massive haemorrhage from an aneurism of the anterior communicating artery. At the acute-care hospital, the patient had post-operatively been hallucinating and had been treated with neuroleptic drugs. When the patient was admitted to the head-injury rehabilitation unit three months post-surgery, he was severely disoriented for time, place and personal information. When interviewed on his personal history, he was prone to confabulate. He could not tell what his present employment was, nor the age of his three children, and he lacked awareness of his own deficits. He had obvious problems with initiation of goal-directed behaviour and remained passive if left alone. Neuropsychological testing revealed general intellectual abilities in the lower normal range. The patient exhibited markedly reduced memory functions, achieving a Memory Quotient of 43 points on the Randt Memory Test (Randt *et al.*, 1980). The patient also suffered a left side homonymous hemianopia.

During the first few weeks in the rehabilitation hospital, the patient reached a fairly adequate level of awareness of his problems in memory and perception but had little ability to cope effectively with his memory difficulties and remained passive on the ward and on visits outside the hospital. The rehabilitation team decided to present the patient with a process-diary programme similar to the one described in the previous case but with more emphasis on orientation and memory functions.

Day-to-day memory was evaluated with a ten-item check-list constructed by the present authors to assess practical day-to-day memory (Table 5.1). The items covered memory for regular activities on the ward, as well as weekend activities which tended to vary more from week to week. The patient's answers were validated against information obtained from the nursing staff and the patient's relatives.

Table 5.1 Memory check-list

QUESTIONS TO BE ASKED ON MONDAY.
1. Have you been in the hospital all weekend?
2. What did you do on Friday?
3. What did you do Saturday morning?
4. What did you do Saturday afternoon?
5. What did you do on Sunday?
QUESTIONS TO BE ASKED ON TUESDAY.
6. What did you do yesterday afternoon?
7. Did you attend physical therapy group this morning?
8. Did you attend group psychotherapy this afternoon?
9. What is the name of your physical therapist?
10. What have you been doing during the last hour?

Table 5.2 Initiative check-list

ACTIVITIES TO BE MONITORED TUESDAY AFTERNOON AND EVENING.
1. Activity immediately before dinner (at 4.00 p.m.).
2. Activity at 6.00 p.m.
3. Activity at 8.30 p.m.
ACTIVITIES TO BE MONITORED ON WEDNESDAY.
4. Activity between 7.00 and 8.00 a.m. — does the patient get up without being reminded?
5. Activity at appr. 9.30 a.m.
6. Activity at appr. 1.30 p.m.
7. Activity immediately before dinner (at 4.00 p.m.).
8. Degree of activity shown when dinner is served.
9. Activity at 6.00 p.m.
10. Activity at 8.30 p.m.

In cooperation with the nursing staff, another ten-point check-list was constructed to measure the degree of goal-directed activities during non-scheduled periods of the day, not the least during early morning, afternoons and evenings (Table 5.2). At set points of time, unknown to the patient, goal-directed activity was scored by nurses assessing whether the patient was passive, participating in activities initiated by another person or occupied in activities initiated by the patient himself.

A baseline registration was carried out for a two-week period, starting a couple of weeks after the patient had been admitted to the rehabilitation hospital. Then a five-week intervention period followed, unfortunately interrupted by a short stay in the neuro-surgical ward for surgical reevaluation. Finally, memory and initiative were assessed during a two-week, post-treatment period.

Figure 5.3 Measures of practical memory pre- and post-treatment.

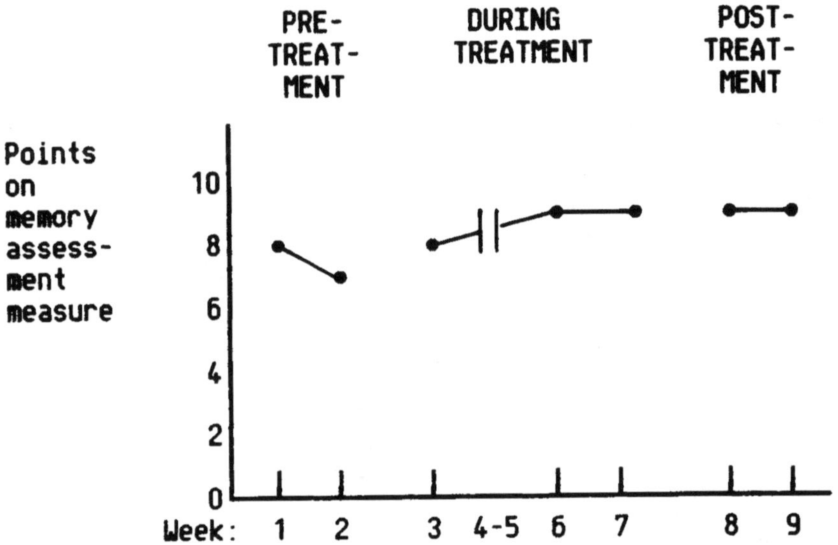

The treatment programme emphasized using the diary as a memory tool and as a systematic reminder to the patient to take initiatives and stay active during his spare time. Important information on what had happened to him, etc., was presented in a special section, daily diary notes were to be written. Awareness of deficits, so important in the treatment of John F., was less emphasized in working with patient B.

As illustrated in Figure 5.3, only a negligible change took place in practical day-to-day memory as assessed by the ten-point check-list during and after the treatment phase. This could possibly have been caused by a ceiling effect of the check-list, as the items chosen tended to be too easy.

The patient reported that he found the process diary helpful to keep up-to-date on what had happened from one day to the next and that it helped fill the holes in his memory for recent events. He also found the diary helped to keep him oriented on details of his own illness. The patient kept writing his daily notes, reading them over each day and bringing his notebook with him to his daily sessions with the psychologist. As the treatment proceeded, there was no need for the nursing staff to remind him to carry out these tasks. Our subjective impression was that the patient's awareness of his memory problems as well as of his visual defect continued to improve, and — not less important — that he was increasingly able to cope actively with his amnesia.

Memory was reassessed psychometrically during the post-line period with a parallel form of the Randt Memory Test. The scores showed a substantial

Figure 5.4 Scores on Randt Memory Test pre- and post-treatment.

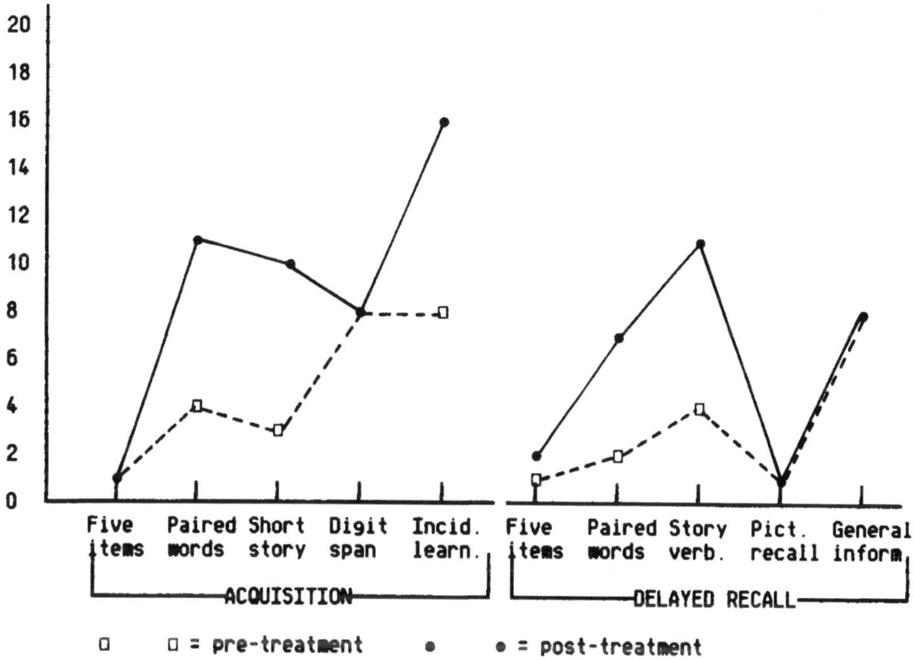

improvement, the patient's memory score now being in the lower normal range (Fig. 5.4), confirming the subjective impression both on the part of the patient and the team that mastery of memory deficits had improved during treatment. It is interesting to note that this progress is revealed on a conventional psychometric memory test, such as the Randt Test. There was also a moderate improvement in tests of psychomotor speed and visuo-constructive performance, as well as a small increase in problem-solving abilities.

On the other check-list, designed to measure ability to initiate behaviour, we found a clear, positive change in goal-directed behaviour from pre- to post-treatment period (Fig. 5.5). Initiative was not assessed during treatment. The improvement included taking more personal initiative in activities of daily living (ADL) tasks, such as getting up in the morning, more participation in group activities and an improved ability to initiate behaviour, such as reading, watching news programmes, etc., in his spare time. The patient also spent more time in social activities with other patients, such as taking walks together with one or two others in the evenings.

There is clearly a need to refine our evaluation methods. The simple single-case design described does not permit us to differentiate well enough between treatment-specific changes, non-specific effects of the treatment programme and the effects of

Figure 5.5 Measures of initiative shown by patient pre- and post-treatment.

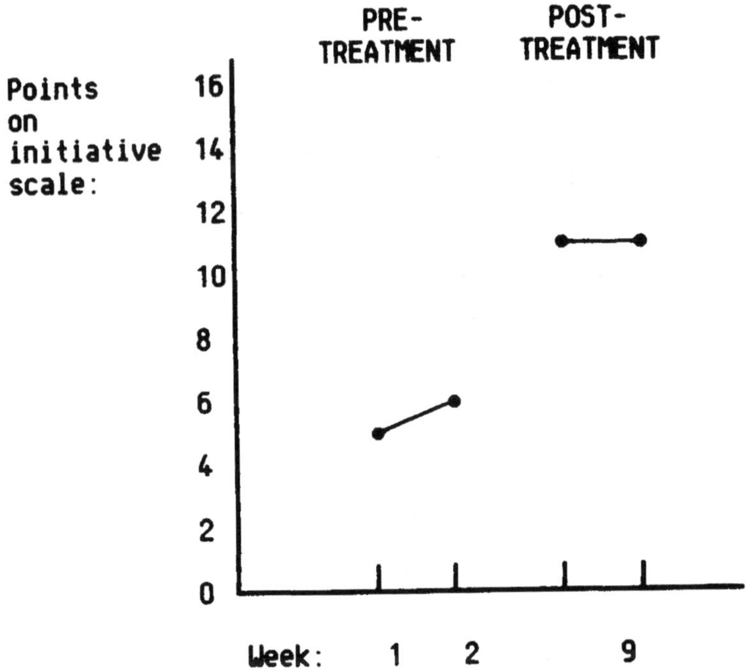

spontaneous recovery. We are continuing our work to develop check-lists designed to assess specific target behaviours on an individual basis. There is an obvious need to develop several individually adjusted check-lists containing items of a varied range of difficulty. Moreover, a multiple baseline design containing a broader range of target behaviours could potentially be a more valid indicator of treatment efficacy.

This case illustration confirms that the measurement of treatment efficacy in brain-damage rehabilitation is a difficult undertaking, especially in areas where conventional neuropsychological tests are of limited validity, such as in measuring initiative and other regulative functions. Moreover, in all assessment of treatment efficacy, there are difficulties in differentiating between programme-specific effects and non-specific recovery.

Concluding Remarks

The process-diary concept is an attempt to apply, in a systematic way, a very common tool in cognitive rehabilitation; the diary or notebook. Each of the interventions described above are variations of techniques used in most centres. The specific merit of our approach may be the attempt to systematize some of these general principles to make them available to the rehabilitation team.

The basic principle of the strategy is to use and build upon the intact abilities of the patients (similar to Deelman *et al.*, see Chapter 6). These abilities may not be used spontaneously because patients experience deficits in behaviour regulation. Through the different assignments and the feedback given by the therapist, the patient should acquire an increasing awareness, both of his deficits and of his intact abilities and skills, hopefully leading to being able to manage daily activities. We have described this process as a cognitive reintegration of function, as the goal is to train the patient to use his intact abilities in developing strategies to overcome his deficits of behaviour regulation (Finset, 1984).

The approach has obvious limitations. The patient must have a certain level of cognitive functioning. Attempts to use the concepts with patients with severe cognitive sequelae have been unsuccessful. The patient must be able to read and preferably write. If patients have these basic cognitive skills, the process-diary concept may prove a useful approach to treatment of memory and regulative functions. However, further development of procedures for assessment of treatment efficacy is needed before more in-depth evaluation of the approach may be reached.

References

CERNY, J. and MCNENY, R., 1983, 'Reality orientation therapy'. In M. Rosenthal, E. R. Griffith, M. R. Bond and J. D. Miller (Eds.), *Rehabilitation of the head injured adult*, pp. 345–53 (Philadelphia: F. A. Davis).

CRAINE, J. F., 1982, 'The retraining of frontal lobe dysfunction'. In L. Trexler (Ed.), *Cognitive rehabilitation*, pp. 239–62 (New York: Plenum Press).

EAMES, P. and WOOD, R., 1985, 'Rehabilitation after severe brain injury: a special-unit approach to behaviour disorders'. *International Rehabilitation Medicine*, **7**, 130–3.

FINSET, A., 1984, 'Re-integrereing av reguleringsfunksjoner som nevropsykologisk behandlingsstrategi'. (Re-integration of regulatory functions as a neuropsychological treatment strategy. English abstract.) *Journal of Norwegian Psychological Association*, **21**, 127–35.

FINSET, A., 1989, *The organization of post-acute head injury rehabilitation in a 17 bed unit: an approach emphasizing program differentiation*. Submitted to 1st World Congress, Int. Ass. for the Study of Traumatic Brain Injury.

GOODKIN, R., 1966, 'Case studies in behavioral research in rehabilitation'. *Perceptual and Motor Skills*, **23**, 171–82.

GRIFFITH, E. R., 1983, 'Types of disability'. In M. Rosenthal, E. R. Griffith, M. R. Bond and J. D. Miller (Eds.), *Rehabilitation of the head injured adult*, pp. 23–32 (Philadelphia: F. A. Davis).

HARRIS, J., 1978, 'External memory aids'. In M. Gruneberg, P. Morris and R. Sykes (Eds.), *Practical aspects of memory*, pp. 172–9 (London: Academic Press).

HARRIS, J., 1984, 'Methods of improving memory'. In B. A. Wilson and N. Moffat (Eds.), *Clinical management of memory problems*, pp. 46–62 (London: Croom Helm).

HOGAN, R. T., 1988, 'Behavior management for community reintegration'. *Journal of Head Trauma Rehabilitation*, **3**, 62–71.

HOWARD, M. E., 1988, 'Behavior management in the acute care rehabilitation setting'. *Journal of Head Trauma Rehabilitation*, **3**, 14–22.

KAZDIN, A., 1982, *Single-case research designs. Methods for clinical and applied settings* (New York: Oxford University Press).

KENDALL, P. C. and NORTON-FORD, J. D., 1982, *Clinical psychology: Scientific and professional dimensions* (New York: Wiley).

LAM, C. S., MCMAHON, B. T., PRIDDY, D. A. and GEHRED-SCHULTZ, A., 1988, 'Deficit awareness and treatment performance among traumatic head injury adults'. *Brain Injury*, **2**, 235–42.

MILLER, J. D., 1983, 'Early evaluation and management'. In M. Rosenthal, E. R. Griffith, M. R. Bond and J. D. Miller (Eds.), *Rehabilitation of the head injured adult*, pp. 37–58 (Philadelphia: F. A. Davis).

MUIR, C. A., HAFFEY, W. J., OTT, K. J., KARAICA, D., MUIR, J. H. and SUTKO, M., 1983, 'Treatment of behavioral deficits'. In M. Rosenthal, E. R. Griffith, M. R. Bond, and J. D. Miller (Eds.), *Rehabilitation of the head injured adult*, pp. 381–94 (Philadelphia: F. A. Davis).

NAUTA, W. J. H., 1971, 'The problem of the frontal lobe: a reinterpretation'. *Journal of Psychiatric Research*, **8**, 167–87.

PRIBRAM, K. H., 1981, 'Emotions'. In S. K. Filskov and T. J. Boll (Eds.), *Handbook of clinical neuropsychology* (New York: Wiley-Interscience).

PRIGATANO, G. P., 1986, *Neuropsychological rehabilitation after brain injury*, pp. 67–95 (Baltimore: Johns Hopkins University Press).

RANDT, C. T., BROWN, E. R. and OSBORNE, D. P., 1980, 'A memory test for longitudinal measurement of mild to moderate deficiencies'. *Journal of Clinical Neuropsychology*, **2**, 184–94.

ROLAND, P. E., 1984, 'Metabolic measures of the working frontal cortex in man'. *Trends in Neuroscience*, 430–5.

STUSS, D. T. and BENSON, B. F., 1986, *The frontal lobes* (New York: Raven Press).

TUCKER, D. M., 1988, 'Neuropsychological mechanisms of affective self-regulation'. In M. Kinsbourne (Ed.), *Cerebral hemisphere function in depression*, pp. 99–132, Progress in Psychiatry series. (Washington: American Psychiatric Press).

WALLS, R. T., 1969, 'Behaviour modification and rehabilitation'. *Rehabilitation Counsel Bulletin*, 173–83.

Chapter 6

Memory Strategies for Closed-Head-Injured Patients. Do Lessons in Cognitive Psychology Help?

B. G. Deelman, I. J. Berg, M. Koning-Haanstra

Introduction

Irritability, memory deficits, slowness and attentional problems are the most frequently reported subjective complaints of closed-head-injured (CHI) patients, months and even years after injury. Complaints about memory score highest in several studies on the effects of brain injury (Oddy *et al.*, 1978, 1985; Tyerman and Humphrey, 1984; van Zomeren and van den Burgh, 1985). According to close relatives, memory deficits after CHI are frequent (McKinlay *et al.*, 1981; Sunderland *et al.*, 1983; Oddy *et al.*, 1985; van Zomeren and van den Burgh, 1985; Brooks *et al.*, 1986; Deelman *et al.*, 1990). The few published longitudinal studies do not show a significant decrease in the percentage of patients complaining about memory at one year (McKinlay *et al.*, 1981), five years (Brooks *et al.*, 1986) or even seven years (Oddy *et al.*, 1985) post-injury.

Objective performance scores on memory tests indicate impairments months and even years post-trauma. Deficits are demonstrated in tasks related to verbal and visual learning, procedural memory, remote memory and access to semantic memory (overviews are given by e.g. Brooks *et al.*, 1984; Minderhoud and van Zomeren, 1984; Levin *et al.*, 1987; Deelman and Saan, 1990). We presently know of only one long-term longitudinal study which included repeated (re)testing of control subjects (Deelman and Saan, 1990). They obtained data on a group of 31 consecutively admitted CHI patients with a coma duration of at least 15 minutes and a Post traumatic amnesia (PTA) duration of at least two hours. Subjects were tested at about

This research is supported by a grant from the Netherlands Organization for Scientific Research (NWO).

30, 90, 180, 360 and 720 days after injury. Only patients whose PTA had ended by the first test session were included in the analysis.

A normal control group of 53 subjects matched to the patients group in age and educational level were tested in the same way, but it was decided to leave out the last (fifth) session as no more test-retest effects were observed. Memory tests included two verbal, multi-trial, free-recall tasks, a recognition test of photographs of faces and two semantic fluency tasks.

The results showed the same pattern for the different tests. One example is given in Figure 6.1, the 15 Words Test, in which words are presented in five learning trials. The acquisition score is the number of items recalled at these five trials; the delayed recall score refers to free recall about 15 minutes after the last learning trial. Because normal distributions of scores were not expected, non-parametric statistical tests were applied (the Wilcoxon rank sum test for within-group comparisons, the Mann–Whitney U test for between-group comparisons). As can be seen, both groups improved in performance up to the third occasion but the large differences between groups remained about the same.

Thus, as yet, neither questionnaires nor tests provide significant evidence of a recovery greater than retest effects in normals. Against this rather pessimistic baseline, any improvement through rehabilitation techniques would be most valuable. We therefore made an attempt to improve memory performance of CHI patients in their daily life by teaching and training memory strategies. This chapter will describe that

Figure 6.1 Development in time of acquisition and delayed recall scores of CHI patients and controls. Differences between groups and occasions indicated by:

* ($p \leq .05$)

** ($p \leq .01$)

*** ($p \leq .001$), two-tailed.

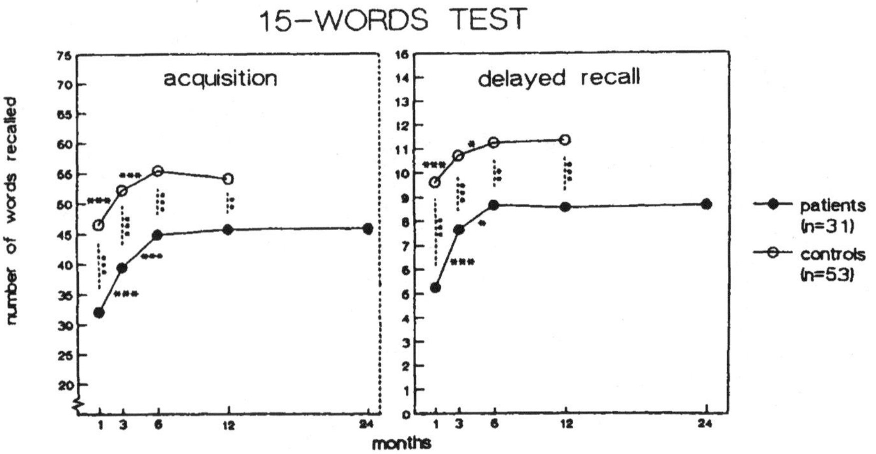

effort. First, the strategies exercised will be discussed and illustrated by three case studies. Next, the design of an evaluation study will be described and the results of the first seven treated patients will be compared with those of seven control patients, retested according to the same time schedule. Subjective ratings of training results, questionnaires for patients and their close relatives and objective test scores will be discussed, followed by a preliminary conclusion based on the first experiences with the strategy programme.

Memory Strategies

Although memory strategies, or mnemonics as they are often called, have been held in high esteem for centuries, they often evoke associations with secret arts and artificiality (Yates, 1966; Wolters, 1985). Over the course of time, authors like Erasmus (1512), Miller *et al.*, (1960), Skinner (1983) and Baddeley (1976, 1982) have tried to fit mnemonics into more general theories on memory, and several authors (Patten, 1972; Glasgow *et al.*, 1977; Crovitz, 1979; Gianutsos and Gianutsos, 1979; Crosson and Buenning, 1984; Grafman, 1984; Wilson and Moffatt, 1984; Schacter *et al.*, 1985; Wilson, 1987a, 1987b) have trained brain-damaged patients to use memory strategies, sometimes with promising results.

This memory-training project considered the potential of these procedures as aides to increase memory performance in patients with CHI. With respect to effective education, theoretical lessons are probably less important than demonstrations and practical exercises. A point to be made in this context is that closed head injury, as a rule, does not cause disturbances in intelligence, general knowledge or verification processes, and usually (with the exception of the so-called frontal syndrome) lack of motivation and self-criticism are not prominent.

We tried, therefore, to translate existing psychological theories of memory functioning into a set of general 'memory rules' for laymen. All patients enrolled in our program of strategy training are given a booklet of about 12 pages. The rules contained in this booklet are presented below, in an abridged form:

1 *It is impossible to cure your memory*. That is, it is not possible to repair or exchange nerve cells, and so far an effective 'memory pill' has not been produced. Yet you can make more efficient use of your remaining capacities. Learning to use more efficient methods, however, takes time and effort.

2 *Acceptance.*Try to accept that your memory is impaired to a certain degree and let others accept this too. Only then is it possible to react calmly when an appeal is made on your memory or to avoid frustration when you have forgotten something. Tension will only make your memory performances worse.

3 *External memory aids*. Use external aids whenever possible. Why try to learn things by heart when they can easily be written down or looked up?

4 *Attention*. Pay as much attention as you can to the information to be remembered. Make sure that you are not distracted by your environment and that you consciously (attentively) focus on whatever you have to remember.

5 *Time*. Spend more time on encoding, Generally, the more time you spend on encoding, the more you will remember. But spend your time economically/efficiently; not too long without a pause, but frequently and little by little.

6 *Repetition*. Whatever you have to remember will sink in more easily if you repeat it. There are several forms of repetition: simple repetition, spaced repetition (with increasing time intervals) and varied repetition (in several ways and situations).

7 *Association*. Making verbal associations (e.g. linking items together in a 'story') and/or visual images will increase the chance of really remembering them later on.

8 *Organization*. Try to categorize or arrange in a logical way the information to be remembered, e.g. when you have to go shopping, try to group your purchases into groceries, dairy produce, vegetables, etc.

9 *Anticipation and retrospection*. Try to link the input and retrieval situations. When you have to remember something in the future, try to anticipate the retrieval situation vividly and link input and retrieval. When you have to retrieve information you have stored in memory in the past, try to think back to the whole input situation. Even seemingly irrelevant details of that situation might facilitate retrieval.

10 *Work in a systematic way*. Whatever method you use to remember or retrieve information, try to use that method systematically. So, if you use a diary, always write all your appointments down. When you use associations to remember people's names, try to do that always. Furthermore, try to arrange your own surroundings in a systematic way, so you do not have to search when you need a particular item.

(In order to make remembering of the rules easier, two examples of a first letter mnemonic are given towards the end of the booklet.)

Use of the memory rules

Treatment always begins with discussing and further explaining the memory rules.

Homework for the first training session(s) consists of asking a patient to study the textbook and try to think up examples of, and experiences with, each described principle. In this way the rules become more concrete and familiar to the patient. During the whole strategy training, the textbook is used again and is commented upon more elaborately each time a new exercise is introduced. Each method of remembering or retrieving information is always explained in terms of the memory rules. Furthermore, the patient gets a 'work book', in which he/she can write down experiences with each particular memory rule and, if necessary, completed by remarks and suggestions of the therapist. So this work book becomes a personal memory book.

Selecting goals

All patients in strategy training are asked which memory problems are the most distressing in their daily life. The patient and the therapist together then make a short priority list, indicating which problem(s) should consecutively be dealt with in the training. Training then consists of both laboratory sessions and homework exercises, such that the patient spends at least two hours a day on training.

Case Studies

Case A

The first patient to be described was a 44-year-old man who sustained a very severe head injury in a motorcycle accident 18 years before treatment. He had been unconscious for three weeks and his post-traumatic amnesia lasted for two months. At the time of his accident, he attended the School for Analytical Chemists; eight years after his injury he finally got a diploma, but at a somewhat lower level than he would have been entitled to had he continued with the same level of education as before his accident. However, even with this lower qualification he soon found a job at an environmental laboratory.

Tested 16 years after the injury in the Neuropsychology department, he appeared to be an intelligent man (IQ of 118) with a poor verbal memory (3rd decile according to normative data of a normal population). He had a lot of problems and still could not accept the consequences of his accident, thinking of his life prior to the accident as a period in which nothing ever went wrong and of his post traumatic life as a chain of misfortune. The poor functioning of his memory caused a feeling of inferiority, especially at work where all his colleagues outdistanced him and no one ever asked him anything about work-related subjects (for 'he never remembers anyway'). He was never allowed to conduct a complicated chemical analysis alone, even after working for years at the environmental laboratory. The advice given to him after this neuropsychological examination was to seek psychotherapy aimed at digesting the consequences of his accident.

Apparently this did not work out as well as was hoped, for when we saw the patient two years later he still had the same complaints and the same feeling of inferiority. He even stated that amelioration of his memory had become his most important goal in life. Problems chosen by this patient to be tackled in the training program were as follows:

1 Work related problems. The first involved remembering the commands to be typed into a computer program to provide a daily working list; the second involved remembering the composition of three, very often used, standard samples for measuring the amount of certain chemical elements in air, water or soil. Looking up this information everyday (and sometimes more than once) was a very time-consuming and interfering activity.

2 How to learn people's names.

3 How to handle distracting activities. This problem had (at least for this patient) two different aspects. Firstly, forgetting what he was doing (or going to do) when a distraction came up; e.g. not going back to the kitchen to finish the dishes after replacing the (distracting) telephone. Secondly, forgetting to carry out a planned activity when this plan or idea occurred to him while he had no time or possibility to execute it immediately; e.g. it often happened that he realized, while at work, that he should make a phone call. If he could not at that moment leave his ongoing activities to execute his plan, he was very likely to forget it altogether.

The training consisted of 20 sessions, 10 in the first and 10 in the second period.

Treatment

Treatment began, as with all other patients, with a discussion and explanation of the memory rules, giving strong emphasis, in this case, on acceptance. In the beginning of the training, this issue was discussed almost every session. The therapist gradually succeeded in convincing the patient that everyone (even the therapist) forgets, that it was not realistic to contrast his post-traumatic and his pre-traumatic life and that his level of aspiration was too high.

Training of the first topic (typing computer demands for a work list) consisted of studying the computer program and trying to understand why something had to be typed in. Originally this analysis of the program was meant for the therapist to get an idea about where it went wrong, but it also served the purpose of helping the patient to remember the proper commands. Having previously only read it on paper, the patient now had to pay more attention to the program in order to explain it himself.

As a consequence, the patient was able to see how the program was organized, assisting the learning process. This process of 'verbal mediation' (see Wood, Chapter 1) helped the patient learn all commands after only two one-hour sessions at our laboratory, backed up by rehearsing the process for two days at home as 'homework'.

The second work-related problem (learning the composition/component parts of three standard samples) took more time to resolve. The mnemonics suggested by the therapist (a combination of first-letter, rhythm and alphabetical order, according to the organization principle) were immediately accepted by the patient as good, working, memory aids. For each sample, the elements were put in alphabetical or rhythmical order and the position of each element in the mnemonic gave an indication about the quantity of that particular element to be used in the sample. (The mnemonics in Dutch are unfortunately not translatable.) It took about two weeks of rehearsing at the lab, at work and at home before he could enumerate all necessary chemical elements in the proper order with the exact quantities for all three standard samples. After that he could almost dream it and never had to look it up again at work.

The next problem tackled was learning people's names. The strategy advised here was to form associations between the name and some characteristic of the person, either visually or verbally. The training material consisted of photographs from magazines, some with a cue (such as the profession of the person) and some without any cue whatsoever; only the face and a neutral background were visible. The patient turned out to be very inventive in finding associations, and much to his surprise he was very capable of remembering people's names once he had a 'fitting' association. Applying this method in his daily life situation (his homework) was a bit more difficult because he felt rather impertinent looking at people so closely and attentively. Nevertheless, the names of his ten colleagues and ten people working at other environmental labs with whom he met now and then were no longer a problem after six sessions of training in face-name associations.

The last major complaint to be handled was coping with distracting activities. During laboratory training the patient was told again and in more detail the principles of anticipation and association and how to use these in his daily life. One exercise, the distracting events exercise, consisted of letting the patient mentally go through a home or work-related task (e.g. collect the car-wash requirements and wash the car) and disturbing him during that imagined action at any one point (e.g. 'the telephone rings, you have to answer it'). After concluding the disrupting activity, he had to realize what he was going to do before his attention was diverted. He managed this by attentively associating (verbally or visually) the car-wash situation and the telephone-call situation, e.g. imagining cold water streaming from the receiver. So, when laying down the receiver, the other situation would pop up as a rule. Another exercise, the distracting thoughts exercise, consisted of mentally going through a certain activity (e.g. making a standard sample) and the therapist (acting as his inner thoughts) telling him an idea, that darted through 'his' mind (e.g. buying postcards). Since in this example the task was imagined to be at work, it was impossible for him to go shopping instantly, so he had to postpone it and make sure that he would think of those postcards again while cycling home from work. The solution here was to direct his attention to the suddenly appearing idea, anticipate doing it on the way home and form an association between cycling home and buying postcards, for which he should make a detour.

In the training sessions, the patient did not forget any of the tasks or activities. Applying the method of anticipation and association to situations in daily life (his homework), however, was much more difficult because it demanded the acquisition of a new style of consciously and attentively reacting to his thoughts. During training sessions he could focus his attention without time pressure, but in real life this is harder to achieve. Nevertheless when he thought of using the strategy in a daily situation (especially when he had to remember something important), it worked very well. He reported several successful applications of the strategy in one week.

After the last training session, in which we recapitulated all the memory principles and the learned mnemonics and strategies, the patient, motivated by the good results during the training sessions, expressed his strong intentions to keep on using and exercising the various methods.

Subjective rating (min = 1; max = 10)

Patient's judgement on the strategy training

Satisfaction	9
Personal fit	8
Applicability: quality	8
Applicability: frequency	7
Effect for now	7
Effect after one year	8
Recommendability	10

Patient's judgement on his functioning

	Before	*After*
Memory capacity	4	5
Insight into memory problems	4	6
Level of tension/irritation	8	6
Possibility to cope	5	6

In the ratings the patient clearly expressed his enthusiasm about the training and the possibilities for using the strategies. He indicated that he believed the effects would grow in the course of time. During training he often stated his conviction that all strategies needed further practice to really become a habit; he seemed to be realistic about his functioning before and after training. He felt his memory was still not up to the mark but he could cope with his problems better than before training. He gained better insight into his problems and became less tense. His wife also reported that since the training the patient reacted with less tension and irritability about his memory failures and had become more cheerful.

Data on the various evaluation tasks of this patient are included in the results.

Case B

This 32-year-old woman sustained a severe head injury in a car accident nine months before treatment. She had been unconscious for five days and her post-traumatic amnesia lasted for 17 days. At the time of her accident, she worked as a family doctor in the practice of a colleague. Seven months after the accident, she resumed work half-time without weekend or night duties.

Tested two months after injury in the Neuropsychology department, her intelligence was still high (IQ 120) with a normal verbal memory (5th decile according to normative data of a normal population). Her verbal fluency (semantic memory) was below the normal level. The speed with which she performed tests was slow. She had complaints concerning her memory, especially about retrieving information. Nevertheless, there had been notable progress in comparison with the results of an earlier examination (three weeks after injury).

When we saw the patient (nine months after the accident) she still had memory complaints, described by herself as 'a somewhat empty recent memory'. Though the memory problems as such were not severe, they were very inconvenient in her work. She mainly had problems with time-orientation, e.g. she did not remember if she had seen a patient a week or a year ago. Although she could look it up (and she usually did), she missed 'a kind of automatic feeling about when things happened' in the period since her accident. Moreover, she sometimes forgot to perform certain actions, e.g. calling a colleague or buying something in town, stating that 'forgetting things like these happened very rarely before the accident'. In her work she realized that remembering the names of her patients was more difficult than before.

In summary, the subjects chosen to be tackled in the training programme were:

1 How to recall when events occurred.
2 How to remember intended actions.
3 How to remember people's names.

The treatment consisted of one three-week period of eight one-hour sessions.

Treatment

Discussing and explaining the memory rules did not take much time. She had already formulated her own strategies in terms of association and attention. She used to talk very frankly about her memory problems, and she had no severe difficulties accepting them. Being acquainted with medical literature and the results of her examination, she felt satisfied with her general recovery, but she very much wanted to improve her memory.

The first problem had to do with difficulty determining the approximate date of events since the accident. It also took a relatively long time to recollect recent activities, and sometimes she failed completely. Both aspects were trained by introducing an active, problem solving, retrieval strategy using retrospection: when you have to retrieve information, try to think back to the input situation. Although she already spontaneously used questions in the recollection process, a more systematic approach was intended in the training. She had to:

(a) try to find a context, by asking herself general questions,
(b) search within that context, by using more specific questions, and
(c) verify the retrieved information.

As an exercise to recollect activities/events from recent days, she was given the instruction to write down daily three more-or-less specific activities of the day, one week before. She had to ask herself the following questions and she had to check if the answers could present points of reference:

(a) General questions: which activities are usual on that day; are you usually at home/ at work/ elsewhere on that day; what are your relatives usually doing on that day; what do you usually do the day before or the day after the day in question?
(b) More specific questions: did something special happen that day; were other people involved in your activities that day?
(c) Verify the answer.

She had no problem with the first few days to be recollected in this exercise. Probably this was caused by the fact that her husband had been absent and she had to settle unusual things (e.g. arranging a babysitter). When 'normal' life restarted, she had more trouble in recollecting specific activities. For example, one day she could only remember that she had worked the week before but could remember nothing of what she had actually done. Gradually she made progress and was able to recollect events from her consulting hour. The systematic approach, as described above, was not always followed exactly, but, as time went by, she was able to select the appropriate questions which could immediately provide a good reference point. The verifying stage was no problem.

To exercise the determination of the date on which remote events occurred, the same approach was used. Events were sampled by the therapist and by the patient's husband, who was asked for a list of personal events of the period since the accident. The list included e.g. the funeral of an uncle, the purchase of a dish washer, a meeting of a committee and the like. The following questions were used as starting points:

(a) General questions: tell something more about the event; is it a unique or a recurring event; did a special reason for this event exist; were other people involved in it; do you remember events related (associated) to the event at hand?

(b) More specific questions: if it is a recurring event, does it have a fixed time pattern; if there was a special reason, does that give information about the date; when did related events occur; did the event in question happen before or after that event?

(c) Verify your answer.

An example and the way she reconstructed a date will illustrate this procedure. The therapist asked her when the third neuropsychological examination had been; her reply was:

> 'I remember the name of the Psychologist, Dr. v.Z. and I remember some tests, a memory test with a list of words and a reaction-time test. I remember the reason was assessing the possible restarting of my work. I restarted in September, so it was done before September. I also remember the examination had to be done before the psychologist went on holidays, so it occurred before the end of July. The second psychological examination was in April just some days after the birthday of my son on April the 15th. So it happened somewhere between the end of April and the end of July. I don't remember other events directly related to this examination. So I guess it was the end of June, yes I think it is right'.

(The exact date was the 7th of July.)

She always succeeded in recalling related events, and she was always sure if it was before or after that occasion and then, rather precisely, how many days or weeks. As described, she soon automatically selected one or a few questions leading directly to the solution instead of following the advice of gradually and systematically 'zooming in'. The verifying stage was never a problem. As far as could be checked, she was right. She liked the exercises and was surprised by her success. 'I have to search more consciously than before my accident, but my time-orientation is better and my memory is less empty than I thought'.

The next subject to be handled was remembering intended actions. With this patient, forgetting was not specifically due to external distraction and/or delay as in the case of patient A. Even when she consciously intended to execute a plan or idea, she sometimes still forgot it. She had already concluded she needed to pay more attention; 'earlier conscious attention was not necessary because I remembered my plans more or less automatically, I did not have to stop at it'. Two kinds of exercises to enhance controlled information processing were introduced:

Firstly, a list of activities was given and she had to remember them by organizing the information and chaining the clusters of activities (e.g. 'I first execute the activities behind my writing desk, studying a medical chapter and writing a letter and then I will buy the book of van Kooten, because after working it is nice to do something pleasant.') Her links were mostly very logical and seldom bizarre. She preferred verbal associations over visual ones. Lists of 12 activities were organized and chained by her very quickly, and she remembered them all, even after some days.

Secondly she was told again the principles of anticipation and association more-or-less on the analogy of the retrospection procedure. In the training she had to describe in detail by mentally going through them tasks mentioned by the therapist (e.g. describe a medical examination of a patient with complaints of dizziness). At any time during her description of the imagined tasks the therapist introduced intended actions as an 'arising idea' or a request from someone else. To provide for real-life examples, her husband was asked to make a list of planned activities for his wife. In the exercise, she had to plan them for the next day, so she had to anticipate the context by overlooking the time schedule for that day. Then she had to make associations between usual activities and intended ones: 'I have to call my friend C. (intended action) and I will do that tomorrow after dinner and after reading the newspaper, because that is the moment I usually relax and that will be a suitable moment.' Then she had to continue describing the imagined tasks. Also in this exercise she arranged activities in a logical way, by using verbal associations. From an exercise consisting of 12 'imagined' and six 'intended' activities, she remembered all in the lab and ten and six, respectively, the next day (homework). She was very satisfied with her achievements, and she judged it a strategy useful in her daily life.

The third aim of the training was learning and remembering people's names by the association strategy (see Case A for the procedure). Material consisted of photographs of unknown people and of names of her own patients. She was inventive in making fitting associations and used a variety of cues. She could still reproduce nearly all the learned names after one week, and she reported some successful applications in real-life practice.

Subjective rating (min = 1; max = 10)

Patient's judgement on the strategy training

Satisfaction	7
Personal fit	9
Applicability: quality	8
Applicability: frequency	9
Effect for now	7
Effect after one year	7
Recommendability	8

Patient's judgement on her functioning

	Before	*After*
Memory capacity	6	7
Insight into memory problems	8	8
Level of tension/irritation	2	2
Possibility to cope	7	8

The patient was satisfied with the training. She learned to apply strategies more consciously. The frequent application of the strategies was probably due to her strong motivation and the kind of laboratory and homework exercises in which much real-life material was used. It became apparent while discussing the memory rules, that the patient had no problems concerning insight and acceptance of the memory problems. The whole training period could therefore be spent on exercises using the memory strategies. Both the patient and the therapist thought there was no need for a second training period in view of the good results. The data from this patient are not included in the results, since the follow-up examination has not yet taken place.

Case C

This 20-year-old man sustained a very severe head injury in a moped accident when he was 16. He had been unconscious for two weeks and his post-traumatic amnesia lasted for at least six weeks. At the time of the accident, he was in the last class of a school for advanced elementary education.

The patient was tested two months and four months after injury in the Neuropsychological department. The second examination revealed an improved intelligence score (IQ 100) in comparison with the first assessment (IQ 80). Four months after the injury, he was taken to be (nearly) back at his assumed pre-traumatic level. Though mental and motor speed had improved since the first assessment, they were still not up to the mark. His memory performance also improved in the course of time but was still far below a normal level at the second examination (1st decile).

Furthermore, he seemed to have little insight into his problems and his self-criticism was noted to be suboptimal. He gave the impression of being childish and unconcerned. The diagnosis of a fullfledged frontal syndrome, however, could not be made. The patient's main complaints concerned his talking (slow and with indistinct pronunciation), incoordination, fatiguability, slowness and forgetfulness, especially for names. He was advised not to restart school too soon for that would probably overload him and lead to great frustration.

When we saw the patient almost four years after the injury he had managed to finish the school for advanced elementary education and was in the second year of a secondary school for economic and administrative education. Though he admitted he had difficulty keeping up with the rest of the class, he thought the poor results were mainly due to an illness earlier that year. Halfway through the year he was already sure he would not be moved up. The complaints spontaneously mentioned were primarily about his physical condition: a disturbance of equilibrium and a spastic clonus in his right arm and leg. Tested on a verbal memory test his performance still seemed to be very poor (2nd decile according to normative data of a normal population). Although he himself did not consider his memory as very problematic, he agreed to participate in the study for the 'sake of science'.

The two memory problems that were identified as appropriate for treatment were:

1 How to remember conversations in general and lectures at school in particular.
2. How to remember what was read.

The training consisted of 14 sessions, seven in the first and seven in the second period.

Treatment

Analysis of the reasons for forgetting conversations and lectures at school revealed two factors of influence: attention and structure. As for the first, the patient stated that his thoughts often wandered in class. As for structure, he had noted that it was very much easier to remember a lecture in which the speaker provided a logical build-up of subjects, e.g. by saying 'firstly . . . , secondly . . . ' or by clearly accentuating the most important issues. With the method used to treat these problems, two birds were killed with one stone. To make sure he listened attentively, he had to bring structure and organization into what he heard by mentally 'high-lighting' important issues, e.g. by asking himself (key) questions and trying to get an answer; relating new information to knowledge already present, e.g. by drawing conclusions about new heard things; and trying to keep track of the chronological order of events.

During training he had to listen as described above to recorded radio interviews and to give a summary right after the presentation, half-an-hour later and some hours beyond that at home for homework. Homework consisted of trying to apply this method of attentively listening in his daily situation and especially at school.

Though he was not always accurate in recalling who said what, he remembered most of the content of the interviews he heard during training sessions (including the long ones (10 minutes) and even after several days). Applying the method at school made sure that he now listened really attentively to the lectures without his thoughts wandering. A test paper at school about the lessons followed since therapy started, yielded a very good result.

His problem with remembering what he read was tackled with the PQRST-method, a well-known way of organizing and structuring the material:

Preview the material to be remembered.
Question — ask important/key questions about the text.
Read the material thoroughly in order to answer the questions.
State the answers, recapitulate the content.
Test at frequent intervals the retention of the information.

The resemblance between attentively listening and attentively reading was apparent to him. He enjoyed reading with this method: 'Even dull articles become fun to read when you ask questions about them and try to find the answers. So you become interested and sometimes even curious and, as a result, attentive.' Newspaper articles read as homework were almost literally recalled 24 hours after reading. The tenor of the articles read, both short and long ones (up to 1 newspaper page), was remembered for weeks.

Since he was able to handle both problems after the first training period, the question arose whether it was useful to go on with a second period. At this point the patient, for the first time expressed his dissatisfaction with his memory functioning. He had noticed, while attempting a broad range of memory tests, that his memory was not as good as he had thought it to be. Even on apparently easy tests, his results (in his eyes) were very poor. This added to the frustration of not being able to play soccer or to skate because of his physical handicaps, making him finally realize how much he was restricted because of his accident. His rating on tension before and after training increased as a result from two to seven (see subjective ratings table), and he displayed a rather depressed manner.

He felt further training would be very useful to him but had no idea which particular problem should be dealt with. It was decided during the second period not to train a particular problem but use some general strategies, especially association and anticipation, on all kinds of material. Association was implemented by learning names to faces and learning routes by linking the various points of recognition. Anticipation was practiced as described with Case A. Though initially he had some difficulty in finding associations, throughout the training period he became gradually more skilful at that and reported some successful attempts of applying the methods in daily life.

Subjective ratings (min. = 1; max. = 10)

Patient's judgement on the strategy training

	After 1st period	*After 2nd period*
Satisfaction	8	10
Personal fit	8	7
Applicability: quality	7	5
Applicability: frequency	7	5
Effect for now	9	7
Effect after one year	7	9
Recommendability	10	10

Patient's judgement on his functioning

	Before training	*After 1st period*	*After 2nd period*
Memory capacity	7	8	9
Insight into memory problems	5	7	6
Level of tension/irritation	2	7	9
Possibility to cope	5	8	8

In retrospect, Mr. C. was very satisfied with both training periods even though the second was not directly aimed at daily problems; his lower rating for personal fit reflects this. Applicability of the methods learned in the first period was also rated higher than that of the second period. However, in contrast to the effects of the first period, which he believed to decrease in the course of time, he thought the strategies learned in the second period would gain in effect. The frustration mentioned during training is also reflected in the ratings: together with the insight into his problems (which he confessed was less before), the level of tension and irritation increased after the first and even further after the second training period. Still, he retrospectively rated his memory capacity as rather high even before training, but at the same time he saw that his ability to cope with his memory problems increased. Fortunately, he stated that the level of tension and anxiety about his memory had decreased two points (from 9 to 7) at the final follow-up, about four months after training. Data of this patient are included in the results.

Evaluation Methods

Design of the Study

The project as a whole focuses on the effects of instructing and exercising memory strategies in comparison with no treatment and repetitive practice with memory tasks. Methodologically, the ultimate goal is to combine a groups design (by which subjects are randomly assigned to the three experimental conditions) with the advantages of a single-case design (by which all consecutive cases are assessed on baseline, first training period, rest, second training period, rest and finally on follow-up). Each of the time periods has a duration of three weeks, with the exception of a follow-up after 12 weeks. Two training periods are intended, but the need of the second one is discussed after results (or disappointments) of the first period have become clear. So the maximal time span is 27 weeks. The maximal number of evaluations is seven (E1-E7). Evaluation tasks are administered in the same way and in the same time schedule for treated and untreated subjects. Because of intra-individual variability of scores, causing 'noise' especially in individual and small group data, scores are pooled over the baseline period (E1-E2), the first post-treatment period (E3-E4), the second post-treatment period (E5-E6) and finally the long-term follow-up (E7).

Conditions

In this contribution we will not dwell on the methods and effects of repetitive practice in which all kinds of memory tasks and memory games are exercised without any suggestion about more efficient strategies. Here we will restrict ourselves to a comparison between the described strategy programme and the no-treatment condition. Patients were randomly assigned to conditions. The control patients voluntarily participated in 'a study on the time course of memory impairments'. They received information about their test results on consecutive examinations. If desired, common consequences of CHI were discussed, and, like the treated patients, their travelling expenses were paid; moreover, the control patients got a small participation fee.

Criteria for Inclusion

Although a group of healthy elderly people was included in the study we will confine ourselves here to the head-injured patients. Criteria for inclusion were (a) closed head injury sustained more than nine months ago, (b) subjective memory complaints in everyday life, (c) objective evidence of memory deficits, (d) no severe (pre- or post-

Table 6.1 *Demographic and neurological data of the treated patients (n = 7) and the untreated patients (n = 7).*

	Age		Level of Education		IQ		PTA in days		Years since injury	
	Mean	s.d.	Median	range	Mean	s.d.	Mean	s.d.	Mean	s.d.
Treated	36.1	12.33	4	3–6	99	9.15	31.3	19.77	5.04	6.09
Untreated	33.1	7.29	4	4–6	104	14.20	32.29	40.34	7.03	5.62
Student-t and Mann Whitney	ns		ns		ns		ns		ns	

traumatic) intellectual, aphasic, apraxic, agnosic or personality disturbances and (e) aged between 18 and 60 years. Of course, motivation to participate in the rather time-consuming study was a decisive factor. Although all patients were tested earlier in the Neuropsychological department, the criteria were checked in a short clinical neuropsychological examination before the baseline assessment took place.

Subjects

In the description of the results, we will confine ourselves only to those patients who have concluded the entire programme including the follow-up evaluation. The two groups of seven patients each did not differ in age, level of education or IQ. Furthermore, they were comparable with respect to the most relevant neurological data, that is length of PTA and time since injury (see Table 6.1).

Evaluation Tasks

Three kinds of data will be discussed here for a first appraisal of the training programme's general effects: subjective ratings of the results of training, memory questionnaires and scores on memory tests. In the questionnaires, estimations of how often 37, every day life memory problems occurred to the patients were given by the patients themselves and by a close relative, using a 7-point scale ranging from 1 = never to 7 = always. Internal reliabilities were shown to be very high (coefficients $\alpha \geq .90$), and the scores differentiate with high probability between head-injured and control subjects (Deelman and Saan, 1990). As a standardized laboratory memory test, a Dutch version of Rey's 15 Words Test was used. (The procedure is described in the introduction of this chapter.) Internal reliability was very high ($\alpha \geq .90$), retest reliability was .80 and the scores differentiate with high probability between head-injured and control subjects (Deelman and Saan, 1990). Three alternate versions of the 15 Words Test were used, version A at E2 and E7, version B (counterbalanced with C) at E1 and E4 and version C (counterbalanced with B) at E3 and E6. At E5 the 15 Words Test was not administered.

Three scores derived from this test (a task not specifically trained in therapy) will be discussed: the sum score of the five learning trials, acquisition score; the delayed recall score approximately 15 minutes after learning; and an index of subjective organization (SO) of the memory, the best measure available at the present time, according to Sternberg and Tulving (1977). This measure is based on the number of response pairs that stay together on two consecutive trials and is corrected for chance.

The SO was computed on the 4th and 5th learning trial and on the 5th learning trial and delayed recall. The SO index is derived from the following formula:

$$SO = ITR - \frac{2c(c-1)}{h.k}$$

ITR = observed number of bidirectional intertrial repetitions
c = number of common items recalled at both trials
h = total number of items recalled at trial t
k = total number of items recalled at trial t + 1

As an 'ecological' memory task, shopping lists were used. In this task the patient had to write down a shopping list of 24 items dictated by the examiner. Each item consisted of three elements, amount, article and specification e.g. '1 bunch of white tulips'. Each correct element scored one point. After a study-time of 90 seconds in which the patient was able to use whatever method he/she wanted in order to remember the list, he/she was asked twice to recall as many items as possible. The delayed recall, about 30 minutes after presentation of the list, seems to be the ecologically most important measure of this test, for this gives an indication of what will happen when the patient is really out shopping. As yet, no psychometric data on this newly constructed task are available.

Seven versions of this test were constructed; at face value all were comparable in difficulty and alternately administered such that the versions were counterbalanced over the seven evaluation moments. Subjective organization was computed on the immediate and delayed recall.

Results

Subjective Ratings

After treatment, patients were asked to rate in retrospect their experiences and feelings in 10-point scales (1 = the lowest possible degree, 10 = the highest possible degree). An overview of mean scores is given in Table 6.2. Satisfaction, recommendability and improved ability to cope in daily life seem to be very high, the frequency with which the learned strategies really can be applied in daily life is rated somewhat lower. Of course these data are subject to all possible biases, especially the need to please the therapists and to favourably assess a rather time- and energy-consuming enterprise.

Figure 6.2 *Memory Questionnaire, mean score per item of treated and untreated patients, according to patients and relatives; before treatment (pre), after first treatment period (p1), after second treatment period (p2), follow-up (f-up).*

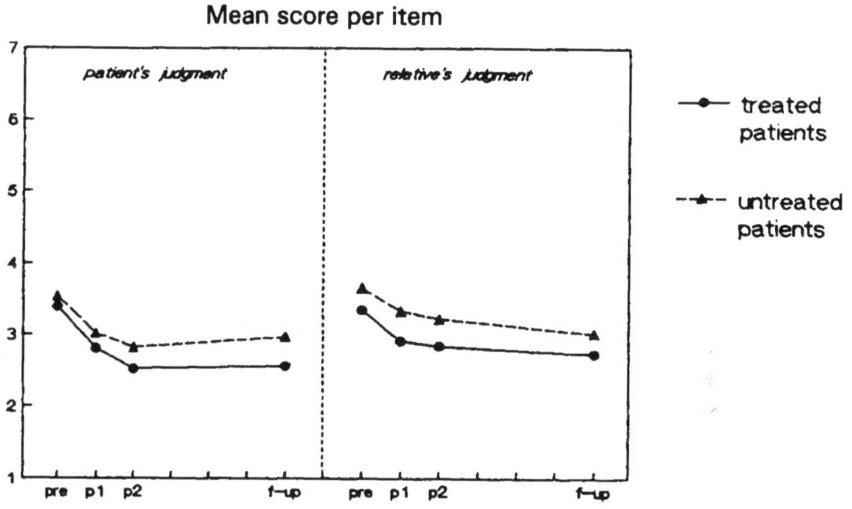

Figure 6.3 *Memory Questionnaire, mean score per item for items related to training and items unrelated to training, according to treated patients and their relatives; before treatment (pre), after first treatment period (p1), after second treatment period (p2), follow-up (f-up).*

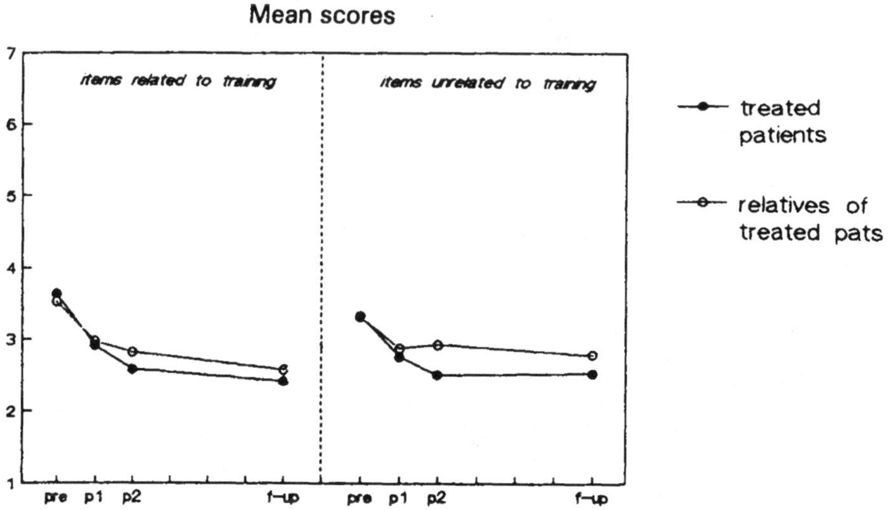

Table 6.2 Subjective ratings of treated patients.

Criteria	Mean score	
– Satisfaction with the training	8.57	
– Personal fit of the training	8.43	
– Applicability of strategies: quality	6.86	
– Applicability of strategies: frequency	6.71	
– Effect of the training for now	7.86	
– Effect of the training after one year	7.83	
– Recommendability to others	9.67	
	Before training	After training
– Memory capacity	5.29	7.43
– Insight into memory problems	5.43	7.57
– Level of tension/irritation because of memory problems	5.14	5.00
– Possibility to cope with memory problems	4.71	7.00

Table 6.3 Memory Questionnaire. Levels of significance for comparisons between pre-treatment, first and second post-treatment and follow-up scores.

Treated patients n=7	Total score		Items related to training		Items unrelated to training	
	pat.	rel.	pat.	rel.	pat.	rel.
pre/post1	**	***	***	***	**	**
pre/post2	***	***	***	***	***	**
pre/follow-up	***	***	***	***	***	*
post1/post2	***	0	***	0	***	0
post1/follow-up	***	0	***	**	*	0
post2/follow-up	0	0	0	0	0	0

Untreated patients n=7	Total score	
	pat.	rel.
pre/post1	*	0
pre/post2	**	0
pre/follow-up	***	*
post1/post2	0	0
post1/follow-up	0	0
post2/follow-up	0	0

Wilcoxon signed rank test,
0: no significant improvement
*: $p \leq .05$
**: $p \leq .025$
***: $p \leq .01$, one-tailed.

Memory Questionnaires

A first look at the curves surprisingly suggests a decrease of memory complaints for both treated and untreated groups, according to both the patients themselves and their relatives (Fig. 6.2). Moreover, the reported improvements within the treatment group seem to be rather generalized and not confined to items referring to the problems explicitly trained in the individual programme (Fig. 6.3).

Statistical tests (Table 6.3) reveal that this improvement is highly significant in most comparisons within the treatment group, but less obvious within the control group, especially with the relatives' ratings. However these differences are too small to conclude with certainty that they are due to the specific effects of the training.

Figure 6.4 15 Words Test, mean scores of acqusition, delayed recall, subjective organization between trials 4 and 5 and subjective organization between trial 5 and delayed recall.

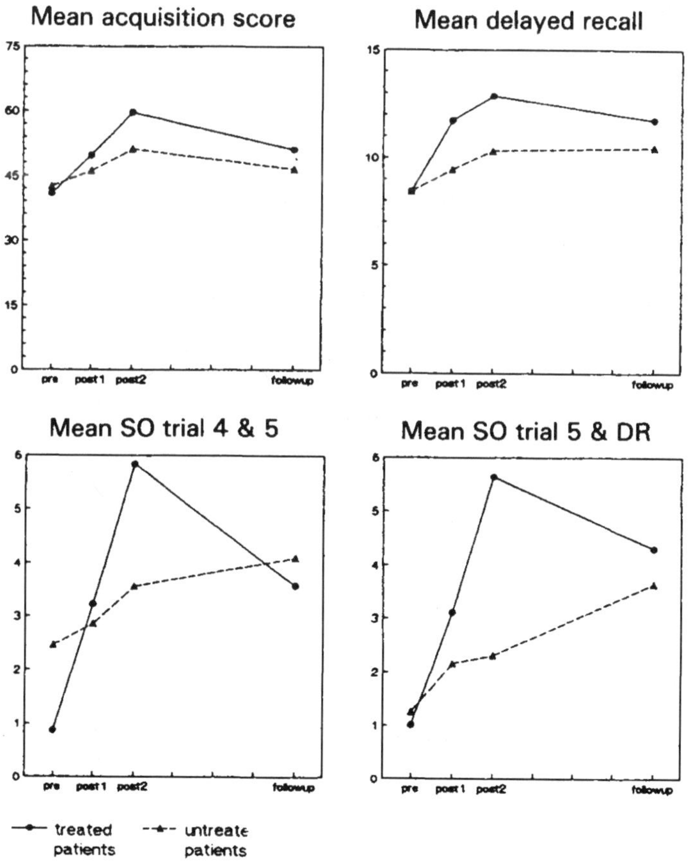

Figure 6.5 Shopping lists, mean scores on delayed recall and subjective organization between immediate and delayed recall.

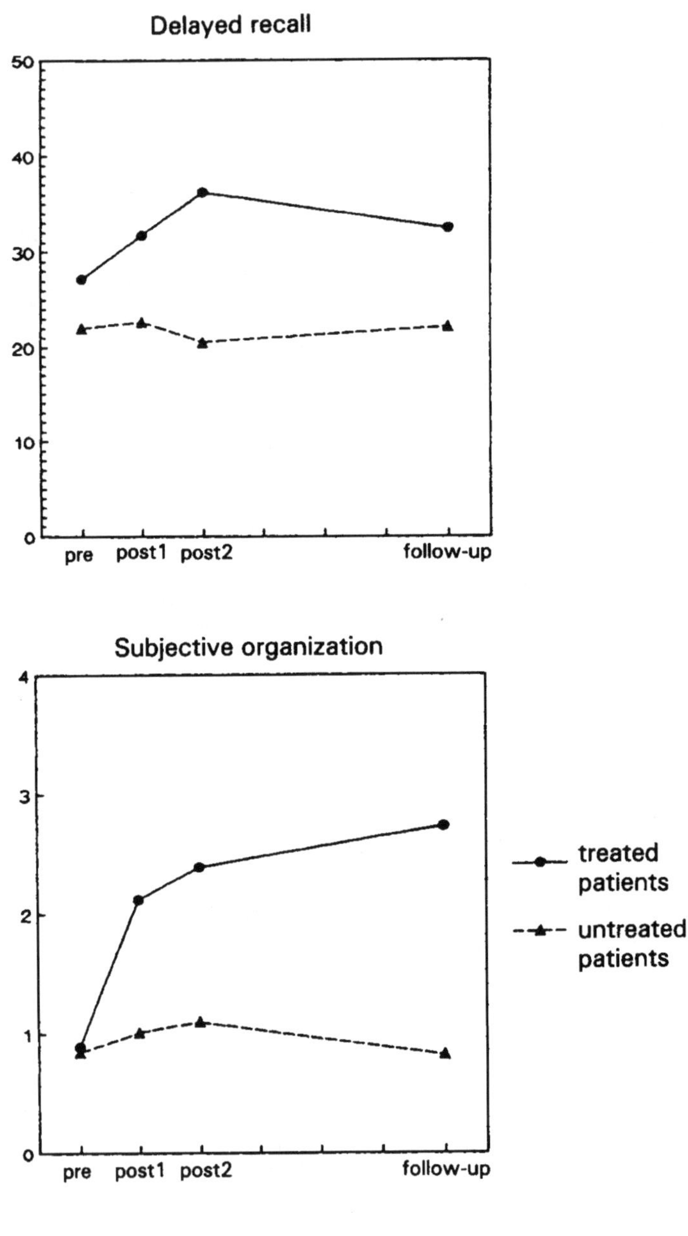

Table 6.4 Levels of significance for comparisons between pre-treatment, first and second post-treatment and follow-up scores.

Treated patients n=7	15 Words Test				Shopping list	
	acquis.	DR	SO–1	SO–2	DR	SO
pre/post1	***	***	**	0	*	0
pre/post2	***	***	***	*	**	0
pre/follow-up	***	***	***	*	*	*
post1/post2	***	0	**	*	*	0
post1/follow-up	0	0	0	*	0	0
post2/follow-up	↓**	↓**	↓***	0	0	0

Untreated patients n=7	15 Words Test				Shopping list	
	acquis.	DR	SO–1	SO–2	DR	SO
pre/post1	0	0	0	0	0	0
pre/post2	**	0	0	0	0	0
pre/follow-up	*	*	0	*	0	0
post1/post2	*	0	0	0	0	0
post1/follow-up	0	0	0	0	0	0
post2/follow-up	0	0	0	*	0	0

Wilcoxon signed rank test, one-tailed.

0: no significant improvement	0: no significant decrease
*: $p \leq .05$	↓*: $p \leq .05$
**: $p \leq .025$	↓**: $p \leq .025$
***: $p \leq .01$	↓***: $p \leq .01$

Several control subjects said that they had experienced the tests as something very positive, and there was no drop out of persons from test sessions. Despite the repeated confrontation with their memory deficits, having the possibility to express their problems and knowing the test results was often felt to be useful and lead, in some cases, to a more conscious 'attitude' (greater awareness) towards their handicap. Before and during the tests, the therapists provided some information about frequently occurring complaints and problematic situations of head-injured patients. Despite our assurance that the study was for scientific reasons only, some patients regarded the test sessions as 'a kind of training'.

Tests

The curves of the results of the (artificial) 15 Words Test and the (ecological) shopping lists all suggest that more improvement occurred within the treatment group compared to the control group. Nevertheless, even with alternate test forms and even after much experience in being tested neuropsychologically, there was a tendency towards gradual improvement within the untreated group (Figs. 6.4, 6.5).

Statistical tests (Table 6.4) reveal, however, that the improvement of the controls did not attain the level of significance in delayed recall and organization of the shopping lists, and only rarely in the delayed recall and subjective organization scores of the 15 Word Test. On the other hand, most of the comparisons within the treated group were highly significant, despite the small number of patients. Disappointingly, however, we observed a significant decline on some measures during the three months follow-up period. It is cold comfort that methodologically this points to specific effects of the training. Nevertheless, on all measures, the treated group still performed at a significantly higher level at follow-up than at baseline.

Conclusions

Our first experiences with the results of memory strategy training are both encouraging and surprising. Most important methodologically seems to be the indications of score improvement, even for untreated patients. These could be attributed to very general psychosocial effects and/or to retest effects even on alternate versions. Furthermore, the results suggest a larger increase in objective test scores for treated patients. Most impressive, however, for the treated patients as well as for the therapists, is the as yet unquantifiable evidence for post-therapy changes in coping behaviour in everyday life memory problems, for improvement in vocational and social activities and for a more 'relaxed' attitude towards what might perhaps be a permanently reduced memory capacity.

References

BADDELEY, A. D., 1976 *The psychology of memory* (New York: Harper and Row Publishers).

BADDELEY, A. D., 1982 *Your memory: A user's guide* (New York: Macmillan).

BROOKS, D. N., CAMPSIE, L. SYMINGTON, C., BEATTIE, A. and MCKINLAY, W. W., 1986, 'The five year outcome of severe blunt head injury: a relative's view'. *Journal of Neurology, Neurosurgery, and Psychiatry*, **49**, pp. 764—70.

BROOKS, D. N., DEELMAN, B. G., VAN ZOMEREN, A. H., VAN DONGEN, H., VAN HARSKAMP, F. and AUGHTON, M. E., 1984, 'Problems in measuring cognitive recovery after acute brain injury'. *Journal of Clinical Neuropsychology*, **6** (1), pp. 71—85.

CROSSON, B. and BUENNING, W., 1984, 'An individualized memory retraining program after closed head injury: A single-case study'. *Journal of Clinical Neuropsychology*, **6** (3), pp. 287—301.

CROVITZ, H. F., 1979, 'Memory retraining in brain-damaged patients: the airplane list. *Cortex*, **15**, pp. 131—4.

DEELMAN, B. G., SAAN, R. J. and VAN ZOMEREN, A. H. (Eds) 1990, *Traumatic brain injury; clinical, social, and rehabilitational aspects*, (Lisse: Swetz and Zeitlinger).

DEELMAN, B. G. and SAAN, R. J. 1989, 'Memory deficits: assessment and recovery.' In B. G. Deelman, R. J. Saan, and A. H. Van Zomeren, (Eds) *Traumatic brain injury; clinical, social and rehabilitational aspects* (Lisse: Swetz and Zeitlinger).

ERASMUS, D., 1512 'De ratione studii'. In the Froben edition of the *Opera*, 1540, **1**, p. 466.

GIANUTSOS, R. and GIANUTSOS, J., 1979, 'Rehabilitating the verbal recall of brain-injured patients by mnemonic training: An experimental demonstration using single-case methodology'. *Journal of Clinical Neuropsychology* **1**, (2), pp. 117—35.

GLASGOW, R. E., ZEISS, R. A., BARRERA, M. and LEWINSOHN, P. M., 1977, 'Case studies on remediating memory deficits in brain damaged individuals'. *Journal of Clinical Psychology*, **4**, pp.1049—54.

GRAFMAN, J., 1984, 'Memory assessment and remediation in brain injured patients'. In B.A. Edelstein, and E.T. Couture, (Eds) *Behavioural assessment and rehabilitation of the traumatically brain damaged* (New York: Plenum Press). pp.151—89.

LEVIN, H. S., GRAFMAN, J. and EISENBERG, H. M. (Eds) 1987, 'Visual imagery as a mnemonic aid for brain injured persons'. *Journal of Consulting and Clinical Psychology*, **45**, (5), pp.717—23.

MCKINLAY, W. W., BROOKS, D. N., BOND, M. R., MARTINAGE, D. P. and MARSHALL, M. M., 1981, 'The short-term outcome of severe blunt head injury as reported by relatives of the injured persons'. *Journal of Neurology, Neurosurgery, and Psychiatry*, **44**, pp.527—33.

MILLER, G. A., GALANTER, E. and PRIBRAM, K. H., 1960, *Plans and the Structure of Behavior* (New York: Holt, Rinehart and Winston).

MINDERHOUD, J. M. and VAN ZOMEREN, A. H., 1984, *Traumatische hersenletsels* (Utrecht/Antwerpen: Bohn, Scheltema and Holkema).

ODDY, M., HUMPHREY, M. and UTTLEY, D., 1978, 'Subjective impairment and social recovery after closed head injury'. *Journal of Neurology, Neurosurgery, and Psychiatry*, **41**, pp.611—26.

ODDY, M., COUGHLAN, T., TYERMAN, A. and JENKINS, D., 1985, 'Social adjustment after closed head injury: a further follow-up seven years after injury'. *Journal of Neurology, Neurosurgery and Psychiatry*, **48**, pp.564—8.

PATTEN, B. M., 1972 'The ancient art of memory: usefulness in treatment'. *Archives of Neurology*, **26**, pp.25—31.

SCHACTER, D. L., RICH, S. A. and STAMPP, M. S., 1985, 'Remediation of memory disorders: experimental evaluation of the spaced-retrieval technique'. *Journal of Clinical and Experimental Neuropsychology*, **7**, (1), pp.79—96.

SKINNER, B. F., 1983, 'Intellectual self-management in old age', *American Psychologist*, March 1983.

STERNBERG, R. J. and TULVING, E., 1977, 'The measurement of subjective organisation in free recall'. *Psychological Bulletin*, **84**, pp.539—56.

SUNDERLAND, A. and HARRIS, J. E., 1984, 'Memory failures in everyday life following severe head injuries'. *Journal of Clinical Neuropsychology*, **6**, pp. 127—42.

SUNDERLAND, A., HARRIS, J. E. and BADDELEY, A., 1983, 'Do laboratory tests predict everyday memory?' *Journal of Verbal Learning and Verbal Behaviour*, **22**, pp. 341—57.

TYERMAN, A. and HUMPHREY, M. 1984, 'Changes in self-concept following severe head injury', *International Journal of Rehabilitation Research*, **7**, (1), pp. 11—23.

VAN ZOMEREN, A. H. and VAN DEN BURG, W., 1985, Residual complaints of patients two years after severe head injury'. *Journal of Neurology, Neurosurgery and Psychiatry*, **48**, pp. 21–8.

WILSON, B A., 1987a, 'Single-case experimental designs in neuropsychological rehabilitation'. *Journal of Clinical and Experimental Neuropsychology*, **9**, (5), pp. 527—44.

WILSON, B. A., 1978b, *Rehabilitation of Memory*, (New York: Guilford Press).

WILSON, B. A. and MOFFATT, N. 1984, *Clinical Management of Memory Problems* (London: Croom Helm).

WOLTERS, G., 1985, 'De kunst van het geheugen', *Psychologie*, **10**, pp. 40—4.

YATES, F. A., 1966, *The Art of Memory*, (Chicago: University of Chicago Press).

PART 4
REHABILITATION OF REASONING AND PROBLEM-SOLVING ABILITIES

Chapter 7

Hypothesis Forming and Computerized Cognitive Therapy

A. Evyatar, M.J. Stern, M. Schem-Tov, and Z. Groswasser

Introduction

Injury to the central nervous system (CNS) brings in its wake a host of cognitive deficiencies concurrent with motor, personality and language impairments. A detailed and comprehensive description of all cognitive deficiencies following traumatic brain injury (TBI) form the basis of every neuropsychology textbook (Luria, 1973, Hecaen and Albert, 1978). It should be noted, however, that these textbooks describe mainly those problems occurring in the acute stage after injury. Stern and Stern (1985), divided cognitive impairments following TBI into those occurring immediately after structural injury and those appearing subsequently, after a period in which the total organism has undergone spontaneous recovery and reached a new homeostasis. In short, it can be said that within the period close to the trauma, cognitive deficits are more 'specific', most noticeably in the forms of agnosia, apraxia and aphasia. In the later stages of the rehabilitation process for TBI, the so-called 'general' deficits, such as a reduction in the capacity of the CNS to process information, the slowing-down of thought processes, difficulties in the ability to shift from one set of data to another, deficits in the organization of units of information and difficulties in analysis and synthesis, are the most common ones.

Because of these deficits in the thought processes, the patient appears to be incapable of coping with cognitive tasks demanding effective use of logical thought. There is a conspicuous inability to apply the rules typifying abstract thought coupled with the tendency to function on a more concrete level. The patient has difficulty in coping with complex cognitive tasks. He/she often simplifies the task, responding only to a few units of information and does not discriminate or distinguish between essential and non-essential information. This prevents the construction of suitable cognitive strategies and leads the person to act impusively or in a trial-and-error way. As a result, the patient reaches the wrong conclusions, based on insufficient analysis of information. Such people also encounter difficulty activating an appropriate control system to regulate other aspects of behaviour that have social adaptivity.

Many training exercises in daily clinical use in a TBI rehabilitation framework have been developed over the past few years for the purpose of improving the cognitive functioning of these patients. It is our view that the capacity to construct hypotheses should be a central and fundamental aspect of every cognitive task. Piaget and Inhelder, in their book '*The Psychology of the Child*', (1969), describe five changes that typify the transition from the concrete thought plane to the formal operational thought plane. First and foremost is the capacity to construct hypotheses. They describe this form of thought as hypothetico-deductive thought.

Piaget's concepts are used here as guidelines. His description of other changes that appear at each specific stage of development can be seen to match our own TBI population description. The stages are: The use of propositional logic; the capacity to dissociate completely form from contents; the capacity to deal with the combinatorial nature of operations; the capacity of being able to insert real cases in the set of all possible cases that can be generated logically.

For Piaget, these five transformations derive from one single identifiable mental structure: the INRC group, where 'I' stands for identity, 'N' for negation, 'R' for reciprocity and 'C' for correlative or dual operation. Piaget's descriptions provide the theoretical and empirical basis which supports the construction of a good working model. It is those same processes, that he describes as normative, that we strive to restore to our patients after brain injury.

Hypothesis construction, among all the complex and abstract thought processes in daily use, is an integrative thought process which demands the capacity to go beyond the given information. This is accomplished by determining our goal and the best and most efficient way of attaining it. Therefore, the process used in constructing a logical thought set demands a methodical approach, involving the correct analysis, of all the component parts of the task, weighing up every single unit of information and its relevance to the goal, comparing them to other simultaneous bits of information and finally, constructing the rules governing their common denominator. This basically complex and integrative thought process mobilizes our total cognitive capacity. Clearly, following cerebral injury, in which many cognitive thought components have been damaged, the patient is unable to exercise this process effectively.

In order to cope with these cognitive deficits, we thought that it would be worthwhile to focus on this particular and integrative aspect of the patients' disabilities, namely, the difficulty they experience when asked to construct hypotheses. The therapeutic approaches that have been developed for this purpose have been mainly based on paper-and-pencil or computer software exercises that have no obvious relevance to hypothesis formation (Bracy, etc.). We felt that it would be more effective, therefore, to write our own software for this training programme.

The Training Task

A way of explaining the exercise is to look at the example in Figure 7.1. The task to be performed is to decide whether the bottom rectangle should be classified 'left' or 'right', using all the available information. This necessitates the formulation of hypotheses in order to find a valid way of differentiating between rectangles on the left and on the right. In the exercise shown, a valid criterion would be the even or odd numbers of forms inside the rectangles. For each new exercise, different criteria would apply. If in one exercise the concept of colour is to be used, in the next exercise it would be form, size, location or number. More complex exercises would require the patient to use different logical rules and the ability to think deductively and analytically.

Figure 7.1 Example of a simple task.

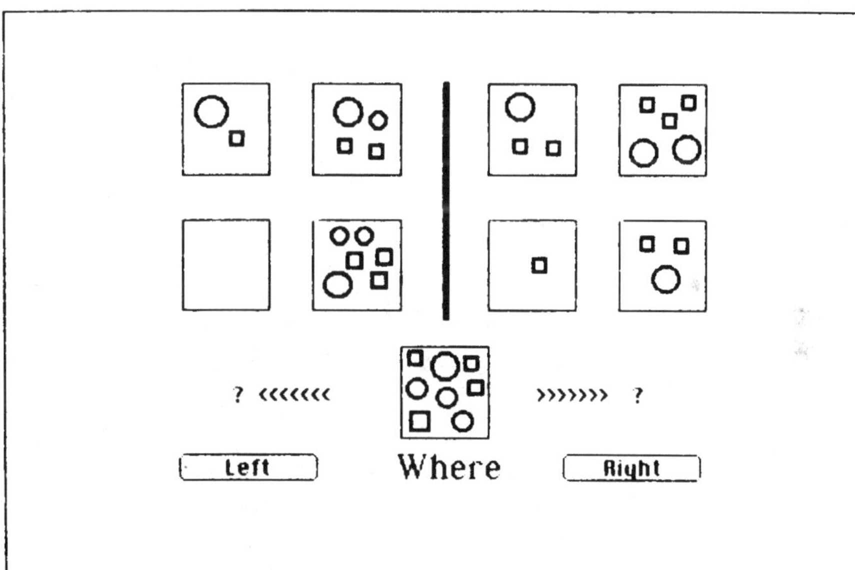

In Figure 7.2. there is an example which involves manipulating both the addition and subtraction forms. In this example the number, form or any other of the simple criteria adopted for the first exercise fails to distinguish between the two sides. A valid procedure for distinguishing between left and right is to realize that, for both sides, the common part of the two top figures on the first line is exactly the figure on the second line on each side. At that point it is easy to decide that looking at the sum (or the union) of the two top figures will give the desired criterion.

Figure 7.2 Example of a complex task.

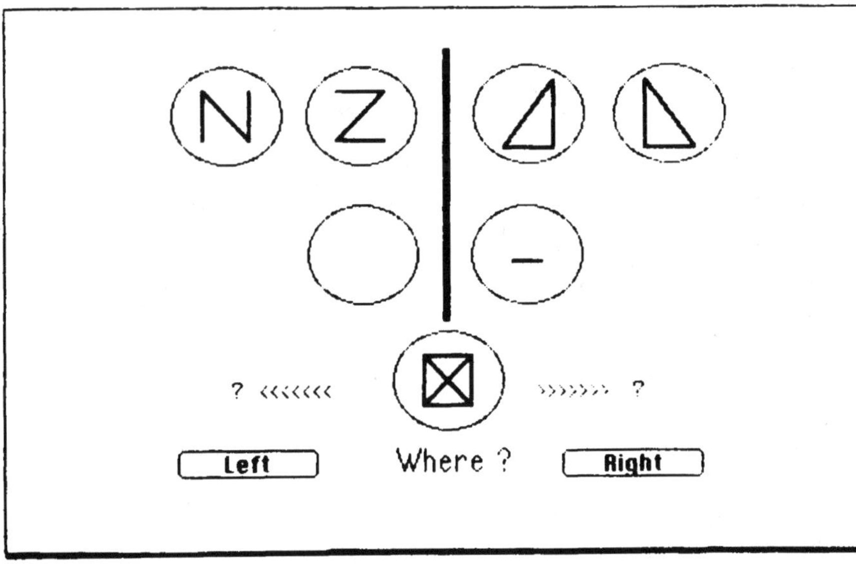

A standard step in the procedure is to always ask the patient to explain his or her choice. Indeed, it is imperative to know if a correct answer is the result of an intuitive perception (based on the cognitive activity of the right hemisphere) which would not be sufficient from the standpoint of therapy. We actually want to teach the patients to translate their perceptions verbally, utilizing the functions of the left hemisphere as well. Of course, this procedure enables the therapist to know if the choice is well-defined and justified.

A few general remarks will help explain how the series of exercises is constructed:

1 The series of exercises is constructed in such a way that the choice of responses is limited at the beginning and slowly increased.
2 Obviously, hypotheses are never conceived *ab initio*, but evolve slowly. The first step, in general, is an analogical argument, taking a clue from an already known structure. Each new hypothesis arises out of the previous one through reconsideration of the total system in an effort to remove discrepancies, while progressively modifying partially successful attempts. Thus, working with our exercise also teaches the idea that complex rules are modifications of simpler ones.
3 Since a single counter example will disallow a hypothesis, the exercises force the patient to look carefully at all possible variables, enabling an increase in the ability to help solve more complex problems by small steps. In order to

check that a patient has a general understanding of the rules, subsequent isomorphic tasks are given. This allows the patient to replicate a previous performance.

4 In the first easy exercises, getting an efficient description of the data will suffice to solve the problem; in the more advanced stages, constructing a model will involve the elimination of irrelevancies and finally, we get to a structure which has alternative descriptions. At this point, when comparing different hypotheses, the patient will have to wrestle with the question of to what extent simplicity is a criterion. (It should also be mentioned that errors are not arbitrary, and this is another reason why the subject is asked to describe his choice verbally.)

Theoretical Background

Three principal theoretical issues relate to the exercises described above. The first problem is to define the notion of structure; the second concerns the cognitive task by which the law relating the configuration at the bottom of the monitor is related to one of the sets of configurations at the left or right side of the monitor. Finally, the third one discusses the possibility that more than one such law exists and which one of these laws should be preferred.

Cognitive and ontological aspects of structures

The first part of the subject's task is to discover organization beyond the apparent chaos of the configurations presented at each side of the monitor so that the additional one will fit within this order, i.e. to discover some inner structure in the presented data. In fact, it is difficult to define the concept 'order' or 'structure'. Jeeves and Greer (1983) wrote that 'structure can be said to exist when there is some form of code or description (verbal or otherwise) which enables the subject to generate all the responses required and which is significantly more efficient, in cognitive terms, than a simple exhaustive catalogue of the contingencies' (p. 11).

This cautious definition demonstrates the ontological problem involved in the concept of structure. Is it an objective property of the phenomenon or does it exist only in the consciousness of the observer? Moreover, we may define the simplifying code itself, which helps the observer to organize the data, as an abstract structure. Our approach is based on the conceptual view that structure is subjective rather than objective. The reason is that different persons often discover different structures in the same data. This is also the view of Simon (1973), Hanson (1958), Harris (1970) and Jeeves and Greer (1983).

Discovery of the structure

Egan and Greeno (1974) suggested two general modes of acquisition of a structure. The first mode is searching a small number of possible hypotheses in an orderly way. The second mode is scanning the features of the available data to form a hypothesis. Brehmer (1976) and Huesmann and Cheng (1973) claimed that since the number of possible hypotheses is very large, or even infinite, the subjects should construct new hypotheses (and test them) rather than using stored pre-existing hypotheses. Jeeves and Greer (1983) described several experiments in which the subject's task was to predict the next stimulus. According to the author's analysis, the results of the experiments should be explained by the hypothesis-testing theory. This conclusion, according to their research, is independent from any developmental factor.

We may, perhaps, infer from the independence of the last conclusion of developmental consideration, that brain-damaged subjects, too, will use the hypothesis-testing method in similar tasks, since no alternative strategy was discovered in the experiments. The cognitive task which we use for our treatment of patients and the tasks of Jeeves and Greer (1983) are similar in the following respect: In both, the subjects are instructed to discover a concealed structure which is common to several configurations. The main difference between our treatment and the experiments of Jeeves and Greer (1983) is that our configurations were presented simultaneously and not consecutively. However, we may infer from the experiment of Jeeves and Greer, in which a memory board was available, that hypothesis testing is also the strategy which our patients used. They found that hypotheses were tested according to their complexity, beginning with the simplest hypothesis possible. This result suits the paradigm of Brehmer (1976) and of Huesmann and Cheng (1973).

Choosing the correct solution

There is, possibly, more than one solution to our exercises. It may be that one solution relates the configuration at the bottom of the monitor to the configurations on the right side, while another solution relates it to the configurations on the left side. Another possibility is that several different solutions relate the configuration at the bottom to the same side (left or right). Therefore, the subjects are questioned regarding the structure which they discovered in the configurations, and we discuss with them the 'amount of correctness' which we relate to this structure. This means that the therapist has to measure the degree of correctness, at least ordinally.

The usual way of ordering two alternative structures is by their relative simplicity and by their predictive power. We saw that a subject usually begins a series of hypotheses testing by looking at the simplest possible structure, until a suitable one is discovered. Therefore, we may, perhaps infer that our patients try to first establish simple criteria by which they can relate the configuration at the bottom to the configuration at one of the sides of the monitor. If they fail, they try more and more complex relations.

However, the problem of defining simplicity of a structure is not simple at all. Authors like Newell and Simon (1972) and Underwood (1978), share the opinion that information theory cannot measure the amount of structure, not even ordinally. Garner (1962) stated that information theory can do no better than a correlation coefficient 0.5 which gives no indication whether we are concerned with an imperfect linear relationship or a perfect curvilinear one. Simon (1972) suggested that this difficulty could be overcome by defining complexity of a structure according to a psychological basis. Such a psychological basis was suggested by Banerji (1969, 1980). We can infer from his work that the complexity of a structure is related to the complexity of a predicate language which is needed to describe it. Another formal linguistic approach to the same problem is that of Chaitin (1975). He defined the complexity of a problem as 'the number of bits that must be put into a computing machine in order to obtain the original series as output' (p.48). If the shortest algorithm is the series itself, it is defined as randomal; thus, not only complexity of a structure is defined, but also the concept 'structure' itself. Another attempt to define complexity of a structure by the length of a lingual description was done by Neisser and Weene (1962). Simon (1972) and Jeeves and Greer (1983) summarized these attempts and concluded that there is no single coding language. The coding depends on the subject and on the conditions of the experiment. Different persons and different conditions may result in different codings.

Bearing these difficulties in mind, we defined simplicity of patients' answers according to two criteria. The first criterion is the shortness of the lingual description; the second is the 'ordinary' character of the concepts involved (following Banerji, 1973). The patients are asked to look for the simplest and natural common denominator of the configurations at either side of the monitor, which suits the configuration at the bottom. The amount of simplicity in their solution indicates their ability to isolate the relevant factors from available data.

Training Procedure

Training was based on a self-contained series of 11 lessons — with about 10 to 12 exercises per lesson — based on hypothesis forming and testing. The training exercises are aimed at gradually and methodically restoring this lost capacity to the patient, starting at relatively simple levels containing a small number of concepts (e.g. colour or shape) and graduating to levels in which attention must be paid to more complicated, abstract and less readily noticeable components.

These exercises can be used regardless of any specific disturbance resulting from TBI. They are constructed in such a way that they demand the simultaneous action of many thought process operations with the objective of utilizing what could be defined as high-cortical functions rather than any special ones, such as perception, psychomotor reaction time, attention, memory, praxis, etc. Because of its need for general cognitive integration, the method can be adapted for use with all types of brain injuries, since it attempts to activate a diversity of functions belonging serially and permanently to both hemispheres. The underlying principle of the exercises is to develop, at different levels of complexity, the integrative thought processes. During training sessions, it is not sufficient that the patient answers correctly (which does not interest us per se, but is rather an indicator of the patient's way of thinking), but he or she is required to explain how any particular problem was solved. It is important to bring the patient to the stage of formalizing answers, or in other words, the patient is forced to conceptualize and verbalize responses and utilize appropriate goal-orientated concepts.

The patient works independently but under the supervision of a therapist. Every exercise aims at activating higher integrative cognitive functions, and, in practice, the following functions are used at all times:

- Identification of visual stimuli
- Collection of all information from the stimuli
- Processing, sorting and categorizing of this information on different levels
- Proper analysis of the material
- Construction of a hypothesis concerning the rules underlying the organization of the given information
- Continual testing of the hypothesis
- Discarding unsuccessful hypotheses and performing a shift to constructing new ones on the basis of different categorizations
- Determination of the relevant rule
- Activation of a new visual stimulus (the next self-contained unit).

Patients and Controls

A total of four groups were examined:

- Two experimental groups: brain-injured patients (TBI) and healthy subjects.
- Two control groups: TBI patients and healthy subjects.

Each group consisted of 10 subjects, eight males and two females. We selected patients whose clinical and neurological state had been stabilized after the acute phase (at least two months after the injury). The healthy subjects were volunteers, either students or hospital staff. The control groups were matched to each of the research groups according to age, sex, education and duration of illness for the patients' group. The patients selected to participate in the project were undergoing therapy following serious penetrating or blunt TBI. Serious TBI is defined as being comatose for a prolonged period (one week to one month), for the experimental and the control groups alike.

The site of cerebral injury was not identical for all patients. A wide range of injury sites were present in our patients, representing several lobes of both hemispheres. At this stage of the project, an attempt was made to select patients suffering from general cerebral damage, rather than to select a homogeneous group from the point of view of the location of the damage. The reason for this was that we wanted to see if treatment would be effective in an undifferentiated population of TBI patients. Therefore, both the experimental and the control groups consisted of patients with injury in various cerebral areas. It should be noted that in all cases there was evidence of structural damage to the CNS, based on computerized tomography (CT) examinations.

Patients included in the experimental group were those whose general condition had stabilized, since it was important to exclude the component of spontaneous recovery which is pre-eminent at the immediate post-traumatic phase in TBI patients. Thus, patients who had been in a therapeutic framework for more than two months after injury were included. All patients showed independence in activities of daily living, were not aphasic and not confused. It was possible to communicate verbally with them and they could express themselves clearly and understand the instructions appearing on the monitor.

Design of the Experiment

The investigation was planned as follows: Each subject, in both groups, first underwent a neuropsychological evaluation (T1 in the figures). Then the whole trial group worked with the exercises, while the controls did not. Going through all lessons lasted between six to eight weeks, at a frequency of two treatment-sessions a week, of one-hour duration each. Once the training was over, each subject again underwent the whole battery of neuropsychological evaluation as before (T2 in the figures). The immediate way to judge the efficiency of the training procedure was to show that, after completing the lessons, the level of performance evaluation by the neurospsychological testing had improved as compared to the controls. On the other hand, all patients were followed for two years after the study. At that time their actual work placement was assessed, as this is considered by us as an integrative criterion for evaluating the outcome including social reintegration and patients' subjective evaluation of quality of life (Najenson *et al.*, 1974, 1980; Melamed *et al.*, 1985).

Evaluation

The evaluation battery was selected out of the complex of tests used for neuropsychological evaluation at the Traumatic Brain Injury Ward at the Loewenstein Rehabilitation Hospital. Assessment included the following tests: Memory Tests (verbal and visual); Rey-Osterrieth Complex Figure (copy and memory); Weigel Test; Block Design; Verbal Logic Tests (examining thinking along three principal channels); Transitive, Inductivo-deductive and Analogic thinking; Raven-Matrix Test and Trail-Making Test (Parts A and B).

Results

The age distribution in the various groups is shown in Table 7.1. Analysis of the results showed no significant difference among the groups according to age and number of school-years of the population (Table 7.1). The mean time elapsed since injury for both brain injured groups was 19 months, with a s.d. of 12.1 months, for the control groups and 21.2 months, with a s.d. of 13.1 months, for the experimental group.

Table 7.1 Mean age and years of education of TBI patients and controls.

Groups	Mean Age (years)	Mean Education (years)
TBI Patients Trial	28.80 ± 13.71	12.20 ± 1.39
TBI Patients Control	34.10 ± 11.05	11.80 ± 1.68
Normal Trial	34.50 ± 11.54	13.00 ± 1.82
Normal Control	31.90 ± 8.77	12.40 ± 1.95

Table 7.2 Interaction between the different groups and the neuropsychological tests.

Tests	Trial/Control	Brain Injury/Normal
	p	p
Block Design	P = 0.0034	n.s.
Sentences Recall	n.s.	n.s.
Story Recall: Short Term	n.s.	n.s.
Story Recall: Long Term	n.s.	n.s.
Words List Recall	n.s.	n.s.
Words List Learning	P = 0.0468	n.s.
Digit Span	n.s.	n.s.
Rey	n.s.	P = 0.051
Weigel	n.s.	n.s.
Trail Making	n.s.	P = 0.0226
Logical Thinking	P = 0.0423	n.s.
Raven-Matrix	P = 0.051	n.s.

The results of the neuropsychological evaluations were examined in two ways: The subjects performing the exercises versus the subjects which did not; and the healthy subjects versus the brain-injured subjects. The results of analysis of variance with two repeated measures are summed up in Table 7.2. We see that in four different tests there are significant changes following the training, and these changes are not related to subjects being patients or controls. Indeed, healthy subjects as well as patients, derived some benefit from the exercises, and to the same extent.

Figure 7.3 Results on the Block Design Test.

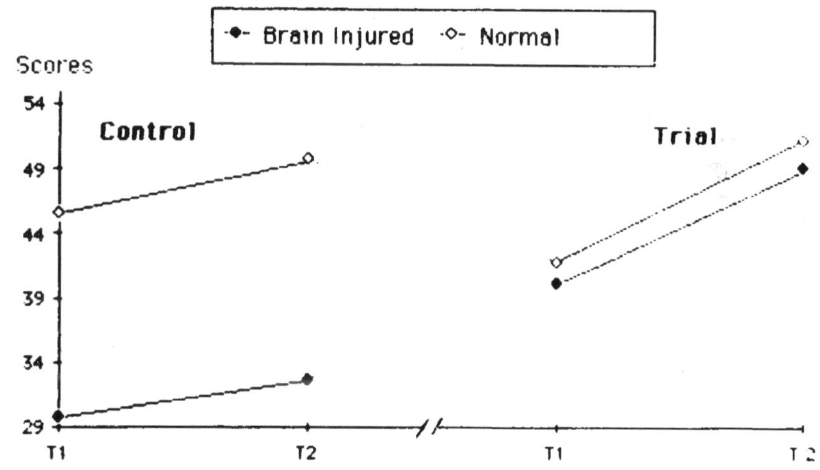

Figure 7.4 Results on the Raven-Matrix Test.

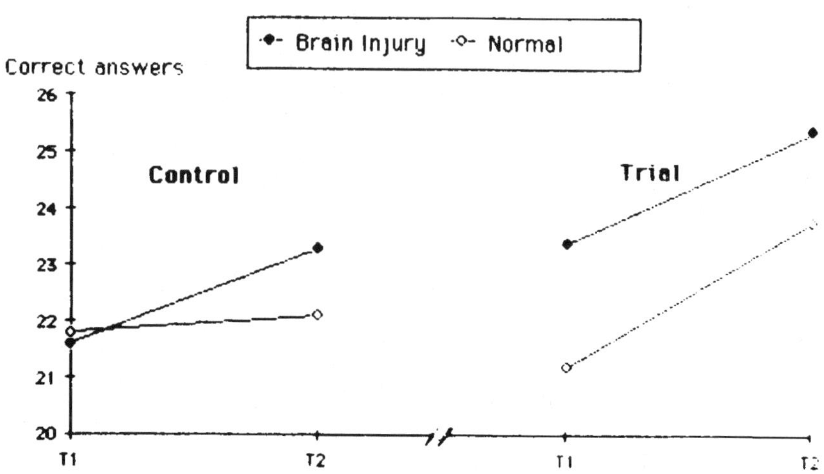

The results of the Block Design Test (Fig. 7.3) show a marked difference between the groups which had done the exercises and those which did not, and the improvement is similar in both the brain-injured and healthy groups. The same can be seen on the Raven-Matrix Tables (Fig. 7.4) and the Logical Thinking Tables (Fig. 7.5). Furthermore, in two tests the results differed as far as healthy or TBI patients were concerned, and these results were not related to the training process. On the Rey-recall Test (Fig. 7.6), the healthy subjects performed better than the patients, while in the Trail-Making Test the patients performed better than their healthy counterparts (Fig. 7.7).

Figure 7.5 Results on the Logical Thinking Tests.

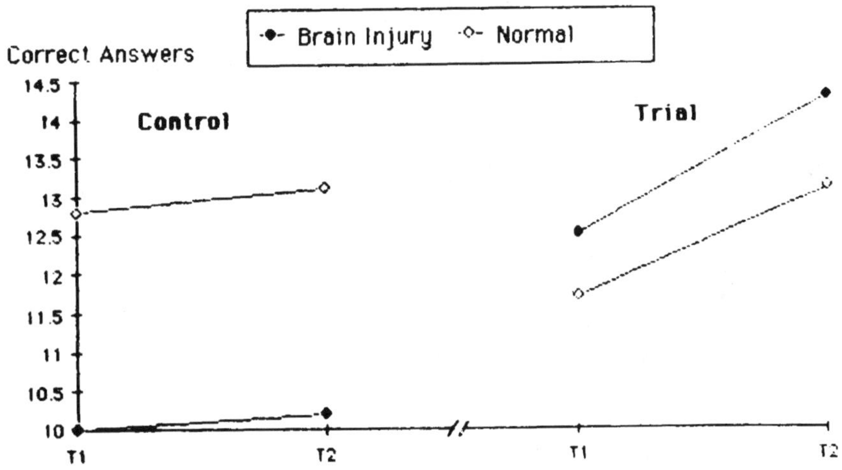

Figure 7.6 Results on the Rey Complex Figure.

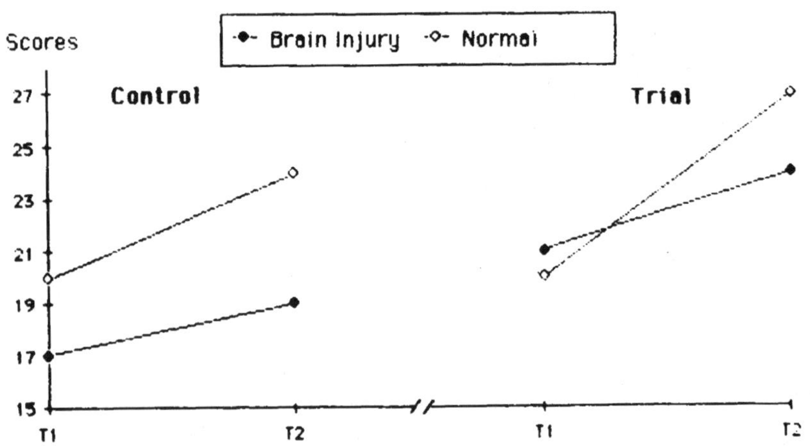

In the follow-up assessment of the patients' actual work, it was found that seven of the trained patients were working in the open market earning their living. The other three patients were working under *sheltered* conditions. In the non-trained group, only two patients were working in the open market, five were working under sheltered conditions and three were not working at all.

Behavioural parameters, such as expressions of low threshold, activity versus passivity and signs of depression and/or anxiety, were examined at the follow-up as well. Each of these symptoms was evaluated on a scale from 1–5 (1 = no pathology: 5 = severe symptoms). In the trained group, we found that the average scoring of each of the above parameters was better in comparison to the non-trained patients (1.3 v. 2.1 for low threshold, 1.9 v. 2.4 for activity/passivity and 1.3 v. 2.6 for depression/anxiety).

Discussion of the Experimental Results

In order to explain the findings, a closer look at the results is needed. As said before, the results of the Block Design Test (Fig. 7.3) show a marked difference between the groups which had done the exercises and those which had not, and the improvement was similar in both the brain-injured and healthy groups. The same is true about the Raven-Matrix tables (Fig. 7.4) and the Logical Thinking Tables (Fig. 7.5).

This means that the effect is not specifically restricted to TBI people; rather, that there exists a learning process from which both groups can benefit, the TBI patients to no less a degree than healthy subjects. On the Rey-recall Test (Fig.7.6), the healthy

Figure 7.7 Results on the Trail-Making Test.

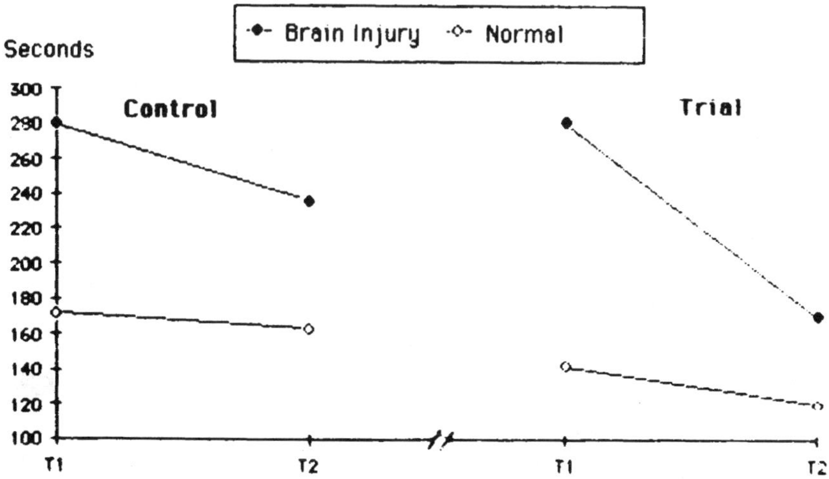

subjects performed better than the patients, while on the Trail-Making Test the patients performed better than their healthy counterparts (Fig.7.7).

This 'learning' can be attributed to having done the test twice. In fact, a difference was found only in the 'recall' part of the Rey's Test and not in the copying part of it. During the first session, having to write down by memory came by surprise to the examined people. It can be assumed, therefore, that during the second evaluation, six to eight weeks later, the subjects already knew they would have to recall the picture and therefore paid more attention to it. What emerges is that the healthy subjects did better in this respect. The difference of scores between the first and second evaluation was smaller with the brain-injured patients, irrespective of having done the exercises or not. They drew no benefit from the first trial, their attention was not drawn to memorizing the picture or they were incapable of doing so.

To give a correct interpretation of the results of the Trail Making Test, we must take the 'ceiling-effect' into consideration because the test requires a short performance time. As the healthy subjects' performance times were very low to begin with, evidently there was little room for improvement. Therefore, comparison between healthy and injured subjects is of low validity in this case. We think one should see the results for themselves, beyond the statistical criteria. In other words, we should watch the results obtained by the TBI patients only and compare those of the trained patients to those of the non-trained. By doing this we can observe a clear-cut significant difference, showing the specific improvement obtained in the performance of those patients who underwent the training procedure.

The manifest changes following training were not only expressed in the results of the neuropsychological tests at the conclusion of therapy (T2) but also in other aspects of the patient's life. On the whole, it can be said that patients subjectively reported differences in their feelings compared to the past. Basically, they felt they were much better equipped to cope when confronting daily problems. This applies to various domains, especially to studies and any occupational framework in which they found themselves. They learned to work methodically, to relate all the information, to consider many different possibilities and not be bound to only one method (not to be rigid). This was clearly shown in the follow-up study as most of the trained patients were actually working on the open market. Acquiring all these traits reinforces self-esteem and increases their faith in their ability to succeed in the tasks which life presents. They also acquired the feeling, which had been lost to them, of mastery in their daily lives (an observation similar to that made by Deelman *et al.*, Chapter 6). As a result they are better able to make decisions and to be more active than in the past. This improvement expressed itself in the better scoring on behavioural parameters by the trained patients.

An important note here is that this training is not the only therapy patients receive during their hospitalization, and therefore it cannot be claimed that all the changes that occur are the exclusive result of training. It would also be grossly incorrect to ascribe general changes to one therapy alone. We can only claim that our exercises constitute a valid contribution to the total treatment existing in the rehabilitation framework. As therapists we are aware of the many obstacles encountered in rehabilitation. Most notable of these is the difficulty of procuring the patient's cooperation in psychological and cognitive treatment, possibly because the significance of deficiencies in these domains is not fully realized. These impairments are substantially more 'abstract' when compared to paralysis or bone fractures. Patients, therefore, often shy away from the 'exercises' they are given, for they do not understand the relevance of these exercises to their outside lives, they do not find them interesting, and they seek excuses to avoid therapy. The advantage of using the computer as a therapeutic tool is that it is appealing, 'magical', powerful. The experimental group was observed to be alert, curious, interested and, above all, cooperative. At the end of training sessions, they asked for more exercises and were disappointed that we could not oblige.

The differences found between the two groups (those receiving training and those not) indicate that our training exercises have a legitimate place in the current overall therapeutic setting. Their contribution to the patient's total cognitive capacity lead to considerably enhanced improvements beyond the spontaneous improvement that occurs without training. Improvement in cognitive ability has far-reaching effects on personality. Skill acquisition and broadening cognitive possibilities allow the patient to regain faith in his or her own ability, a trait that is lost as a result of the injury. Self-respect is reinstated as a result of this training; the patient feels less anxious and threatened by the outside world and is able to introspect and thereby to understand more fully the motives underlying behaviour. Self-image also undergoes positive changes. The patients are consequently better able to relate adequately to their surroundings and to regain the personal respect which was once their birthright.

Conclusions

Problems similar to our exercises are used in psychometric tests, and it is well known that scores on their solution are positively and significantly correlated with academic achievements. Therefore, we expect that developing the patient's ability to discover structures by our treatment may transfer to the ability to discover structures in other areas. An interesting point is that paradoxically, the number of mistakes decreased when the exercises became more complicated, which implies that a learning process is indeed taking place. We hope that the exercises will help patients suffering from TBI improve their cognitive capacity by teaching them to work in a systematical way. They will be able to apply rules when confronted with cognitive tasks, as it is needed in daily life, and by that to improve their functional capacity in solving problems.

Acknowledgement

The authors wish to thank the Dr. J. Isler Foundation, The Neta-Bucksenbaum Foundation and the Neaman Institute for their support.

References

BANERJI, R. B., 1969, *Theory of problem solving; An approach to artificial intelligence* (New York: Elsevier).

BANERJI, R. B., 1973, 'Simplicity of concepts, training and the real world'. In A. Elithorn and D. Jones (Eds) *Artificial and human thinking* (New York: Elsevier).

BANERJI, R. B., 1980, *Artificial intelligence: A theoretical approach* (New York: North Holland).

BREHMER, B., 1976, 'Learning complex rules in probabilistic inference tasks'. *Scandinavian Journal of Psychology*, **17**, 309–12.

CHAITIN, G. J., 1975. 'Randomness and mathematical proof.' *Scientific American* **232** (5), 47–52.

DIENES, Z. P. and JEEVES, M. A., 1965, *Thinking in structures*, (London: Hutchinson).

EGAN, D. E. and GREENO, J. C., 1974, 'Theory of rule induction: Knowledge acquired in concept learning, serial pattern learning, and problem-solving'. In L. W. Gregg (Ed.) *Knowledge and cognition.* (Maryland: Lawrence Eribaum).

GARNER, W. R., 1962, *Uncertainty and structure as psychological concepts* (New York: Wiley).

GLAZNER, M. and CLARK, W. H., 1963, 'The Verbal Loop hypothesis: Binary numbers'. *Journal of Verbal Learning and Verbal Behaviour*, **2**, 301–9.

HECAEN, H. and ALBERT, M. L., 1978, *Human Neuropsychology* (New York: John Wiley and Sons).

HANSON, N. R., 1958, *Patterns of discovery: An inquiry in the conceptual foundations of science* (Cambridge University Press).

HARRIS, E., 1970, *Hypothesis and perception: The roots of scientific method* (London: George Allen and Unwin.)

HUESMANN, L. R. and CHENG, C. M., 1973 'A theory for the induction of mathematical functions'. *Psychological Review* **80**, 126–38.

JEEVES, M. A. and GREER, G. B., 1983, *Analysis of structural learning* (London: Academic Press).

LURIA, A. R. 1973, *The working brain* (New York: Penguin Books).

MELAMED, S., STERN, J. M., RAHMANI, L., GROSWASSER, Z. and NAJENSON, T., 1982, 'Work congruence, behavioural pathology and rehabilitation status of severe craniocerebral injury'. In M. Lahav (Ed.), *Psychological research in rehabilitation* (Tel Aviv, Israel: Ministry of Defence Publishing House).

NAJENSON, T., GROSWASSER, Z., MENDELSON, L. and HACKETT, P., 1980, 'Rehabilitation outcome of brain damaged patients after severe head injury.' *International Rehabilitation Medicine*, **2**, 17–22.

NAJENSON, T., MENDELSON, L., SHECHTER, I., DAVID, C., MINTZ, N. and GROSWASSER, Z. 1974. 'Rehabilitation after severe head injury'. *Scandinavian Journal of Rehabilitation Medicine*, **6**, 5–12.

NEISSER, U., 1976. *Cognition and reality: Principles and implications of cognitive psychology* (San Francisco: Freeman).

NEISSER, U. and WEENE, P., 1962, 'Hierarchies in concept attainment'. *Journal of Experimental Psychology*, **64**, 640–5.

NEWELL, A. and SIMON, H. A., 1972, *Human problem solving*. (New Jersey: Prentice Hall, Englewood Cliffs).

PIAGET, J. and INHELDER, B., 1969, *The Psychology of the child* (New York: Basic Books.)

SIMON, H. A., 1972, 'Complexity and the representation of patterned sequences of symbols'. *Psychological Review* **79**, 369–82.

SIMON, H. A., 1973. 'Does scientific discovery have a logic?' *Philosphy of Science*, **40**, 471–80.

STERN, J. M. and STERN, B., 1985, 'Neuropsychological outcome during late stage of recovery from brain injury: a proposal'. *Scandinavian Journal of Rehabilitation Medicine*, Supplement, **12**, 27–30.

UNDERWOOD, G., (Ed.) 1978, *Strategies of information processing* (London: Academic Press).

Chapter 8

Frontal Lobe Dysfunctions in Patients — Therapeutical Approaches

D.Y. von Cramon and G. Matthes-von Cramon

Introduction

About 40 per cent of brain-damaged in-patients admitted to our clinic display serious planning and problem-solving disabilities which prevent them returning to a productive private and vocational life. Although patients with problem-solving disturbances represent a heterogeneous group with respect to etiology, extent and localization of brain lesions (Cramon, 1988), there is a certain agreement among researchers that 'executive function' is mainly impaired due to frontal lobe damage.

Contrary to the host of studies and case reports dealing with the clinical picture and the most frequently used diagnostic approaches, only a few controlled studies have tested the possible effects of a cognitive remediation programme in these 'frontal' patients (c.f. Goldstein and Levin, 1987). At present some rehabilitation centres, especially in the United States, try to elaborate a therapeutic management for these patients as the studies of Prigatano and co-workers (1984, 1986), Ben-Yishay *et al.* (1985) and Scherzer (1986) demonstrate. Their 'holistic' approach includes cognitive as well as psychotherapeutic interventions, and their remediation programmes are set up for periods of several months or more. They mainly treat chronic patients with high level cognitive problems affecting judgement, awareness and self-monitoring ability; these patients are selected according to rather strict criteria.

The aim of our study was to investigate the effects of a much shorter (six week), cognitive training programme for unselected in-patients, admitted 'ad hoc' at a stage of their rehabilitation process when explicit cognitive training procedures had not yet taken place. The primary intention of our problem solving training was to provide 'frontal' patients with techniques enabling them to reduce the complexity of a multi-stage problem by breaking it down to more manageable proportions (an approach similar to that reported by Wood, 1990). A slowed-down, controlled and stepwise processing of a given problem should replace the rash and unsystematic approach 'frontal' patients spontaneously choose. It was hoped that in establishing certain, simple problem-solving techniques, the handicap of these patients in every day life would also diminish.

The most challenging task was to make the patients understand that they had a 'problem', relevant enough to cope with. For this reason we tried to reinforce their effort towards a critical (i.e. more realistic) evaluation of their problem-solving ability. (The same problem has been addressed from a neurobehavioural perspective by Burgess and Alderman, Chapter 9, and the reader may wish to refer to this as an alternative strategy). It was hoped that the training programme described here might help us to improve our judgement on a patient's available rehabilitation potential (Cicerone and Tupper, 1986); the results of the training would provide arguments for the decision as to whether further cognitive training might be reasonable and, if that were the case, to decide on the kind of programme that should follow.

The study was based on a quasi-experimental design as proposed by Campbell and Stanley (1963). Given the constraint that in a clinical setting it is not acceptable to assign patients randomly to treatment groups or to have control groups, small quasi-experimental group studies with good pre-treatment and post-treatment assessments seem to be a powerful alternative to classical group studies.

Outcome measures

Table 8.1 gives a short survey of the routinely applied neuropsychological tests measuring attentional as well as memory and learning functions. It is beyond the scope of this paper to discuss the patients' performance in these tests.

In Table 8.2 tests are shown that appear to examine more specifically frontal lobe dysfunction. From standardized German Intelligence Tests we selected those subtests which presumably measure inductive and analogical reasoning as well as verbal abstraction. The patients' capacity to form concepts and to shift from one category to another was assessed by the 'Modified Card Sorting Test', using the version of Nelson (1976). Test performance was evaluated by the number of categories reached and the total error score which is calculated as the percentage of perseverative errors in comparison with the total number of errors.

For an assessment of the patients' ability to learn from experience and observation, we used the 'Tower of Hanoi' puzzle. The 'Tower' comprises one of the best-known transfer problems currently available in neuropsychology (Simon, 1975; Kotovski *et al.*, 1985). We used a computerized version of the four-disk problem with fixed start and target positions (Matthes, 1988). The patient was to optimize his/her solution strategies across five consecutive trials. The test score consisted of the added numbers of moves of the fourth and fifth trial.

Table 8.1 Survey on the routinely administered tests for the assessment of attention, memory and learning function.

Attention

Zahlen-Verbindungs-Test: Oswald and Roth, 1978

DR 2 (simple choice reaction time task):
Bukasa and Wenninger, 1986a

RST 3 (complex choice reaction time task):
Bukasa and Wenninger, 1986b

PASAT (paced auditory serial addition task):
Gronwall and Wrightson, 1974

Memory and Learning

Digit Span
Block Span (Corsi's Block-Tapping-Test: Lezak, 1983)
Free recall of a word list[1]
Free recall of a 57-unit story[1]
Free recall of a 57-unit story (48 hours delay)[1]
Recall of 8 face-name-associations (48 hours delay)[1]
Learning of paired-associates (words, faces-names, objects)[1]
Buschke Selective Reminding Test (Vorländer, 1987)
California Verbal Learning Test (Ilmberger, 1989)

1) c.f. Schuri (1988)

Table 8.2 Survey on the Intelligence subtests and problem-solving tasks administered to assess frontal lobe dysfunction.

Intelligence Tests:

- Leistungs-Prüf-System (LPS; Horn, 1983)
  Inductive Reasoning
- Intelligenz-Struktur-Test (IST 70; Amthauer, 1973)
  Categorizing
  Analogies
  Similarities
- Wilde-Intelligenz-Test (WIT; Jäger and Althoff, 1983)
  Proverbs

Problem-solving tasks:

- Modified Card Sorting Test (Nelson, 1976)
- Tower of Hanoi Puzzle (computerized version)
- Planning Test (Stoltze and Matthes-von Cramon, in preparation)

The 'Planning Test' was developed by ourselves as a standardized instrument with high ecological validity (Stoltze and Matthes-von Cramon, in preparation). The patients scheduled several items on an agenda which they were to carry out within a certain time limit. Thus, they had to utilize information such as various opening hours, fixed appointments, time required for a certain affair, time needed for the transfer from one location to another, etc. The test score was defined by the number of correctly scheduled items.

In addition to these cognitive measures, a rating scale was devised (Matthes-von Cramon and von Cramon; unpublished data) comprising 17 operationally defined variables relating to different aspects of behaviour relevant for 'frontal' patients. These included 'social behaviour', 'drive (Antrieb)', 'goal-directed ideas', 'cognitive and action style', 'verification and judgment'. Each item was rated on a three-point scale (0 = normal, 1 = occasional, 2 = frequent). Only the item 'unawareness of deficits' was rated on a four-point scale according to the operational definitions shown in Table 8.3.

In a multi-disciplinary clinical team, raters will not be strictly independent in their judgments because of a multitude of common discussions about a certain patient. On

Table 8.3 List of operationally defined behavioural categories included in the Rating Scale for Frontal Lobe Dysfunction (c.f. Matthes-von Cramon and von Cramon, in preparation).

Behavioural categories	
Inflexibility	Emotional indifference
Concrete thinking	Euphoric mood
Lack of ideas	Violent outbursts
Inconsiderate decisions	Tactless behaviour
Lack of determination	Tangentiality
Inadequate monitoring	Talkativeness
Impaired self-corrections	Apathy (A-/Hypobulia)
Premature actions	Poverty of speech
Perseverations	Narrowed exploration
Rule breaking	Lack of mental effort
Action slips	Loss of standpoint
Utilization behaviour	Augmented libido
Imitation behaviour	Reduced libido
Awareness of deficits	
— complete unawareness (with or without explicit denial)	
— unspecified awareness	
— learned awareness	
— adequate awareness	

the other hand, raters, who are not part of the staff, have no chance to reliably assess the patient's behaviour because they have not seen him/her in a sufficiently large number of relevant situations. For that reason we had to be content with a 'collective rating' (Lienert, 1969). Observations by nurses and other therapeutic personnel, as well as reports from the patient's family were integrated into a 'consensual judgment', at least on the basis of an acceptable compromise. The raters were not given any details on the patients' performances in the psychometric tests or during the training programme.

The Patient Sample

Forty-eight, consecutively admitted patients, with various aetiologies of brain damage were examined. Patients with significant aphasic disorders or visuo-spatial neglect were excluded from the study since they could not cope with the above-mentioned tests. The sample was dichotomized by using, as cut-off scores, the medians of those tests which are supposed to be sensitive to frontal lobe dysfunction. Twenty-seven patients scoring below average in at least two of the three problem solving tasks were classified as 'poor problem solvers' (indicated as PS –) whereas the remaining 21 patients who scored above average were classified as 'good problem solvers' (indicated as PS +).

PS + and PS – did not significantly differ as to age, sex, education, aetiology and time since lesion (see Table 8.4). However, poor problem solvers tended to be older and to have longer post-onset intervals in comparison with good problem solvers. These patients also obtained significantly lower scores in their attention and memory performances.

Table 8.4 Sample of the 48 brain-damaged patients included in the study. PS + : good problem solvers; PS – : poor problem solvers (for detailed explanation see text).

	PS +	PS –	p[1]
Number	21	27	
		Median (range)	
Age (y)	34 (19–60)	45 (19–59)	ns
Sex (m,f)	13, 8	19, 8	ns
Education (y)	10 (9–18)	9 (9–18)	ns
Aetiology			
–closed-head injury	12	13	
–cerebro-vascular acc.	6	7	
–cerebral hypoxia	1	2	
–others	2	5	
Time since lesion (m)	4 (2–60)	8 (3–120)	ns

1) Mann-Whitney-U-Test.

Table 8.5 Localization of brain lesions. The numbers in brackets refer to the number of patients with visible frontal lobe damage on CT/MRI Scan.

Site of lesion	PS + (n = 21)	PS – (n = 27)
Right brain damage	6 (0)	6 (6)
Left brain damage	3 (1)	3 (3)
Bilateral brain damage	0	12 (11)
Unknown	12	6

As for the brain lesions (as far as CT and MRI scans can reveal them), patients with bilateral brain lesions were exclusively allocated to the poor problem solvers (Table 8.5). The large number of unknown brain lesions in the PS + group is due to traumatic brain damage no longer visible in later neuroimaging examination. As a matter of fact, 20 out of 21 patients with problem-solving deficits and visible brain lesions revealed frontal lobe damage in comparison with only one in ten 'good problem solvers'.

Comparing the PS + and PS – groups, significant differences were found in most of the intelligence subtests, except for the 'Similarities Subtest' in which 'good problem solvers' also scored below-average. According to our selection criteria (c.f

Table 8.6 Test scores of good (PS +) and poor (PS –) problem solvers in Intelligence subtests and Problem Solving Tasks.

	PS +	PS –	p[1]
Intelligence Tests			
IQ (LPS)	105 (84–120)	100 (79–115)	*
	T-values: Median (range)		
Reasoning (LPS)	50 (40–60)	48 (25–60)	**
Categorizing (IST)	50 (41–60)	40 (20–66)	*
Analogies (IST)	52 (41–59)	44 (27–55)	***
Similarities (IST)	42 (33–68)	36 (22–56)	ns
Proverbs (WIT)	52 (45–67)	44 (20–52)	***
Problem-solving tasks	Median (range)		
MCST (Nelson, 1976)			
–number of categories	7 (5–7)	3 (0–7)	***
–total error score	0 (0–33)	39 (0–98)	***
Tower of Hanoi			
–moves (T4 + T5)	30 (30–42)	56 (39–107)	***
Planning Test (von Cramon 1988)			
–raw score	15 (13–15)	0 (0–13)	***

1) Mann-Whitney-U-Test: * $p<0.05$; ** $p<0.01$; *** $p<0.001$.

Table 8.7 Behavioural rating (collective rating) of good (PS+) and poor (PS−) problem solvers. Asterisks indicate a significant predominance of behavioural alterations in the PS− group

	PS+ (n=21)	PS− (n=27)	p[1]
Awareness (of deficits)			***
Social behaviour			**
—emotional indifference			**
—violent outbursts			*
—tactless behaviour			*
—placidity			*
Drive ('Antrieb')			**
Goal-directed ideas			***
Cognitive style			***
—inflexibility			***
—concrete thinking			***
—insufficient problem identification			***
—lack of heuristics			***
—impaired reasoning			***
Action style			***
—premature actions			**
—perserverations			**
—rule breaking			***
—action slips			*
Verification/judgment			***
—inconsiderate decisions			***
—inadequate cognitive control			**
—impaired self-corrections			***

1) Mann-Whitney-U-Test: * $p<0.05$; ** $p<0.01$; *** $p<0.001$.

above), the group medians differed considerably for the three problem-solving tasks (see Table 8.6). The two groups could also be distinguished by their behaviour. There were highly significant differences in all aspects of social and cognitive behaviour collectively rated by members of the ward personnel and the family (Table 8.7).

Six out of 27 patients with problem-solving deficits (PS−) dropped out for reasons which had nothing to do with the planned-training programme. The remaining 21 patients were allocated to either an explicit problem-solving training (PST) or to a memory training (MT); the latter was expected to have, at most, implicit effects on problem-solving abilities. Memory-training patients were taught reductive as well as elaborative coding strategies in order to improve their learning ability. (The tendency of the PST group to perform less efficiently than the MT group in the problem-solving tasks, especially in the 'Tower of Hanoi' puzzle, would reinforce the result if, in fact, the PST ought to bring about better therapeutic effects than the MT).

Table 8.8 Main clinical data of the PST and the MT group.

	PST	MT	p[1]
Number	12	9	
		Median (range)	
Age (y)	47 (19–59)	37 (23–53)	ns
Sex (m,f)	10, 2	5, 4	ns
Education (y)	9 (9–18)	9 (9–13)	ns
Aetiology			
—closed-head injury	7	4	
—cerebro-vascular acc.	2	2	
—cerebral hypoxia	1	1	
—others	2	2	
Time since lesion (m)	9 (3–120)	8 (3–36)	ns

1) Mann-Whitney-U-Test: * $p > 0.05$.

Table 8.9 Paralleled cognitive performances of the PST and the MT group regarding attention, memory and learning functions.

	PST (n = 12) MT (n = 9)
Speed of information processing	ns[1]
Sustained attention	ns
Free recall of a (56-item) story	
—without delay	ns
—with delay of 48 hours	ns
Paired-associates learning	
—word association test	ns
—faces/names association test	ns
—object association test	ns
Auditory-verbal learning	
—cluster score (California Verbal Learning Test)	ns

1) Mann-Whitney-U-Test: $p > 0.05$.

The PST and the MT group were equivalent in respect of their demographic data (Table 8.8) and their main cognitive performances (Table 8.9). This increases the probability that any changes in outcome measures reflects a treatment effect. Both training programmes were carried out over a period of six weeks with an average of 25 sessions per patient per programme.

Table 8.10 Taxonomy of Problem Solving Behaviours adopted from H. A. H. Rowe (1985).

1. Directions/instructions/stimulus
   Passage-related activity:
   - survey of given information
   - identification of problem/or its parts from given information
2. Solution-directed activity:
   - heuristics
   - reasoning
3. Critical evaluation/judgment:
   - critical assessment/verification
   - judgment/evaluation

Treatment Goals

Our treatment goals were formulated on the basis of Rowe's (1985) taxonomy of problem-solving behaviour (Table 8.10). The first stage was one of problem analysis. Patients were to survey information by reading and rereading directions and formulating questions to increase their understanding of instructions.

The next stage, solution-direction activity, includes the application of heuristics and reasoning. Patients were trained to divide a multi-stage task into smaller, more manageable proportions. We gave them immediate feedback on the suitability of their operations and prompted hypotheses on alternative solutions. At the stage of critical

Table 8.11 Pre-/post-treatment comparison of behavioural abnormalities (collective rating) for the PST (n = 12) and the MT (n = 9) group. Asterisks represent a significant decrease in behavioural abnormalities.

	PST	MT
Awareness	.0679	.1797
Social behaviour	.0277*	.1797
Drive (Antrieb)	.0431*	.3173
Goal-directed ideas	.0117*	1.0000
Cognitive style	.0051**	.1797
Action style	.0679	.1797
Verific./judgment	.0431*	.3173

Wilcoxon Matched-pairs Signed-ranks Test: * $p<0.05$; ** $p<0.01$; *** $p<0.001$.

evaluation and judgement, we tried to elicit a greater sensitivity to errors and discrepancies based on a means-end relationship. Patients learned to recognize wrong moves or failures and to correct errors.

The PST programme consisted of four modules which were all put into action during the course of a week. This was an indispensable pre-requisite because, for organizational reasons, we had to admit new patients at the beginning of each week. We felt it was important for patients to become actively involved in their therapeutic programme. Compliance with treatment could be significantly raised by using a great variety of tasks and exercises closely related to their every day experiences.

The exercises of the first module referred to the problem of generating goal-directed ideas. Initially, this implied a kind of 'brainstorming' to produce alternatives to a given problem (e.g. what can be done when the employees of the Italian Railroad go on strike and you have to return to Germany immediately). Secondly, these alternatives had to be weighed by pondering the premises for their realization and by anticipating their positive and negative consequences.

The second module aimed at a systematic and careful comparison of information. Patients were to recognize discrepancies in two strings of items by carefully comparing, for instance, positions in a want list with those of a delivery note. Another set of tasks required the patients to detect one particular sales offer out of six to ten similar ones. Wrong offers were to be cast out by gradually augmenting the amount of information to be considered. A third type of task asked for the patients' ability to discern relevant from irrelevant information. We presented them brief descriptions of daily life situations. They were to extract the relevant information in the form of a want ad for a newspaper.

The third module consisted of tasks where multiple information needed to be processed simultaneously. For that purpose we used time tables, schedules and tariffs. Patients, for instance, compared the catalogues of several tourist offices in order to find the most favourable two-week trip to England for a family of four.

In the fourth module we paid attention to the patients' difficulties in drawing inferences. For that reason we worked with short detective stories. Patients enjoyed cracking the problems by uncovering discrepancies between different declarations and statements of suspects, or by detecting hints of how a crime could have been committed. They were encouraged to make sketches to illustrate the scene in question.

Both PST and MT were conducted as group-training sessions. We arranged the PST either in parallel or in project groups (c.f. Mosey, 1986). Patients suffering from a marked apathy (abulia) or a lack of mental effort ('Verlust der Anstrengungsbereitschaft') can only be treated in a parallel-group setting because no consistent group interaction of the kind needed can be expected in a project group. The therapist is compelled to continually prompt each patient in order to maintain effort and participation.

In the project-group setting — suitable for about half of the patients — two or three group members cooperated on a task as a team for a limited time. Working together, they had to adapt to individual differences in efficiency and speed of performance. It was hoped that when confronted with their partners' problems in one or another task, a more realistic stance towards his/her own incapacity would be established. Generating goal-directed ideas was not an easy task for the 'frontal' patients. Even after more than 20 sessions, the majority produced only few reality-oriented ideas. The brainstorming within the group, however, helped to disguise the individual lack of ideas. Patients also learned from this experience that there are various options for a given problem, other than the one they might have thought of.

Comparing information in pairs seemed to be relatively easy provided that they were clea.ly organized. The patients ran into trouble, however, when the information to be compared was interspersed in a text with additional distracting facts. For this reason, patients found working with time tables, schedules and tariffs rather demanding. They showed great difficulty in surveying rows and columns simultaneously because of their obvious incapacity to cope with more than one piece of information at a time. As for drawing inferences, patients mostly failed when the relevant propositions were not concrete and /or not closely connected to each other.

Results

We retested the two experimental groups (PST and MT groups) with the diagnostic tools we mentioned before. Only the Modified Card Sorting Test could not be administered twice for fear that patients had remembered the right solution. In the following preliminary data, the pre-/post-treatment effects of the PST for some Intelligence Subtests, the Planning Test and the Tower of Hanoi Puzzle are demonstrated.

Pre-/post-treatment comparisons (Fig. 8.1) between the two experimental groups indicated an increase of five or more T-values for the reasoning subtest in seven out of twelve patients of the PST group; the median of the T-values rose from 45 to 50 (Wilcoxon Matched-pairs Signed-ranks Test: $p = .0180$). In contrast, only one in nine patients of the MT group markedly improved on this test. The group median dropped from 50 to 45 (Wilcoxon Matched-pairs Signed-ranks Test: $p = .5930$). As for the subtest 'categorizing' the entire PST-group improved significantly (Wilcoxon Matched-pairs Signed-rank Test: $p = .0229$); eight subjects showed an increase of five or more T-values. The performance of the MT group in this test did not significantly change; only two patients had better post-treatment performances (Wilcoxon Matched-pairs Signed-ranks Test: $p = .7353$).

The PST group also performed better in the analogies subtest (Wilcoxon Matched-pairs Signed-ranks Test: $p = .0440$); however, a marked improvement could

Figure 8.1 Intra-individual pre-/post-treatment comparison of the intelligence subtests, reasoning and categorizing (T-values) for the PST (n = 12) and the MT group (n = 9). For details see text.

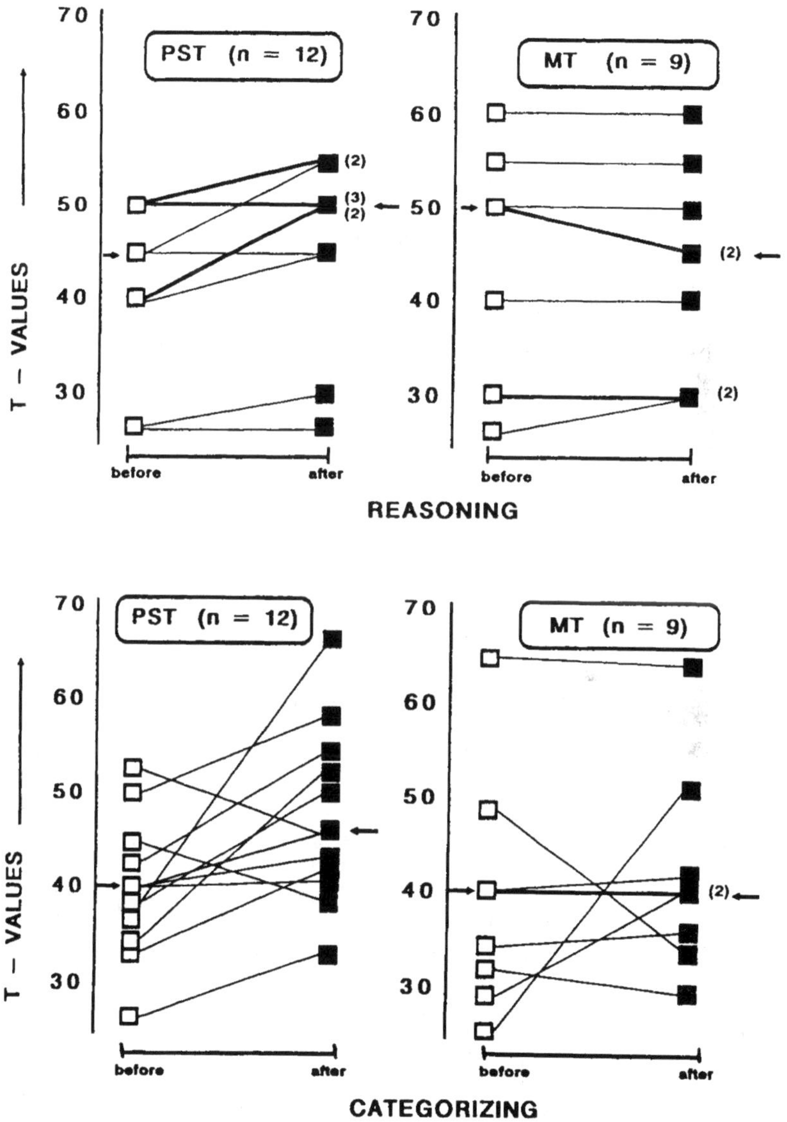

Figure 8.2 Intra-individual pre-/post-treatment comparison of the Planning Test (raw scores) for the PST ($n = 12$) and the MT ($n = 9$) group. For details see text.

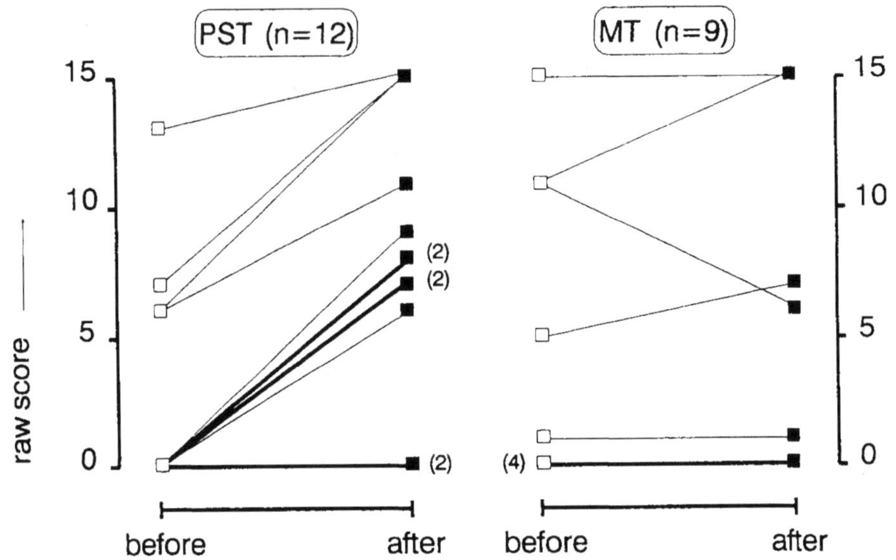

Figure 8.3 Intra-individual pre-/post-treatment comparison of the Tower of Hanoi puzzle (added moves of the fourth and fifth trial) for nine patients of the PST and eight patients of the MT group. For details see text.

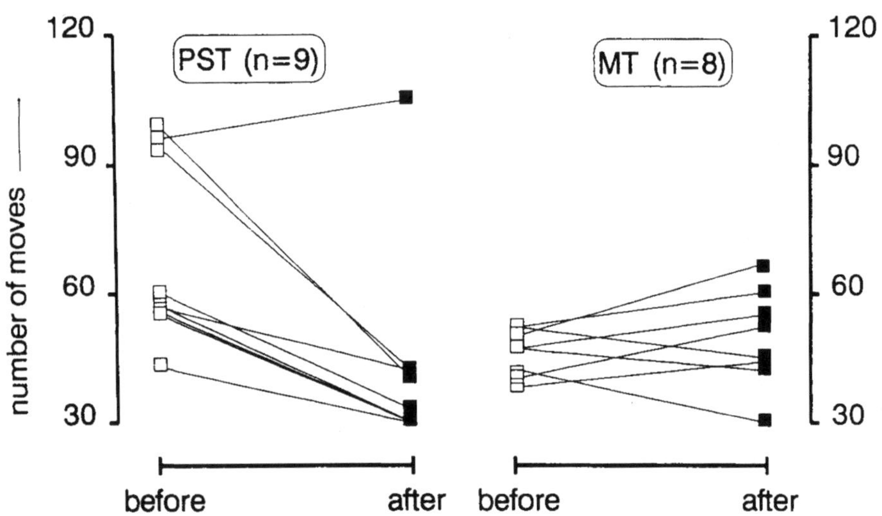

be demonstrated for five patients only. As for the similarities and proverbs subtests neither the PST nor the MT group gained significantly better scores.

For the two problem-solving tasks, the effects of the PST were still more obvious. Figure 8.2 presents the pre-/post-treatment raw scores of the Planning Test both for the PST and the MT group. Whereas only two patients in nine of the MT group improved in this particular task (Wilcoxon Matched-pairs Signed-ranks Test: $p = .6547$), ten out of twelve patients of the PST group had considerably better performances after the training (Wilcoxon Matched-pairs Signed-ranks Test: $p = .0051$). The median of the raw scores rose from zero up to 8.5.

Figure 8.3 shows the results of those patients in both groups for whom we had complete pre- and post-treatment data on the Tower of Hanoi puzzle. Eight in nine patients of the PST group required significantly less moves in the fourth and fifth trial (Wilcoxon Matched-pairs Signed ranks Test: $p = .0109$). In contrast, only three out of eight MT patients did better after the training (Wilcoxon Matched-pairs Signed-ranks Test: .4017). These results cannot easily be attributed to a simple retest effect as the PST and the MT group did not substantially differ in their baseline data. (It should be mentioned here that the MT group also improved significantly, but in associate learning and not problem-solving tasks.)

According to our behavioural rating scale, the PST group showed a significant decrease in behavioural abnormalities, particularly for the item groups goal-directed ideas and cognitive style. The effect was mainly due to less concrete thinking, better problem identification and enhanced reasoning in everyday activities, whereas the items inflexibility and lack of heuristics remained unchanged. As for unawareness of deficits and inappropriate action style (including the behavioural items premature actions, perseverations and rule breaking), which were only implicitly addressed, no significant change could be rated. It should be emphasized that the MT did not reveal any favourable influence on goal-directed ideas and cognitive style, at least during this six-weeks training interval.

As for the subsequent rehabilitation programme, seven in twelve PST patients began with a graduated work trial in their previous jobs. Three patients who, according to the behavioural rating, were still unable to generalize acquired problem-solving strategies (to a less well-structured environment) were allocated to a conjoint cognitive and vocational programme. In contrast, seven in nine patients of the MT group had to remain in residential care after the six-week training programme; only two of them entered a graduated work trial. Because of their marked behavioural disturbances and still very poor cognitive functions, two patients of the PST group had to be considered non-responders. They suffered from a dense anterograde amnesia, were completely apathetic and unaware of their conspicuous cognitive deficits. For these patients cognitive training seemed no longer justified. They were allocated to a family counselling programme instead.

Conclusions

The following points were concluded from this study: An intensive six-week remediation programme consisting of cognitive interventions seems to be helpful to 'frontal' patients; Explicitly occupying the patient's mind with certain aspects of problem solving is obviously superior to a more unspecific cognitive training; The effect of explicit cognitive training apparently generalizes, at least to a certain extent, to everyday activities; and Non-responders can be singled out, and patients with unsatisfying improvements can be allocated to further training programmes.

Acknowledgements:

We thank Dr. Wolfram Ziegler and Dr. Norbert Mai for their helpful comments and their methodological support. We are especially grateful for the assistance of Dr. Nicole von Steinbüchel in testing our patients.

References

AMTHAUER R., 1973, *I-S-T 70 Intelligenz-Struktur-Test*. Handanweisung (Göttingen, Toronto, Zürich: Hogrefe).

BEN-YISHAY, Y., RATTOCK, J. and LAKIN, P., 1985, 'Neuropsychologic Rehabilitation: Quest for a holistic approach' *Seminars in Neurology*, **5** (3), 252–9.

BUKASA, B. and WENNINGER, U., 1986a, *DR2, Test zur Erfassung des Entscheidungs- und Reaktionsverhaltens*. Kuratorium für Verkehrssicherheit, Wien.

BUKASA, B. and WENNINGER, U., 1986b , *RST3, Test zur Erfassung der reaktiven Belastbarkeit*. Kuratorium für Verkehrssicherheit, Wien.

CAMPBELL, D. and STANLEY, J., 1963, *Experimental and quasi-experimental designs for research* (Chicago: Rand McNally College Publishing Co).

CICERONE, K. D., TUPPER, D. E., 1986., 'Cognitive assessment in the neuro-psychological rehabilitation of head-injured adults'. In B. P. Uzzel and Y. Gross (Eds) *Clinical neuropsychology of intervention* (Boston, Dordrecht, Lancaster: Martinus Nijhoff).

GOLDSTEIN, F. C. and LEVIN, H. S., 1987, 'Disorders of reasoning and problem-solving ability'. In M. J. Meier, A. L. Benton, L. Diller (Eds) *Neuropsychological rehabilitation* (Edinburgh, London, Melbourne and New York: Churchill Livingstone) pp. 327–54.

GRONWALL, D. and WRIGHTSON, P., 1974, 'Delayed recovery of intellectual functions after minor head injury'. *Lancet*, **2**, pp. 995–7.

HORN, W., 1983, 'Leistungsprüfsystem L-P-S. Handanweisung' (Göttingen, Toronto, Zürich: Hogrefe).

ILMBERGER, J., 1988, *Deutsche Version des California Verbal Learning Tests*. Institut für Medizinische Psychologie der Universitat München.

JÄGER, A. O. and ALTHOFF, K., 1983, *Der WILDE-Intelligenz-Test*. Ein Strukturdiagnostikum. Handanweisung (Göttingen, Toronto, Zürich: Hogrefe).

KOTOVSKI, K., HAYES, J. R. and SIMON, H .A., 1985, 'Why are some problems hard? Evidence from Tower of Hanoi', *Cognitive Psychology*, **17**, 248–94

LEZAK, M. D., 1983, *Neuropsychological assessment (2nd edn)* (New York, Oxford University Press).

LIENERT G. A., 1969, *Testaufbau und Testanalyse*. 3.Auflage (Weinheim, Berlin, Basel: Verlag Julius Beltz) pp. 255–313.

MATTHES, G., 1988, ' Der Einsatz des 'Turm von Hanoi' -Computer-programms zur Diagnostik von Störungen des problemlösenden Denkens bei Patienten mit erworbenen Hirnschädigungen'. *Biomed*. **19**, 10–3.

MOSEY, A. C., 1986, *Psychosocial components of occupational therapy* (New York: Raven Press) pp. 274–93.

NELSON, H. E., 1976, 'A Modified Card Sorting Test sensitive to frontal lobe defects'. *Cortex*, **12**, 313–24.

OSWALD W. and ROTH, E., 1978, *Der Zahlen-Verbindungs-Test* (ZVT) (Göttingen: Hogrefe).

PRIGATANO, G. P. and FORDYCE D. J. 1986, 'The neuropsychological rehabilitation program at Presbyterian Hospital'. In G. P. Prigatano (Ed.) *Neuropsychological rehabilitation after brain injury* (Baltimore London: Johns Hopkins University Press) pp. 96–118.

PRIGATANO, G. P. FORDYCE, D. J., ZEINER, H. K., ROUECHE J. R., PEPPING, M. and WOOD, B. C. 1984, 'Neuropsychological rehabilitation after closed head injury in young adults'. *Journal of Neurology, Neurosurgery, and Psychiatry*, **47**, 505–13.

ROWE, H. A. H., 1985, *Problem solving and intelligence*. (Hillsdale, New Jersey, London: Lawrence Erlbaum Associates).

SCHERZER, B. P. 1986, 'Rehabilitation following severe head trauma: results of a three year program'. *Archives of Physical Medicine Rehabilitation*, **67**, 366–73.

SCHURI, U., 1988, 'Lernen und Gedächtnis'. In D. von Cramon and J. Zihl (Eds) *Neuropsychologische Rehabilitation*. Grundlagen — Diagnostik - Behandlungsverfahren (Berlin, Heidelberg, New York, London, Paris, Tokyo: Springer-Verlag) pp. 215–247.

SIMON, H. A., 1975, 'The functional equivalence of problem solving skills'. *Cognitive Psychology*, **7**, 268–88.

STOLTZE, A. and MATTHES-VON CRAMON, G. *Der Planungstest: ein Test zur alltagsnahen Untersuchung von Störungen des problemlösenden Denkens* (in preparation).

VON CRAMON, D., 1988, 'Planen und Handeln'. In D. von Cramon and J. Zihl (Eds) *Neuropsychologische Rehabilitation*. Grundlagen — Diagnostik — Behandlungsverfahren (Berlin, Heidelberg, New York, London, Paris, Tokyo: Springer-Verlag). pp. 248–63.

VORLÄNDER, T., 1987, *Konzeption eines klinischen Kurzzeitgedächtnis-Tests für hirngeschädigte Patienten*. Diplomarbeit des Psychologischen Institutes der Universität Trier.

WOOD, R. Ll., 1990, 'A neurobehavioural paradigm for brain injury rehabilitation'. In R. Ll. Wood (Ed.) *Neurobehavioural Sequelae of Traumatic Brain Injury* (London: Taylor and Francis).

PART 5
COGNITIVE APPROACHES TO THE REHABILITATION OF BEHAVIOUR DISORDERS

Chapter 9

Rehabilitation of Dyscontrol Syndromes Following Frontal Lobe Damage: A Cognitive Neuropyschological Approach

P. W. Burgess and N. Alderman

It is by now well established that neurological damage may lead to loss of supervisory or attentional control structures, the symptoms of which may vary from relatively mild deficits in higher cognitive skills, such as organization and planning (Shallice, 1982; Duncan, 1986), through to severe loss of supervisory control structures (as for example in utilization behaviour [Lhermitte, 1983; Shallice *et al.*, in press]). This loss of control over subordinate cognitive skills is most commonly attributed to frontal lobe dysfunction (Goldberg and Bilder, 1987) producing deficits in what Luria (1966) described as the programming, regulation and verification of behaviour.

These deficits are most frequently characterized in terms of patients' performance on neuropsychological tests (Milner, 1982; Stuss and Benson, 1984), and the constellation of characteristics seen in these patients has been described by Baddeley and Wilson (1988) as the 'dysexecutive syndrome'. In some patients, individual cognitive skills themselves may be preserved, but the ability to initiate their use, monitor their performance and use this information to adjust their behaviour is impaired. Such deficits are notoriously difficult to characterize because most neuropsychological investigation methods are designed to measure discrete skills — the building blocks of cognition — rather than the structures that control them (Shallice and Burgess, in press). Patients with these deficits are often problematical for rehabilitation professionals because the first step towards the formation of a rehabilitiation programme is the adequate characterization and assessment of the deficit. But few methods of assessment exist, and most that do are unreliable and seem so far removed from real-life skills that extrapolation from test scores to their consequences in activities of daily life (for instance) seems impossible. This situation has arisen because of a lack of a coherent interpretive framework for these deficits. Often the behavioural disorders that are seen following frontal lobe damage are interpreted in terms of 'change in personality' or 'lack of insight', 'poor social awareness' and so forth. Whilst on one level, these descriptions are of course true, they do not help when trying to form a rehabilitation programme. But by placing these sorts of disorders within a cognitive neuropsychological framework and interpreting the deficits in information-processing terms, one can begin to set a firm ground for programme planning.

We will be using Norman and Shallice's (Norman and Shallice, 1980; Shallice, 1988) model of cognitive control to explain the treatment rationale behind the intervention approach used with two patients who presented with similar symptoms but with different causes. This will be done in three stages. Firstly, we will present the model: secondly an attempt will be made to explain how the model helps characterize behaviour disorders in terms of damage to control structures. Finally two case studies will be presented to illustrate how such an approach can lead to a therapeutically effective treatment strategy. These case studies will include sufficient neurological and neuropsychological data to support the hypothesis that the patients' disorders were due, at least in part, to frontal lobe dysfunction, since this will form the basis for the theoretical interpretation of the disorders and their treatment.

Shallice's Information Processing Model

Shallice (Norman and Shallice, 1980; Shallice, 1982, 1988) details a model of the organization of levels of cognitive control that relies essentially on the interaction of four processing levels: (1) cognitive units, (2) schemas, (3) contention scheduling and (4) supervisory attentional system (see Fig. 9.1). These will be explained in turn.

Cognitive units

These are basic cognitive abilities that relate to specific neuroanatomical or neuropsychological systems, for example perceptual abilities, memory, language and so forth.

Schemas

Schemas (which can exist either in the thought or action domain) are units which control specific overlearned actions. Shallice (1982) cites, as examples of these overlearned skills, drinking from a container, doing long division, making breakfast, or finding one's way home from work. These schemas can be activated in two ways — either by triggering by perceptual input or by the output of other schemata. Shallice *et al.*, (in press) use the analogy of driving a car as an example of a hierarchically

Figure 9.1. The Norman/Shallice model of action control. Dotted lines represent activating input, hatched lines represent the primarily inhibitory function of contention scheduling. Reproduced from Shallice et al., *1989, with permission.*

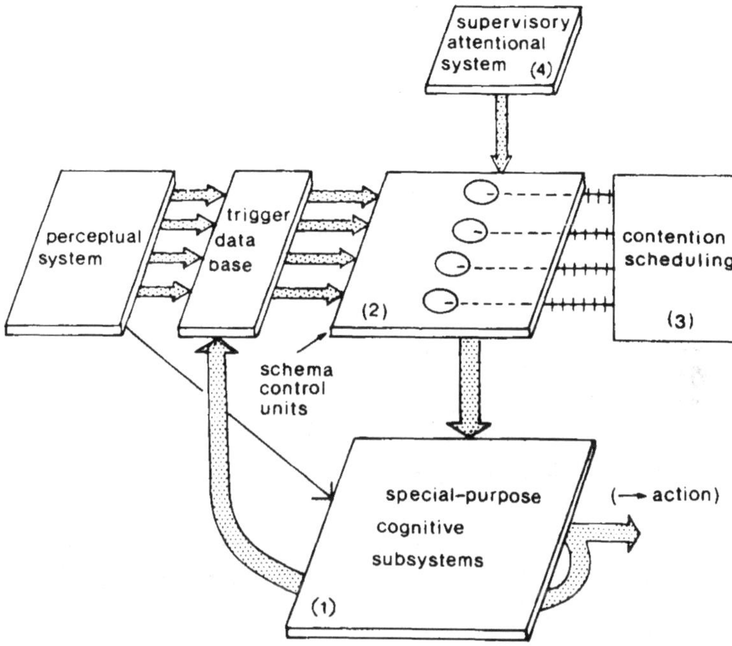

organized set of schemata. A low-level schema might be a very basic behavioural routine, for example the control of the movement of the head and eyes to look in the mirror. A higher-level schema might be a whole complex action routine, such as one's actions on approach to some traffic lights. This would include slowing down, indicating, and so forth, and would be triggered by the sight of the lights turning red. An example of the triggering of one schema by another might be that when this 'approaching traffic lights' schema has been activated, this might activate other related sub-schemas — for instance gear changes, checking the mirror, looking at road signs, etc.

Contention scheduling

This process has the function of selecting the most efficient set of schemas which will fulfil the task demands. This is a routine function and is designed to deal with familiar situations. It works by selecting a limited number of compatible schemas so that they can successfully control the available resources until the goal is achieved, or alternatively until a higher priority schema is activated (as would be the case in the situation where one is doing something fairly routine and suddenly some unexpected event happens which necessitates one's immediate attention). Contention scheduling is a rapid triggering and selection process for familiar situations with clear rules and guidelines.

The supervisory attentional system (SAS)

The SAS has the job of dealing with unfamiliar or novel situations where routine schemata selection is not sufficient to fulfil the task demands. This it does in a much slower and deliberate fashion than the contention scheduling process, and it works by altering the likelihood of certain schemas being selected. Its most common function is that of monitoring. In the situation where contention scheduling fails or there is no known appropriate behavioural routine, or where the schemas are so weakly activated that they cannot trigger other schemas, the SAS is activated. This process is held to be part of the functions of the frontal lobes. Shallice (1982) characterizes his model as an information-processing analogue of Luria's (1966) unit for the programming, regulation and verification of behaviour and predicts that damage to this system will lead to many of the characteristics of the 'frontal lobe syndrome', including disturbances of attention, concreteness, lack of flexibility, perseveration and so forth.

The Implications of the Model for Rehabilitation

The term 'cognitive rehabilitation' is the most commonly used to refer to rehabilitation aimed at ameliorating deficits in basic cognitive skills, for instance memory, reading and language and so forth. These individual cognitive abilities are what Shallice refers to in his model as 'cognitive units'. However, it is plain that damage following neurological trauma may also affect systems that are higher in the 'cognitive hierarchy'. Damage to the SAS may lead to deficits in the ability to utilize those basic cognitive skills and to loss of control over emotional aspects of behaviour and thinking as well. Of course in practical day-to-day terms, an inability to use, control and monitor an intact skill may be just as debilitating as if one had lost that skill altogether. However, the symptoms of damage to these control structures are often discussed as if they were beyond the remit of 'cognitive rehabilitation' because patients who present with symptoms of SAS breakdown (which may include frontal adynamia, disinhibition, perseveration, impulsivity, lack of social awareness and insight), have these problems interpreted using a frame of reference such as the 'personality changes' that may follow neurological trauma. This is true at one level of course, but it says little about how one might go about changing that patient's behaviour. We argue that interpreting these dyscontrol syndromes in terms of information-processing deficits may help the rehabilitation professional to understand how the processes of change might occur. In order to do this further, explanation of the practical implications of Shallice's model is required.

Luria's (1966) conception of the frontal lobes as being concerned with the programming, regulation and verification of behaviour has many implications in the social situation. Loss of the ability to select the right behaviour in the first instance, to monitor feedback from others and adjust one's behaviour accordingly will clearly lead to inappropriate social responding. If we assume that in Shallice's model, schemata not only control behaviours appropriate to situations such as driving, but also more complex social situations, one can begin to see the implications of damage to the SAS. We all know that we behave differently in different social situations; one doesn't act in the same way at, for instance, a job interview as one might at a party with one's friends. Yet mostly we are not aware of having to *try* to change our behaviour — our contention scheduling process routinely selects appropriate behavioural schemas. But consider the situation where one is in a bar with friends and unexpectedly one's boss turns up. It is quite conceivable that the sight of the boss might be a strong enough stimulus to trigger a different set of schemata which may mean different behaviour now that s/he has walked through the door.

It is well known that lesions of the frontal lobes can lead to changes in social behaviour, with increased impulsivity, lack of concern for social rules, disinhibition, decreased insight and an inability to monitor one's own behaviour often quoted as examples (Stuss and Benson, 1986). Within Shallice's model, if the SAS failed to increase the likelihood of competing schemata being activated, a person's behaviour may be dominated by the first impulse (or stimulus) that comes to mind or those schemata which are currently activated. The decreased monitoring that results from damage to the SAS means that the output of the activated schemata is not necessarily inhibited or modified, which may lead to inflexibility, perseveration and those characteristics often described as unconcern and inability to appreciate the consequences of one's actions.

Thus, it is possible to see how dyscontrol syndromes of the frontal type may be characterized in terms of cognitive neuropyschological theory. The implications for rehabilitation that follow from the use of this model predict three methods for management of these disorders:

1 Ensure that the patient is never in a situation where inappropriate schemata will be activated, i.e. remove the patient from situations where the patient has to exercise behavioural control.
2 Somehow, either increase the effectiveness of the remaining SAS system or else subsume its function with something else.

3 Modify the schemata and contention scheduling process so that previously existing behavioural routines no longer exist or new competing routines (schemata) are established which are more likely to be selected (by the contention scheduling process) in a given situation than the old ones.

Clearly the problem with option one is that unless one isolates the patient permanently from all social contact, this method is neither realistic nor practicable. Obviously, any diminishment in social contact would be undesirable, and so this is not an attractive or realistic option.

The problems associated with option two are methodological as well as practical. It is becoming increasingly accepted amongst rehabilitation professionals that the 'mental muscle' approach to treatment is largely unhelpful (Giles and Fussey, 1988, p. 17). That is to say that treating brain functions as muscles that will somehow get stronger with practice ignores all we know about neurological and neuropsychological recovery. It is extremely unlikely that one could somehow 'exercise' the SAS thus leading to recovery of function (it would also be conceptually difficult). It is perhaps more acceptable that, as in the case of a densely amnesic patient, it is better not to try to improve the lost ability per se, but to think of ways of structuring the environment and establishing new behaviour patterns that mean the patient no longer has to rely on the impaired ability.

Option three is clearly the most attractive treatment approach to arise from the model. It may also be the mechanism by which traditional 'cognitive therapy', which uses verbal mediators of behaviour to change a person's beliefs (i.e. cognitive or thought schemata) and therefore their behaviour, works (see Alderman and Burgess, Chapter 10). In order to answer the obvious question of how to put this into practice, two detailed case studies will now be presented. These will take the form of first describing the patient's neuropsychological and neurological state, then the behavioural disorder followed by the treatment. Lastly, the case will be discussed in terms of Norman and Shallice's (1980) model. Obviously in treatment an understanding of the behavioural disorder will come *before* treatment, but hopefully the usefulness of the model will be more easily understood if the treatment is discussed first.

Case 1

SJ, a twenty-four-year-old man was admitted to the Kemsley Unit, St. Andrew's Hospital, Northampton, UK. At the age of 17, he had been involved in a motor vehicle accident; he was found unconscious and showing no response to stimulation. A CT brain scan at the time of the accident showed a shallow collection of blood in the right hemisphere with blood along the falx and in both lateral ventricles and evidence of contusion. There was marked damage to the right temporal lobe. He now has a left hemiplegia and requires a wheelchair for independent mobility. He needs physical assistance with all transfer activities but is otherwise largely independent. An EEG at the time of his admission showed no clear evidence of paroxysmal activity.

There were no significant changes in SJ's drug regimen throughout the treatment period to be described.

Neuropsychological Assessment

SJ's verbal IQ as measured on the WAIS-R (Wechsler, 1981) fell within the borderline defective range, whilst his non-verbal scores were generally lower, his overall performance falling at the top of the defective range. He had problems with visual scanning and with complex visual material, but his analysis of perceptual material when single items were used was intact (20/20 fragmented letters; Warrington and James, 1988).

Verbal memory was generally good (Recognition Memory Test [RMT] words: scaled score 13 (Warrington, 1984); Wechsler story recall low average). By contrast visual recognition memory was weak (faces: scaled score 4 (Warrington, 1984); Complex Figure recall very poor). There was no suggestion of prosopagnosia. SJ's naming skills were average and his reading was low average. There was no difficulty reading text; spelling was at the low average range which was probably commensurate with his pre-morbid level.

SJ's performance on a range of tests thought sensitive to frontal lobe function was extremely poor. Thus, he scored at or below the 5th percentile on tests of Verbal Fluency, Cognitive Estimates (Shallice and Evans, 1978), Proverb Interpretation, Colour-Form sorting (Weigl, 1941), on the Wisconsin Sorting Task (Milner, 1982) and on Petrides and Milner's (1982) Self-Ordered Pointing Task.

In conclusion, SJ's overall level of verbal skills fell at a borderline defective level while his non-verbal skills were at the top of the defective range as measured on the WAIS-R. His verbal memory performance was satisfactory, but his visual memory was selectively impaired. In addition his performance on a range of frontal lobe tests was extremely poor. These findings are consistent with maximal non-dominant, fronto-temporal involvement, which occurred in the context of a more generalized weakness in cognitive performance.

Presenting Difficulties

A number of previous rehabilitation attempts over a six-year period had failed because of the level of SJ's behavioural disturbances. On admission to the Kemsley Unit, he presented with two main forms of behavioural disorder. One was a problem with general sexual disinhibition; he would frequently masturbate in public, make lewd comments to female members of staff and would touch others inappropriately. His second problem was that he would shout and swear excessively over a wide range of situations throughout the day. His sexual disinhibition was successfully treated with a two-minute seclusion Time-Out programme (Wood and Burgess, 1988). SJ's inappropriate shouting and swearing was then targeted for treatment, and the initial stage of this programme will be described in detail.

Treatment Procedure

SJ's behavioural disorder was treated in the following way: Before instituting a programme, his shouting and swearing episodes were baselined using a time-sampling

Figure 9.2. Patient SJ: three-week time-sampling baseline of shouting and swearing episodes. Failure to earn tokens (FTE) occurred if SJ shouted or swore. These tokens were paid at 15 min intervals.

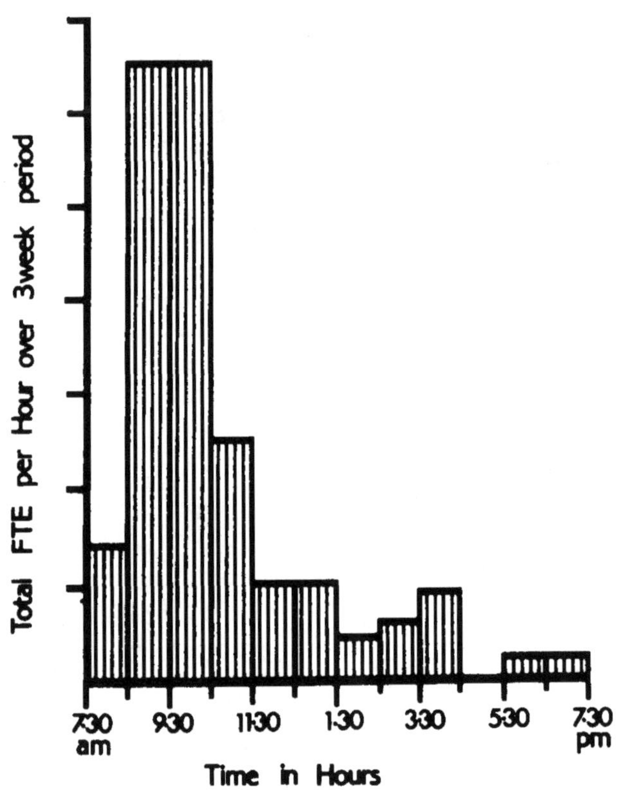

method (Wood, 1987) over a three-week period. The results of this baseline are shown in Figure 9.2.

The baseline clearly revealed that SJ's shouting behaviour occurred considerably more frequently at certain times of the day, with a tendency to peak between the hours of 8.30 and 11.30 am. Retrospective analysis of the ward programme showed that the first morning peak corresponded to his morning washing programme and that the second peak occurred during his conductive education (Giles and Gent, 1988) sessions. An ABC analysis over a two-week period was then conducted (see Fussey *et al.*, 1988 for an explanation of this method) in order to identify the antecedents to the behaviour. This analysis revealed three primary antecedents to his noise-making: (1) In response to provocation from patients; (2) when confronted with tasks he was reluctant to do; and (3) during or immediately preceding tasks which SJ found anxiety-provoking. The behaviour at these times would begin with repeated stereotyped requests for instructions (for instance 'Tell me how?') which quickly increased in frequency and volume until the point where even if the therapist did answer his requests, he would be shouting so loudly that he would be unable to hear anyway. It should be mentioned at this point that his questioning conveyed no real request — the things he was being asked to do were quite straightforward and he knew exactly how to do them.

SJ's shouting led to two main consequences: Either he would be 'Timed-Out-On-The-Spot' (TOOTS) (Giles *et al.*, 1988) by some or all of the staff or he would be assisted by staff to complete the task. At these times he attracted a great deal of attention from the other patients. Obviously these inconsistencies in the consequences of his behaviour leaves scope for a number of reinforcement paradigms to be operating, but there were only two types of trigger to SJ's shouting. A proportion of the screaming was attributable to anxiety, leading to avoidance behaviour which was being negatively reinforced. The remaining noise was due to his reduced tolerance to frustration. It appeared that the shouting during the morning programme was primarily due to the former factor.

It was decided that the shouting would, as a starting point, be treated context-specifically, so another baseline was conducted which concentrated on his behaviour during his morning washing programme (one of the times of most frequent responding, as mentioned before). Over a five-day period, he spent between 8 and 76% of his time during the morning programme engaged in shouting. An ABC analysis of the events surrounding his episodes of shouting showed that they were associated with two particular events within the morning programme: showering and transferring. When asked why he screamed (during a pre-treatment assessment interview), he said that he felt a little anxious when transferring and showering. When he was being put into the shower (since he was wheel-chair bound he was reliant on others), he felt that the shower would be cold. He would actually start shouting before the water was turned on and continue no matter what the actual temperature turned

Figure 9.3. Patient SJ: Treatment for shouting during his morning ward washing and dressing programme.

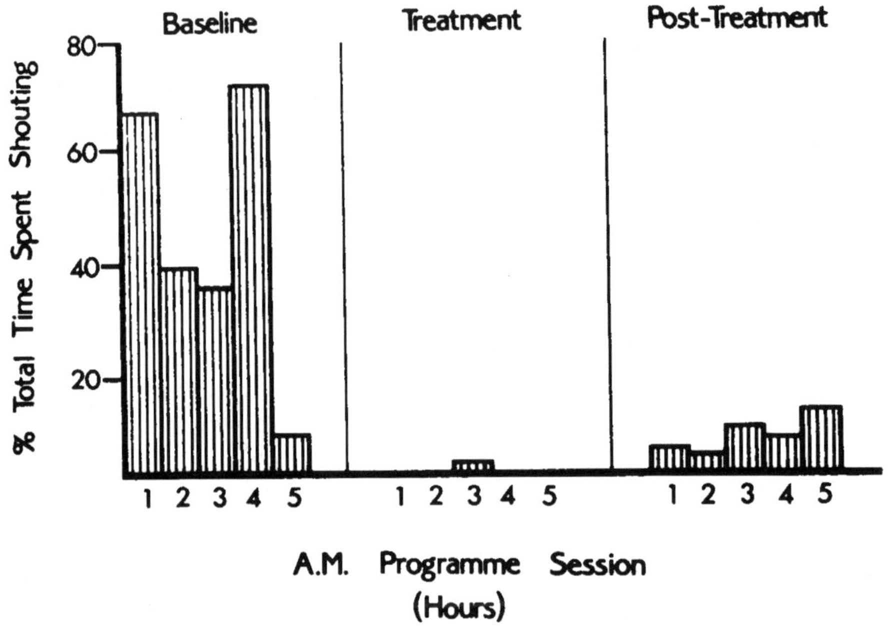

out to be. He said that, left to his own devices, he would either wait to see that the water was warm enough, or, preferably, avoid having a shower at all. His clinical records described an incident at a former rehabilitation centre where he had been suspended above a bath in a hoist and had been left there when the staff were called away on an emergency. This had made him very anxious. With prompting he was able to recall this experience. When asked, as he approached the shower, he did not report any anxiety and denied that he would feel anxious at all. However, once actually in the situation, he freely reported feeling physical/somatic symptoms. In order to verify this lack of insight, three self-report questionnaires were administered immediately after a shower session. On the Zung Subjective Anxiety Scale (Zung, 1971) he scored 29/80; on the MAPQ, 33/132 and on the Automatic Thoughts Questionnaire (Hollon and Kendall, 1980), he rated himself 19/56. These scores are very low, indeed the MAPQ score is the minimum possible and suggested a gross lack of insight, a characteristic often accorded to frontal lobe damage.

A baseline was conducted in the morning programme over five days before treatment began, and then treatment was for one hour per day for five days. SJ was then baselined again over a further five-morning sessions. The results can be seen in Figure 9.3.

Figure 9.4. Patient SJ: Reported Subjective Units of Discomfort (SUDs) indicating his levels of anxiety during his showering programme.

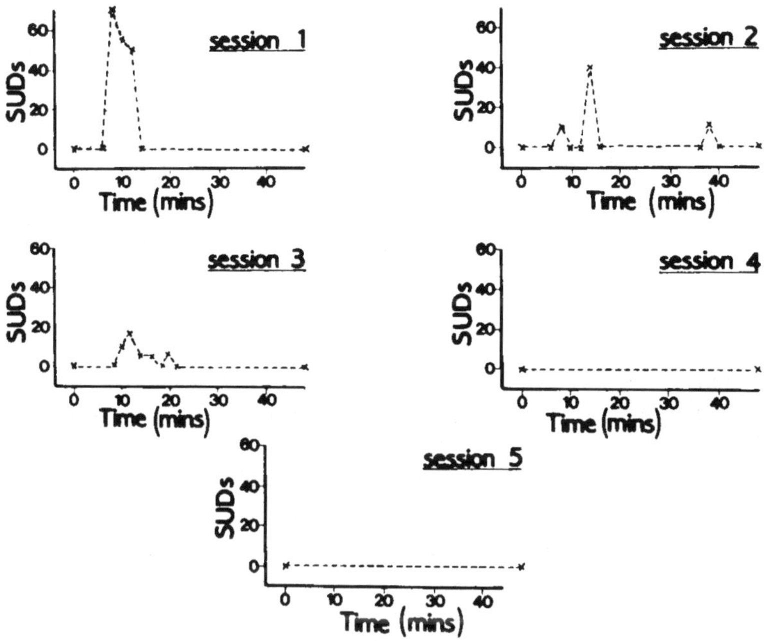

Treatment sessions were conducted in addition to, and at a separate time from his regular washing and dressing programme. During each of these treatment sessions, SJ was taken through his showering programme. Every two minutes he was asked to rate his level of experienced anxiety on a 'Subjective Units of Discomfort' (SUD) scale of 0-100 (100 being the most anxious he had ever felt in his life). If he reported feeling anxious, he was asked to repeat a phrase (that he volunteered himself using a simplified form of cognitive restructuring) which aimed to modify his cognitions ('the water is going to be warm enough because its already been warmed up') and asked to rate himself again on the SUD scale. This was continued until he reported no discomfort. The next stage of the showering programme was then undertaken, and the rating/cognitive restructuring cycle was repeated. In addition, over the five sessions he was encouraged to acquire 'mastery' skills by being taught to adjust the shower temperature himself and to put his hand under the shower to check the water temperature. The successive changes in the levei of his reported anxiety are shown in Figure 9.4.

Referring back to Figure 9.3, we can see that during the treatment sessions SJ shouted considerably less than in the baseline levels. Immediately after the treatment phase was started his shouting decreased. This was interpreted at the time as the effect of acknowledging his anxiety together with the effect of intensive personal input as a distractor. However, this effect continued beyond the programme phase, as can be seen from the post-treatment baseline in Figure 9.4. A repeated baseline at three months demonstrated maintenance of this level.

This programme clearly succeeded in its aims, and when subsequent reports were made of SJ's shouting, it was no longer associated with his showering but with other aspects of the ward programme and usually in response to frustration. This was then treated with a ward-based token programme followed by a satiation training programme, which proved successful.

Understanding SJ's Disorder and its Treatment in Terms of Norman and Shallice's Model

At the simplest level, we can conceptualize SJ's problem as an increased irritability following his injury. But it is apparent that there was more than just this. He had a marked lack of control over his own behaviour. In terms of Shallice's model, the damage to the SAS leads to a situation where inappropriate behavioural sets or routines cannot be inhibited. Once activated, a behavioural schema becomes more likely to be automatically selected by the contention scheduling process (given the same triggering stimuli) in the future. Thus, a behavioural pattern establishes itself. In SJ's case, his immediate response to an anxiety-provoking situation (of which showering was one of the two most salient) was to shout. Most of us (and no doubt SJ before his accident) would inhibit this immediate reaction in favour of a more reasonable way of dealing with the situation. This inhibitory function is performed by the SAS which is believed to be held primarily in the frontal lobes. SJ has major frontal lobe dysfunction (assuming consequent SAS damage) so his ability to stop himself from shouting was severely diminished. One of the effects that the programme had was to modify SJ's 'thought schema' involving the showering situation (obviously there were 'action schemas' involved as well, but the main point is to be made about 'thought schemas'). It did this by repetition and replacement until the schema that was most likely to be automatically triggered by the shower situation was no longer that of shouting, anxiety and avoidance, but was one involving checking the temperature of the water and repeating the set phrase to himself and so forth. So the 'cognitive restructuring' element of the programme can be seen as the active ingredient in the modification of that 'thought schema'.

Case 2

BM, a 60-year-old male with a Master's degree in chemistry, sustained a severe head injury in a road traffic accident. He was taken to hospital unconscious and started responding to painful stimuli after two days. A CT scan 37 days post-trauma showed rather prominent, but not displaced, fourth, third and lateral ventricles, with atrophic changes in both frontal lobes. No focal area of abnormal attenuation was identified. He suffered a severe injury inside his mouth and upper part of the pharynx. Laryngoscopic examination revealed gross oedema and laceration secondary to trauma. This caused difficulty in breathing and swallowing, and he underwent tracheostomy operation.

Eleven weeks post-injury, he was transferred to a rehabilitation unit. Physical examination at this time revealed no external injury, and he could stand and walk around without difficulty. All aspects of the neurological examination were unremarkable. However, the staff began to complain of a behavioural disturbance. He was confused and uncooperative and at times was noisy and restless. His major problem was his irritability, and he had outbursts of temper towards his wife and the medical staff. For some time he refused to swallow food. Soon it became obvious that his behavioural disturbance was proving a significant handicap to his rehabilitation, and he was referred to the Kemsley Unit.

Neuropsychological Assessment

BM's general behaviour throughout assessment was markedly impulsive and perseverative. Nevertheless, he scored within the borderline defective level on verbal subtests of the WAIS (Wechsler, 1958) and within the dull average range on non-tests. He showed marked expressive and word-finding difficulties and variability in his ability to perform simple arithmetic operations. In contrast, his digit-span performance fell within the lower average range. Basic perceptual skills were intact, but there was some suggestion of a mild associative agnosia.

BM's memory skills were very poor; he was able to give his date of birth but then perseverated on this once asked subsequent questions about the present date, the time of his accident and so forth. He was unable to give any information as to his whereabouts. It was not possible to give formal tests of memory because of his severe tendency towards perseveration, but he appeared unable to give any information about anything he had done that morning, or on any other recent occasion.

BM demonstrated a significant dyslexia and dysgraphia and read at an eight-year-old level. Irregular word reading was very poor indeed. Naming of low frequency items was significantly impaired, and his overall level of verbal expression and ability to communicate in syntactic sentences was severely limited by his nominal aphasia. Word-picture matching fell at an eight-year-old level, but his repetition of multi-syllabic words was intact.

On tests of frontal lobe function, his performance was severely handicapped by his other general cognitive difficulties, but was nevertheless extremely poor and grossly perseverative. He was completely unable to grasp the requirements of the Weigl sorting task (Weigl, 1941) or perform satisfactorily on a simple rule-finding task (Chorover and Cole, 1966). On Shallice and Evans's (1978) Cognitive Estimates test, he estimated the Post Office Tower to be 20ft high, and then went on to answer '20ft' to any other question asked him.

In conclusion, BM suffered marked intellectual deterioration, and his memory functions were considerably impaired. In addition, he had multiple language deficits and exhibited a severe 'frontal syndrome'.

The Presenting Problem

BM's main behavioural difficulty was with the volume of his voice. His speaking volume was excessively loud and would extend to a shout if he became anxious, which he was prone to do. The volume of his normal speaking voice was so loud that he was completely unmanageable in a group setting. This problem occurred in the context of normal hearing on clinical testing. He could occasionally be heard to speak at an appropriate volume, but this was rare. Speech therapy assessment highlighed hyperkinetic dysphonia and mild dysphagia, but no apparent physical cause could be found which might explain his excessively loud voice. Since BM showed a marked tendency to become anxious, and at these times his voice would become louder, medication changes were made on admission in an attempt to reduce his levels of anxiety. These did decrease his apparent agitation and his blood pressure, but his excessively loud speech volume remained the same.

Speech therapy techniques were tried but failed to produce any significant change. At this point the speech therapist requested a psychological treatment intervention.

Treatment Procedure

The first method used was a simple behavioural programme where the patient was prompted to speak more quietly (when his voice volume was excessive to questioning) and if he did not, the staff would TOOTS him until such time as he did speak appropriately. Unfortunately, it soon became clear that this approach was not effective. Clinically, it appeared that BM's problem was that the cognitive mechanisms that might enable him to benefit from such feedback were not working. This was attributed to three symptoms of one underlying problem, all of which are regularly quoted as common sequelae of frontal lobe damage: reduced insight and social awareness, behavioural dyscontrol and an inability to use one's knowledge to correct one's actions. As explained in the section describing Shallice's (1982) model, damage to the SAS would predict such problems. The treatment procedure, therefore, would have to assume that he no longer had this process intact and would have to change his behaviour at the level of contention scheduling selection of the behavioural schemas.

A relatively objective measure of BM's speech volume was obtained by using a microphone and VU meter placed a fixed distance from the patient. The equipment was calibrated for the appropriate speaking volume by a male therapist reading a list of 50 high frequency words several times. The dial was marked as to the highest level that was subjectively felt to represent appropriate speech volume. The words were then presented to BM on cards, and he was then required to read the words aloud (the words were presented with a picture as an aid since BM does have difficulty reading). The first baseline was thus collected and can be seen as B1 of treatment phase 1 in Figure 9.5. BM read none of the words at or below the acceptable level.

Figure 9.5. Patient BM: Treatment of inappropriate speech volume.

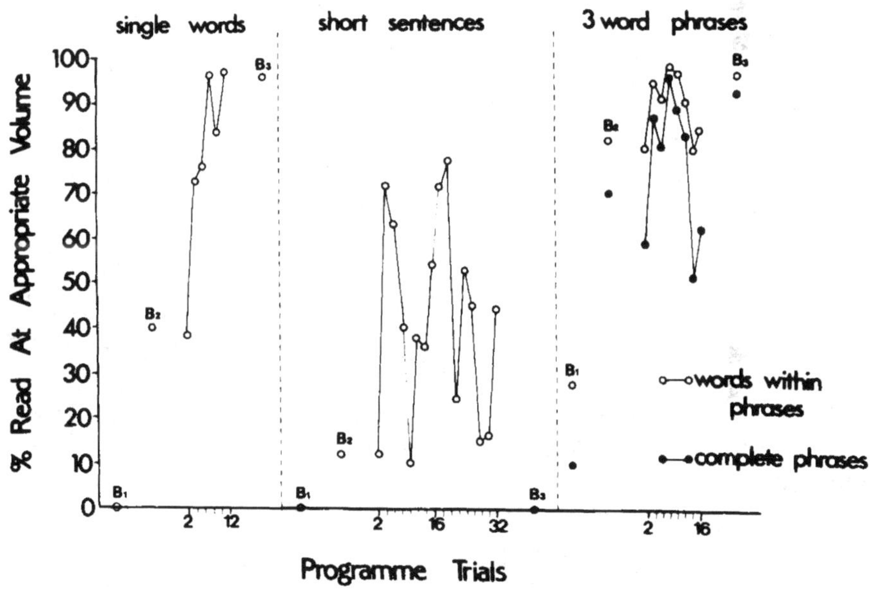

Two types of feedback were used to make BM aware of when he was speaking at the appropriate volume. Firstly, a therapist sat next to him, monitored the VU meter and told him whether he had spoken at an appropriate volume. Secondly, at the beginning of the session, he was given 50, one-pence pieces and was required to give the therapist one of these every time he spoke a word too loudly. Initially, in order to collect baseline data on the effect of merely introducing a structured programme rather than additionally introducing any reinforcement contingencies, the loss of the pennies was not linked to any longer term consequence or secondary reinforcer. Under these conditions, BM read 20/50 words at the appropriate volume (B2 of phase 1 in Figure

9.5). This served as the baseline for the feedback that was inherent in the programme structure. A target was then introduced that was two above the baseline. If he failed to reach this level, it remained the same. If he achieved it or exceeded it, the next target level was two more than the highest level reached so far. The only reinforcer that could be found for BM was that he was keen to leave sessions, so when he achieved his target he was permitted to go to his room. However, with practice BM became well motivated towards achieving his treatment goals, and he usually wanted to stay in the session and increase his target.

The sessions were run once a day, five days a week. There were two runs of word reading in each session. The programme was run 12 times, and on the last session, he read all the words at an appropriate volume. The 50 words were then rebaselined (without feedback) and he managed to read 48/50 words appropriately (B3 of the first treatment phase in Figure 9.5).

Clearly BM had established the ability to read single words at a correct volume. The next stage of the programme, therefore, aimed to establish the ability to read short sentences at an appropriate volume. Fifty, six-word sentences were constructed with high-frequency words, and each was accompanied by a picture. The above procedure was repeated; he was baselined with no feedback, and under these conditions he read none of the sentences at an appropriate volume. He was then baselined under the conditions of the programme structure, but with no secondary reinforcers and was treated over 32 sessions with two 'runs' within each session before being rebaselined.

Unfortunately, as can be seen from the graph, this phase of the programme could not be described as a success. BM did not significantly improve in his ability to read the six-word sentences at an acceptable volume, and when baselined post-treatment, he did not read any of the sentences appropriately. Since he had demonstrated the ability to improve when single words were used, there was obviously something about this task which made it qualitatively different. Consideration of the neuropsychological scores confirmed the clinical impression that the task was simply too difficult (at least at this early stage of treatment). BM found the task too effortful to monitor his speech volume *and* perform the task simultaneously, and as a consequence he would become anxious and agitated. He would tend to slip into a cycle of perseveration and then try to break out of this, resulting in increased anxiety, leading to increased volume.

The solution was to devise a task half-way between that which had been shown to be effective and that which had proved too difficult. So in the third-treatment phase, BM was required to read three-word phrases which were constructed with high-frequency words and were unfamiliar to the patient. The pre-treatment baseline was 10% (of the sentences read at the appropriate volume). With the introduction of the programme structure, this rose to an initial 66% level. Treatment then ran for 16 sessions with the reinforcement schedule described above (i.e. he had to give the therapist a penny each time he did not read a complete phrase within the desired volume limits), after which he was rebaselined. As can be seen in Figure 9.5, after treatment BM managed to read 92% of the phrases and 96% of the words within those phrases at an appropriate level.

This programme showed that BM could adjust his speech volume himself, which was by no means certain at the beginning of treatment. It also demonstrated that he could make use of feedback if that feedback was made particularly salient and the task was within his capabilities. In the sessions, he picked up the habit of looking at the VU meter himself and adjusting his voice accordingly. This immediate feedback increased his motivation and in turn led to a greater understanding of his problem and a desire to modify his behaviour. Clinically, however, the problem of his excessive speech volume remained. Whilst he had learned how to control his speech in sessions, outside these sessions he still spoke too loudly. The aim of the next stage was, therefore, to explore the potential value of a 12-hour-a-day feedback system using a microphone headset to aid generalization. The role of the initial programme had been to establish that BM could, in fact, exercise control over his speech, and this had been proven.

Understanding BM's Problem and its Treatment in Terms of Norman and Shallice's Model

Unlike patient SJ, BM's problem did not appear to be context-specific — his speech was too loud in all situations throughout the day (although it was worse when he was anxious). The problem was not amenable to usual speech-therapy methods and seemed to stem from a problem with regulation: one of Luria's three 'programming, regulation and verification' characterizations of the functions of the frontal lobes. He appeared to have diminished ability to monitor and modify his own behaviour, even though once he was helped to realize that he had a problem, he was well motivated to do so. In terms of the model, a degraded SAS had led to decreased ability to inhibit the selection of certain schemas and activate others within the contention scheduling process. In other words, people choose whether to speak loudly or softly depending on the circumstances, but BM could not because he had a diminished ability to make use of feedback to regulate his behaviour. For example, imagine you are talking to a friend while walking down a very busy and noisy street on the way to a library. You will have to talk very loudly, or even shout, to your friend in order to make yourself heard. At this point, your currently activated 'action schema' governing the volume of your speech is the 'speak loudly' schema. Of course if you were to enter the library with this schema still activated you would disturb everyone around you. So, as you approach the library, two things may happen. Either your SAS, which is monitoring the environment, will 'notice' that you are drawing nearer to the library and will override the currently activated ('speak-loudly') schema in favour of the set of schemas associated with 'library behaviour', one of which will be a 'speak-quietly' schema. Or else, as might happen if you are very pre-occupied with your conversation (i.e. your SAS is currently being used largely for this), you may walk into the library still talking loudly and then suddenly become aware that you need to talk more quietly. At this point, your SAS will have to switch its 'attention' momentarily from the conversation you are having to assessing the environment and activating the 'library behaviour' schemas. This happens so quickly that one is rarely aware of it. Although this is a highly simplified example, and indeed there are some intellectual problems with its use, it serves as a simple illustration of an explanation of BM's problem. In his case, he had lost this SAS-monitoring capacity and so had a diminished ability to inhibit the 'speak loudly'-type schema once it had been activated (presumably this schema is originally activated through the contention scheduling process either when BM became anxious or when he was trying to break out of one of his perseverative cycles). The programme subsumed the functions of the SAS in providing the necessary environmental feedback, and modification of the action schema/contention scheduling process was achieved in this way (within the confines of his other neuropsychological difficulties).

Discussion

These cases presented with superficially similar behavioural disturbances — that of excessive verbal 'noise'. In addition the behavioural difficulties in both cases stemmed from a loss of control most likely to have resulted from damage to the frontal lobes. However, the similarity between the two cases goes little further, and it is possible to learn a great deal from consideration of the treatment approaches that proved effective (and equally those that did not) when they are seen within an adequate theoretical framework.

It is worth noting that in both cases limited generalization was achieved. This is exactly what would be predicted by the model. If the SAS is the structure involved in the implementation of a rule abstracted from one learned situation to another, damage to this system will lead to problems with generalization. There is considerable evidence that the frontal lobes are involved in processes of abstraction and reasoning and also in the regulation of behaviour. One can predict that frontal lobe damage might result (amongst other things) in an inability to extract a general principle from a single exemplar of a given set and apply it to others of that set. This is in accord with the authors' own clinical observations, but evidence remains, for the moment, anecdotal. This does not mean, however, that rehabilitation is necessarily more problematic, only that the patient's behaviour may have to be changed in a progressive fashion, taking each problem behaviour and each new context in which it occurs as the target of a new programme. To expect one small programme, aimed at one characteristic of a more general problem to have great effect upon that problem as a whole, may be too much to expect (although see Craine, 1982, p. 256).

The advantages of the cognitive neuropsychological approach

Many of the techniques and problems described here will be familiar to rehabilitation professionals, and in most cases therapists will be familiar with describing them in terms derived from other therapeutic frameworks. For instance, many aspects of the discussion of how behavioural schemas are established and modified will be familiar to behavioural therapists, who are used to understanding the emergence of behavioural disturbances in terms of conditioning events and subsequent maintenance in terms of reinforcement paradigms. This is a useful framework and is completely compatible with the cognitive neuropsychological approach. However, its flaw is that it has difficulty explaining the origin of behavioural dyscontrol syndromes. In the case of patient BM, for instance, how does learning theory explain his (or any other patient's) loss of control immediately following an injury? Clinically, disinhibition and loss of control are often first seen as the patient emerges from unconsciousness — before any 'conditioning' could have occurred. Are we to say then that the brain injury has somehow led to that patient losing past conditioned associations? That the patient's social behaviour, which is a complex network of conditioned responses, is immediately lost following brain insult? Certainly this makes little sense in terms of what we know about other forms of conditioned responses following brain injury. If it were the case that head injury led to conditioned associations being 'lost', the head-injured person would present very differently. It is obvious that brain injury does not lead to a simple loss of the wealth of established conditioned responses. An argument which suggests that some brain damage may lead to the loss of control over the selection of these conditioned responses rather than the loss of the responses themselves is much easier to support.

An additional advantage of the model described above is that it does not deny the role of cognition in behaviour. That humans do not respond to reinforcement paradigms in the same way as animals has been known for some time (Davey, 1981; Wood and Burgess, 1988). These differences are largely due to the role of cognition and language in the establishment and maintenance of behaviours. Shallice's model postulates both 'thought' and 'action' schemas. In this way it suggests that sets of 'thought schemas' (i.e. well-rehearsed sequences of cognitions) exist alongside 'action schemas'. Obviously, the two are not independent, and the output of one type may provide the trigger for a different type. Thus, there is an interaction between the two types as well as within the forms themselves. In the same way that damage to the SAS may lead to the inability to inhibit behavioural schemas (see Shallice *et al.*, in press), it may also lead to the inability to inhibit or modify thought schemas; hence perseveration of thought, concreteness, lack of insight, inflexibility, deficits of reasoning and problem solving and other cognitive phenomena which are seen following frontal lobe damage. Thus, the model satisfies some of the criteria required by cognitive therapists, who work to change the patient's understanding of his or her problems, often despite the patient's continuing relative lack of insight.

The success of the rehabilitation programmes described here obviously depended upon many factors. But what they particularly emphasise is the importance of a sound, theoretical framework for the understanding of the problem before treatment is attempted. This is particularly true in the case of dyscontrol syndromes, and hopefully the described cases go some way in demonstrating how useful a theoretical model can be in the understanding of some of the phenomena seen following brain injury.

Acknowledgements

The authors wish to thank the staff of the Kemsley Head Injury Rehabilitation Unit, St. Andrew's Hospital, Northampton, UK. Thanks are also due to Doreen Baxter for neuropsychological assessment data, Heather Youngson, Georgina Slater and Mary Lees and to Dr Martyn Rose for permission to report on patients under his care. Particular thanks are due to Tim Shallice and Jane McNeil.

References

BADDELEY, A. and WILSON, B., 1988, 'Frontal amnesia and the dysexecutive syndrome'. *Brain and Cognition*, **7**, 212–30.

CHOROVER, S. L. and COLE, M., 1966, 'Delayed alternation performance in patients with cerebral lesions'. *Neuropsychologia*, **4**, 1–7.

CRAINE, J. F., 1982, 'The retraining of frontal lobe dysfunction'. In L. E. Trexler (Ed.) *Cognitive rehabilitation, conceptualization and intervention* (New York: Plenum Press).

DAVEY, G., 1981, 'Conditioning principles, behaviourism and behaviour therapy'. In G. Davey (Ed.) *Applications of conditioning theory* (London: Methuen).

DUNCAN, J., 1986, 'Disorganisation of behaviour after frontal lobe damage'. *Cognitive Neuropsychology*, **3**, 271–90.

FUSSEY, I., CUMBERPATCH, J. and GRANT, C., 1988, 'The application of a behavioural model in rehabilitation'. In I. Fussey and G.M. Giles (Eds) *Rehabilitation of the severely brain injured adult: A practical approach*, (Kent: Croom Helm).

GILES, G. M. and FUSSEY, I., 1988, 'Models of brain injury rehabilitation: from theory to practice'. In I. Fussey and G. M. Giles (Eds) *Rehabilitation of the severely brain injured adult: A practical approach* (Kent: Croom Helm).

GILES, G. M. and GENT, A., 1988, 'Conductive education and motor learning'. In I. Fussey and G.M. Giles (Eds) *Rehabilitation of the severely brain injured adult: A practical approach*, (Kent: Croom Helm).

GILES, G. M., FUSSEY, I. and BURGESS, P. W., 1988, 'The behavioural treatment of verbal interaction skills following severe head injury: a single case study'. *Brain Injury*, **2**, (1), 75–9.

GOLDBERG, E. and BILDER, R. M., 1987, 'The frontal lobes and hierarchical organisation of cognitive control'. In E. Perecman (Ed.) *The frontal lobes revisited* (New York: IRBN Press).

HOLLON, S. D. and KENDALL, P.C., 1980, 'Cognitive self-statements in depression: Development of an automatic thoughts questionnaire'. *Cognitive Therapy and Research*, **4**, 383–95.

LHERMITTE, F., 1983, 'Utilization behaviour and its relation to lesions of the frontal lobes'. *Brain*, **106**, 237–55.

LURIA, A. R., 1966, *Higher cortical functions in man* (London: Tavistock).

MILNER, B., 1982, 'Some cognitive effects of frontal lobe lesions in man'. *Philosophical Transactions of the Royal Society of London B*, **298**, 211–26.

NORMAN, D. A. and SHALLICE, T., 1980, *Attention to action: willed and automatic control of behaviour*. Center for Human Information Processing Technical Report No. 99. (Reprinted in revised form in R.J. Davidson, G.E. Schwartz and D. Shapiro (Eds.), 1986, *Consciousness and self-regulation, Vol. 4* (New York: Plenum Press).

PETRIDES, M. and MILNER, B., 1982, 'Deficits on subject-ordered tasks after frontal- and temporal-lobe lesions in man' *Neuropsychologia*, **16**, 1–13.

SHALLICE, T., 1982, 'Specific impairments of planning'. *Philosophical Transactions of the Royal Society of London B*, **298**, 199–209.

SHALLICE, T., 1988, *From neuropsychology to mental structure* (New York: Cambridge University Press).

SHALLICE, T. and EVANS, M. E., 1978, 'The involvement of the frontal lobes in cognitive estimation'. *Cortex*, **14**, 294–303.

SHALLICE, T. and BURGESS, P. W., 1990, 'Deficits in strategy application following frontal lobe damage in man'. *Brain*. (In press.)

SHALLICE, T., BURGESS, P. W., SCHON, F. and BAXTER, D. M., 1989, 'The origins of utilisation behaviour', *Brain*, **112**, 1587–98.

STUSS, D. T. and BENSON, D. F., 1984, 'Neuropsychological studies of the frontal lobes'. *Psychological Bulletin*, **95**, 3–28.

STUSS, D. T. and BENSON, D. F., 1986, *The frontal lobes* (New York: Raven Press).

WARRINGTON, E. K., 1984, *The recognition memory test* (Windsor, Berks: NFER-Nelson Publishing Co. Ltd.).

WARRINGTON, E. K. and JAMES, M., 1988, 'Visual apperceptive agnosia: A clinico-anatomical study of three cases'. *Cortex*, **24**, 13–32.

WECHSLER, D., 1958, *The measurement and appraisal of adult intelligence* (New York: Williams and Wilkins).

WECHSLER, D., 1981, *Wechsler Adult Intelligence Scale-Revised*. (Cleveland: The Psychological Corporation).

WEIGL, E., 1941, 'On the psychology of so-called processes of abstraction'. *Journal of Abnormal and Social Psychology*, **36**, 3–33.

WOOD, R. Ll., 1987, *Brain injury rehabilitation: a neurobehavioural approach* (London: Croom Helm).

WOOD, R. Ll. and BURGESS, P. W., 1988, 'The psychological management of behaviour disorders following brain injury'. In I. Fussey and G. M. Giles (Eds) *Rehabilitation of the severely brain injured adult: A practical approach* (London: Croom Helm).

ZUNG, W. W. K., 1971, 'A rating instrument for anxiety disorders'. *Psychosomatics*, **12**, 371–9.

Chapter 10

Integrating Cognition and Behaviour: A Pragmatic Approach to Brain Injury Rehabilitation

N. Alderman and P. W. Burgess

Introduction

Recent application of behavioural techniques to brain injury rehabilitation have led to the emergence of methods for controlling or reducing post-traumatic behavioural sequelae, allowing therapies aimed at increasing functional independence to take place (Wood, 1987).

However, despite the reported efficacy of a behavioural approach, it has been subjected to a number of serious criticisms (e.g. Baer *et al.*, 1968; Keeley *et al.*, 1976). These may be summarized as follows:

1 A behavioural programme may fail to change or have no significant impact on the frequency or severity of a target behaviour whilst it is in operation.
2 A programme may successfully reduce the frequency or severity of a target behaviour whilst it is running, but behaviour may return to pre-treatment levels when the programme is withdrawn.
3 Similarly, treatment gains may only survive within the environment in which the treatment was conducted and fail to generalize to other settings, individuals or situations.

Considering the cognitive deficits and learning problems produced by brain injury, such criticisms have serious implications for the value of using behavioural techniques with this group of patients. Clinical experience has shown that some members of this population do not benefit from the range of behavioural techniques described in the brain injury literature. (e.g. Wood, 1987) and, despite a thorough behavioural analysis and consideration of the neuropsychological deficits which underlie certain behaviour problems, some treatment programmes have no lasting impact.

Given that a sub-group of patients exist who show limited response to traditional behavioural techniques alone, it is necessary to consider alternative treatment methods capable of tackling this problem. One alternative lies in the application of recent cognitive neuropsychological theory (see Chapter 9) which predicts that changing cognitive schemata simultaneously with behavioural responses leads to increased generalization and maintenance of responses. The next section will introduce the theory behind these methods, and later in the chapter, four cases will be presented which demonstrate this point.

Combining Cognitive and Behavioural Approaches

Recent years have seen the development of the 'cognitive-behaviour modification' movement which is seen by some as a way to address the limitations of current behavioural approaches. There are a number of therapies which fall within the umbrella of cognitive-behaviour modification. Examples include rational emotive therapy (Ellis, 1962), self-instructional training (Meichenbaum, 1977) and cognitive therapy (Beck, 1976). The common link between these different therapies lies in their theoretical roots. They attempt to not only modify observable behaviour, but also internal, covert variables such as thoughts, beliefs, attitudes and other private events which have been labelled cognitive. Such events are believed to play a significant role in the determination of behaviour because changes in cognition tend to have a controlling effect on action. This change is believed to promote generalization of behaviour because changes in cognitive schemata, especially the verbal mediators of behaviour, alter the individuals perception of (and interaction with) the environment.

Empirical evidence exists which suggests that maintenance of behaviour change is superior in programmes which attempt to directly modify internal cognition as well as overt behaviour. For example, Lowe *et al.*, (1979) found greater generalization of behaviour change in different groups of long-stay chronic schizophrenics using self-instructional training. Other examples showing how the modification of cognition may facilitate generalization and maintenance can be found in Lowe and Higson (1981) and Jones *et al.* (1989). This might suggest that an improved probability of generalization and maintenance of behaviour change would be possible in the brain injured if covert cognition, as well as behaviour itself, was manipulated by a treatment programme.

The failure of some brain-injured patients to respond to cognitive therapy may be attributable to two factors. Firstly, patients who actively deny problems and have poor insight may fail to appreciate the need to change and will lack the necessary motivation to participate in therapy. Secondly, it may reflect the severity of their neuropsychological deficits. A central requirement for participating in any form of cognitive therapy is the need for the client to play an active role in treatment, whereby changes in cognition are facilitated through reflection and meaning acquired through the synthesis and internalization of new, adaptive cognitions (Meichenbaum and Cameron, 1973).

Brain-injured patients, particularly those who have sustained damage to the frontal lobes and their afferent and efferent connections, may not have the necessary cognitive skill to facilitate this process. Such patients may be concrete in their thinking, be unable to change between competing response sets or perseverate with set patterns of thoughts and ideas. When questioned about their behaviour, many severely brain-injured patients are able to comment and agree on the unacceptability of their behavioural disorders. However, they are still unable to change their behaviour to match their attitudes about it; in many ways this resembles the dissociation between knowing and doing which Teuber (1964) noted in frontal patients. Individuals who present with such patterns of deficit are more likely to revert to automatic, stereotyped behaviour and will lack the skills necessary to be able to change their behaviour or engage in the cognitive therapies.

Applying Cognitive Behaviour Modification in Severe Brain Injury

Wood (1988a) has described severity of brain injury as being the variable which will determine whether verbal psychotherapy can be conducted with this group of patients. He has stated that methods, such as counselling or group therapy, can improve the behaviour and social adaptability of individuals with minor damage, but that they will often fail to achieve success with more severely damaged patients. Patients admitted to the Kemsley Unit, St Andrew's Hospital, Northampton, fall into this category, with duration of coma (one frequently used measure of severity) typically lasting months, rather than the weeks or days reported by investigators describing patients who attend day or outpatient centres.

A descriptive analysis of the presenting characteristics of thirty recent admissions to this Unit was made by two raters who examined case notes and quantified information about patients from their initial six-week assessment. Information regarding behavioural disorders was derived from the results of a behaviour rating scale that had been completed by staff; from this it was possible to gather data about the prevalence and severity of positive, negative and other psychosocial behavioural disorders. Similarly, the results of neuropsychological testing were used to obtain information about language, perceptual, memory, frontal lobe and intellectual functioning. Finally, the occupational therapist's report was used to determine what problems patients had with a range of physically oriented activities of daily living, including mobility, continence, feeding, washing and dressing. In each case, a four-point rating scale was filled in for each item and, from this, information obtained regarding the frequency and severity of these problem areas in the sample (see Appendix 1). The results are displayed graphically in Figure 10.1.

Figure 10.1. Severity of behavioural disorders, cognitive impairment and physical/ADL problems in a sample of 30 patients on admission to the Kemsley Unit (figures above the bars indicate the percentage presenting with that problem/impairment).

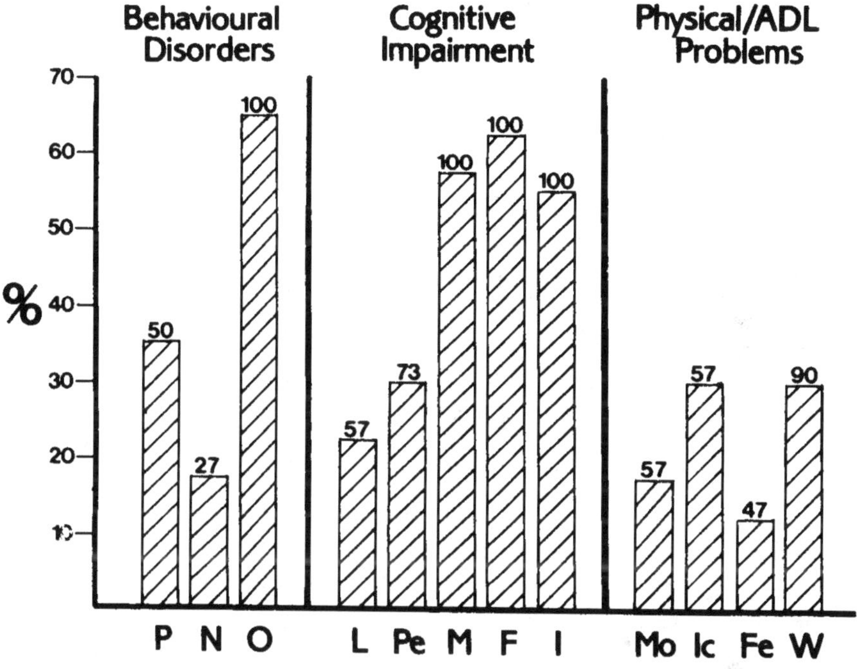

Obviously, there are methodological issues associated with an analysis of this kind. It should be noted that while Figure 10.1 appears to imply that comparisons across measures can be made, in reality, they are independent from each other and not equivalent. Just because a patient may be behaviourally disturbed does not mean that s/he will necessarily have a pattern of severe underlying cognitive impairments accompanied by physical or activities of daily living (ADL) difficulties.

As can be seen, on the whole our patients tend to have severe problems with memory, organization and planning ability and intellectual functioning. In addition, half the sample presented 'positive' behaviour disorders (mainly in the form of verbal and physical aggression), whilst all the patients had some form of psychosocial disturbance. The distribution of physical and ADL problems was more variable; most patients required some form of training for washing and dressing, and others had difficulties in the areas of mobility, continence and feeding, although on the whole, these tended to be less severe. Such individuals characteristically present with severe deficits in the very skills required to engage in and benefit from the cognitive therapies.

Response Cost

Some types of behavioural techniques can be applied to the brain injured which are capable of both modifying action and changing the content of cognition.

Our experience has suggested that this can be achieved through the use of a particular method, that of response-cost. This is a behavioural technique based on the operant principle of negative punishment, whereby the loss of something pleasant immediately following a target behaviour subsequently leads to a reduction in the frequency of that behaviour. The 'something pleasant' may consist of anything which is valued by the individual, such as money, food or tokens (plastic discs or points which can be exchanged for actual goods). Response-cost has been used successfully in the treatment of a number of behaviour disorders with a variety of different client groups (e.g. Wulfsohn and Barling, 1978; McLaughlin *et al.*, 1987), but, as yet, it does not appear to have been extensively used with brain-injured patients as a method to promote behavioural control.

Response-cost is a behavioural technique which incorporates important cognitive components, providing a paradigm that addresses the need for behavioural control on the one hand and greater awareness of behaviour on the other. At one level, response-cost is a straight-forward conditioning technique, but the nature of the interaction between behavioural event and its consequence involves a cognitive operation because the procedure encourages the patient to verbalize the reason for losing a token (or some other form of reward). What starts out as an opportunity for pure associational learning, ends up as an opportunity to utilize language to improve awareness and understanding of the event. This offers an opportunity for verbal mediation in the understanding and control of similar situations which could lead to response-cost.

One reason for preferring response-cost as opposed to reinforcement procedures has been provided by Levine and Fasnacht (1973). They maintain that rewarding a behaviour leads to an inevitable decline in a person's intrinsic motivation to engage in that behaviour, known as the 'overjustification effect' (Lepper *et al.*, 1973). Very generally, their rationale is that when reinforcement is given for a behaviour that the patient finds intrinsically rewarding, there is a resulting change in that patient's control (which an individual holds when engaged in a behaviour which has intrinsic rewards) to an external locus of control which occurs when the behaviour is maintained only when rewards for that behaviour are present. As the change from internal to external occurs, the patient's perception of why s/he is engaging in that behaviour changes — they no longer see themselves as engaging in the behaviour for its own sake, but for the external reward associated with it. So when the reward is removed, then the individual has no further reason to persist in that behaviour.

While there are serious criticisms of the validity of interpreting behavioural treatments in terms of the overjustification effect (see Ogilvie and Prior, 1982), we wondered whether, for a certain class of patients, the process of rewarding them for behaving appropriately might actually decrease their own motivation to do so. This could account for our inability to produce lasting changes in the behaviour of these patients.

What we required, therefore, was a behavioural method that did not have the effect of changing the patient's locus of control from internal to external. If possible, we needed a method which would emphasize the patient's own responsibility for control over his/her behaviour. We felt that if we could find such a method, it would serve the purpose of involving the patients more in their own treatment. One solution was the use of response-cost as a method in which a patient gives 'us' something whenever an inappropriate behaviour occurs, rather than us *doing* something to them. This would serve the purpose of emphasizing an internal locus of control.

Our clinical observations suggest that the subgroup of patients who fail to respond to behaviour techniques are those who present the most severe difficulties with frontal lobe functioning. The frontal lobes have been described as having an executive function which allows attention to be focused and sustained, enabling the patient to select and interpret information from the environment from which he can assess the impact of his behaviour and modify his subsequent actions.

Cognition, as a product of executive function, also has an executive role (Belmont and Butterfield, 1977), the content of which is modified and updated on the basis of feedback received from the environment. The ability to change cognition (in the form of the verbal mediators of behaviour) is dependent in turn on the ability of the frontal lobes to allow accurate interpretation of the effect of an action and to use this feedback to modify intervening cognitive schemata. However, damage to the frontal lobes has been shown to produce increased distractibility, leading to difficulties in monitoring performance or utilizing the feedback available from environmental changes (Wood, 1988b). This inhibits the ability of the individual to perceive cues in the environment that signal a certain kind of behaviour and to use this feedback to evaluate the appropriateness of an action. Under such conditions, an individual will fail to modify behavioural strategies. In these circumstances patients may be able to make accurate statements regarding the inappropriateness of their behaviour but fail to use this knowledge to change it under the conditions in which it occurs. As such, their behaviour is not under any form of control, internal or external. Behaviour is, therefore, a response which occurs impulsively, according to ideas or environmental contingencies that happen to be present in any given situation.

A result of this inability to make use of normal feedback is that brain-injured individuals adopt verbal mediators for behaviour which are stereotyped in manner and unresponsive to changes in the environment. At the same time, individuals no longer possess the faculties necessary to modify verbal mediators through participation in cognitive therapy. What is required, therefore, is a form of behavioural intervention which will modify the verbal mediators of behaviour to facilitate maintenance following treatment withdrawal. We believe that response-cost is a technique which can achieve this aim.

In addition to improving awareness and locus of control, response-cost procedures also facilitate learning of appropriate behaviour by attempting to obviate problems imposed by memory impairment or attentional deficit. Under ordinary token economy conditions, a fixed interval reinforcement procedure operates, which means that a patient may not actually lose tokens for some undesirable behaviour until token payment times are arranged which maybe 15, 30 or even 60 minutes after the event. By this time, many patients with memory problems or attentional difficulties are not able to associate previous behaviour with current reinforcement, therefore, no contingency is established and conditioning, if it takes place at all, is slow and unreliable. The immediate and overt nature of response-cost allows contingencies to be established more easily, and the association between a response and its consequences is further reinforced by the verbal explanation or translation of the event that occurs at the same time.

Case Studies

The following four case studies demonstrate the use of response-cost with patients who did not respond to treatment using traditional time-out and positive reinforcement programmes. All of the cases were treated using variations of response-cost programme; additional improvement was obtained in one of the four cases when cognitive overlearning (see Wood, 1987; pp. 113–114) was added to the basic intervention.

Case One

CE, a 26-year-old male, had sustained a very severe head injury in a road traffic accident two years prior to treatment. A computerized tomography (CT) scan shortly after injury demonstrated the presence of multiple petechial haemorrhages. Post-traumatic amnesia was estimated as lasting approximately one year. He remained wheelchair-dependent due to lower limb weakness.

CE attended a number of hospitals for medical treatment and rehabilitation before being discharged. However, he proved to be unmanageable in the community due to behavioural problems, making it necessary to admit him to the Kemsley Unit. Neuropsychological assessment revealed multiple cognitive handicaps including global impairment of memory and a short attention span (only three digits forward being reliably recalled). An expressive dysphasia and dysarthria were evident. Particular difficulties with non-verbal reasoning, visual inattention and an inability to monitor his performance were also found.

Behaviour during the early part of CE's rehabilitation was characterized by disinhibited and attention-seeking behaviour. In particular, he remained intolerant of other patients and would make inappropriate responses to staff requests. He frequently engaged in verbal outbursts, characterized by shouting and swearing, which disrupted therapy activities. An epileptiform basis to this behaviour was not convincingly demonstrated, and a behavioural analysis suggested that it was attributable to CE's poor ability to tolerate frustration.

Initial attempts at treatment were carried out by use of a general token system (see Wood, 1987). CE would fail to earn tokens for periods during which he engaged in verbal outbursts. The consequence of this was that he had fewer tokens to exchange for back-up rewards. In addition to receiving or not receiving a token every 15 minutes, specific verbal feedback was given regarding his behaviour for that period. If it had been appropriate, CE was given verbal praise; if it had not, he was told that his verbal abuse had led to token loss. In this way it was hoped that, over time, CE would learn to control his behaviour and increase his ability to tolerate frustration.

Unfortunately, this did not work. Despite 10 weeks of treatment, a review of his progress using time-series analysis techniques (Jones *et al.*, 1977; Tyron, 1982) demonstrated no downward trend in the weekly number of tokens lost for verbal abuse ($C = -0.137$; $Z = -0.518$).

Staff felt that the lack of improvement in CE's behaviour may have been due to verbal abuse being reinforced by attention when he was told why he had not earned his token for a 15-minute period. This observation was plausible because much of CE's behaviour appeared to have an attention-seeking quality. If this was the case, then any behaviour which resulted in staff attention would be reinforced and thereby maintained.

In order to test this hypothesis, a change was made in the way that the token system was administered to CE. Whilst CE continued to receive his tokens and praise for appropriate behaviour, he was given no feedback for the periods in which inappropriate behaviour had occurred. In this way, if staff attention was reinforcing, then a reduction in the number of tokens lost for verbal abuse would be expected to occur.

In fact, the opposite was found. Instead of a downward trend in the weekly number of tokens lost for verbal abuse, time-series analysis demonstrated an increase in this behaviour ($C = 0.339$; $Z = 1.769$; $p < .05$). These results suggested that verbal feedback enabled CE to control his abusive behaviour to a greater extent then when such feedback was not given. However, even when this occurred regularly at 15-minute intervals, it was not sufficient to eliminate the behaviour altogether, and it continued to be inappropriate within the rehabilitation setting.

The problem still remained of how to elimate or reduce further the frequency of

Figure 10.2. Patient CE: Effect of the token system (with and without verbal feedback) and response-cost on the frequency of verbal abuse.

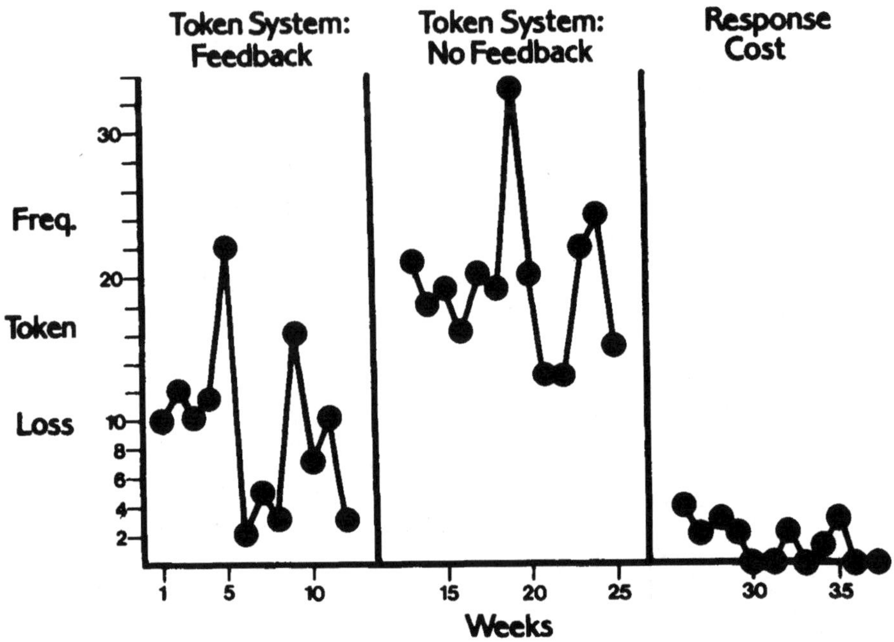

verbal abuse. Reference to CE's neuropsychological deficits, especially his poor attention, memory, self-monitoring ability and his concrete thinking style, suggested that it was necessary to give feedback immediately upon observation of the target behaviour and that it needed to be exaggerated if effective learning was to take place.

It was felt that this could be achieved by implementing a response-cost programme which would remain in operation throughout the day and which would replace the normal token system for CE. Instead of being given a token for every 15 minutes of appropriate behaviour, CE was given a number of tokens which could subsequently be exchanged at a later time during the day for a variety of back-up reinforcers. However, when CE engaged in verbal abuse, staff would immediately intervene, tell him he had been 'verbally abusive' and prompt him for one of his tokens. In this way, CE lost a token every time he exhibited the target behaviour. At fixed times during the day, CE exchanged his tokens for a reinforcer; the quality of this was dependent on the number of tokens that remained in his possession. He was then given the next pre-designated number of tokens which would cover the period up to the next time he could exchange those remaining for a reward, and so on.

Before the programme began, time-sampling observations were used to calculate the number of tokens CE was given at fixed points during the day. The length of time between these token-exchange points ranged from 30 minutes to 165 minutes.

Figure 10.2 demonstrates the reduction in the frequency of CE's verbal abuse over 12 weeks. The significance is confirmed by statistical analysis; analysis of variance by ranks (Kruskal-Wallis) over the three treatment conditions shows a significant difference between group means ($H = 27.4$; $df = 2$; $p < .01$). Further analysis, using Neuman-Keuls, demonstrates that the feedback condition of the token system (mean weekly token loss = 9.25) was superior to the no-feedback condition (mean = 19.46; $q = 10.212$; $p < .01$); however, the response cost programme (mean = 1.42) was, in turn, superior to this ($q = 7.833$; $p < .01$).

Case Two

GM, a seventeen-year-old male, sustained a very severe head injury at the age of twelve in a road traffic accident. He was in a coma for some months following injury and subsequently developed a right-sided hemiplegia which left him wheelchair-dependent. In addition to his physical disability, GM also presented with a number of behavioural disorders. He was difficult to manage both at home and in a residential college. His main problems were described as failure to tolerate his peer group, aggression and sexual disinhibition. As a consequence, he was admitted to the Kemsley Unit for a period of assessment and rehabilitation.

Neuropsychological assessment revealed a number of cognitive deficits. His attention span was severely limited, and he had difficulty monitoring his own performance on tests of frontal lobe functioning (performance on these measures was noted to improve when he was encouraged to self-verbalize what he was doing). His problem-solving and organizational skills were poor, and he had major problems with verbal and non-verbal memory functioning. Verbal skills were generally poor compared to non-verbal abilities.

Behaviour following admission was characterized by GM's very low ability to tolerate frustration. It was noted that when he was asked to perform activities by staff, or when other patients were near him whom he disliked, he would undergo rapid mood change. As a result he would become verbally and physically aggressive, attacking the object of his frustration. In addition, he was observed to be very attention seeking and would use a wide range of unsuitable social skills to get others' attention, as well as making inappropriate comments, laughing and grinning for excessively long periods.

As with CE, the general token system was used as the initial form of treatment. GM would frequently not earn tokens for poor social skills. When he was informed of this, he would often lose his temper and physically attack members of staff which in turn led to frequent use of the time-out room. Time-series analysis techniques showed

Figure 10.3. Patient GM: Effect of the token system, response-cost and combined response-cost/verbal prompting on the frequency of poor social skills.

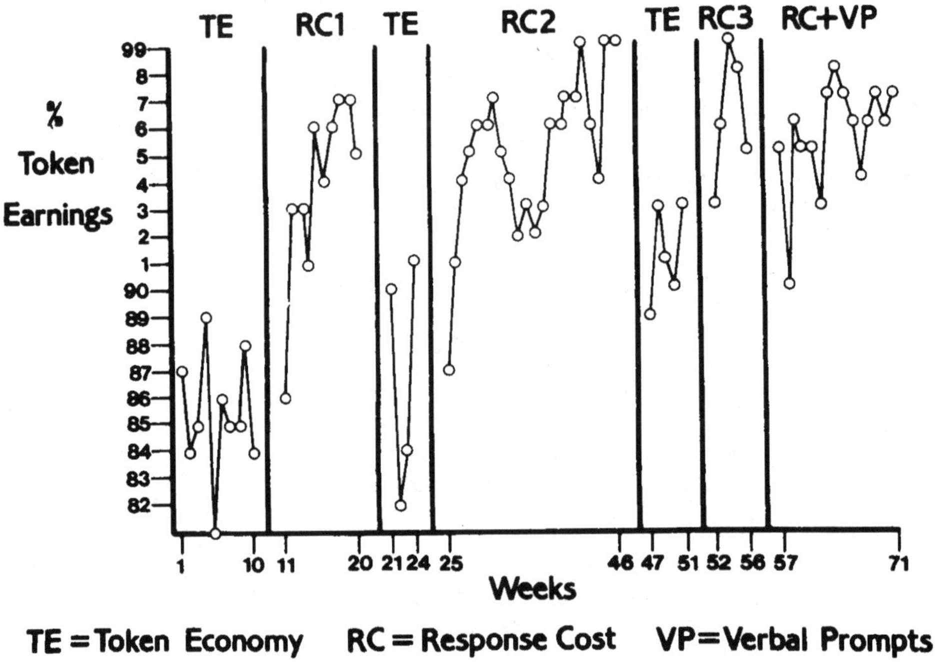

that after 10 weeks on the token system, the trend in GM's weekly token earnings was falling ($C = 0.519$; $Z = -1.827$; $p < .05$), suggesting that his behaviour was deteriorating rather than improving. Subsequent behavioural analysis suggested that this lack of improvement may have been partly due to learning constraints caused by his underlying neuropsychological impairments. Memory impairment, difficulties in monitoring his own behaviour and an inability to make cognitive abstractions appeared to combine in such a way that he could not relate his behaviour to its consequences. This, in turn, would frustrate him and typically escalate into a time-out situation.

In order to facilitate associational learning, the normal token system was replaced by a response cost programme, the mechanics of which were similar to that instigated with CE. However, GM had to forfeit tokens to staff for a variety of target behaviours. Most tokens lost were for poor social skills, but staff requests for his tokens usually precipitated an aggressive outburst for which further tokens would be lost. As a result, behavioural training was aimed at shaping GM's social skills and increasing his ability to tolerate frustration by providing specific verbal feedback, together with the loss of a token immediately following observation of any target behaviour; this loss decreased the probability that he would subsequently obtain a tangible reward. Recordings of behaviour were obtained every 15 minutes, as with the token system, in order that the two different treatment methods could be compared. Figure 10.3 shows the improvement in overall control of behaviour following implementation of the programme. The average number of token recordings increased from 85.6 a week, using the token system, to 94.8 per week when response cost was used.

The programme was then withdrawn to allow a further baseline to be made of GM's target behaviour; during this time he was put back on the token system. After four weeks this was, in turn, replaced by a more demanding version of the original response cost programme and continued for a further 22 weeks. Five weeks were then spent back on the token system.

This alternation between the two programmes was conducted in order to determine if the greater control acquired over his behaviour whilst on the token system would maintain following its withdrawal. Although it will be noted from Figure 10.3 that behavioural recordings made whilst on the token system were not as high as when on the response cost programme, comparison of the three successive baselining periods shows an increase over time in the average number of tokens earned per week (85.6, 86.8 and 91.2, respectively) which also reached statistical significance ($H = 6.345$; $df = 2$; $p < .05$).

Further maintenance of treatment gains were obtained in the most recent intervention which used a system of verbal prompts in addition to response cost. The quality of GM's response to staff intervention improved to the extent that, for the most part, he tolerated their interaction without resorting to physical aggression. This enabled the programme to be changed so that GM was given verbal feedback only when target behaviours were seen (e.g.'G, it's a poor social skill to shout across the room'); a token would only be removed if he persisted with the target behaviour. To date, as can be seen in the last part of Figure 10.5, GM's high level of behavioural control has been successfully maintained, mainly by using occasional verbal feedback without the necessity of having to frequently remove a token.

Case Three

A further variant of response cost and its effectiveness in maintaining behaviour change will be made with reference to SJ, a 24-year-old male who had sustained a very severe closed-head injury six years before admission to the Kemsley Unit. He developed a left-sided hemiplegia and, as a result, was confined to a wheelchair. The reader is referred to Chapter 9 for a more detailed description of this case.

During the first few weeks of admission, SJ was noted to be frequently incontinent of urine during the day, despite being able to take himself to the toilet and use a bottle. Medical examination did not suggest that this was due to any physical abnormality or the presence of infection. Observation suggested that an attentional factor may have been involved as SJ was usually engaged in some form of activity at the time he was incontinent, which he would frequently continue despite acknowledging that he was wet.

As with the previous cases, initial attempts at behavioural management were carried out through application of the token system. SJ did not earn his token for any 15-minute period during which he had been incontinent; he was informed why he had not earned at token payment times and instructed to go to his room to change his soiled clothing. After eight weeks of treatment, no decrease in the weekly trend of incontinence was found ($C = 0.03$; $Z = 0.097$). Examination of token recordings made during this time showed that he remained incontinent on average 14.5 times per week (range = 4 – 29).

Given his poor attention and other neuropsychological deficits, it was felt that response cost would be a more appropriate form of treatment. A simple intervention was consequently designed and implemented, alongside the token system. SJ was given five distinctive tokens at the beginning of each day (he named these his 'pleasure tokens'). As soon as he was observed to be incontinent of urine, staff directed his attention to this by informing him that he was wet and then asking him to give up one 'pleasure token'. He was then told to go to his room to change his clothing as before. In the evening, SJ was prompted to hand in his remaining tokens which he could exchange for an additional reward of his choice, providing he had retained a minimum target number of tokens.

As the programme progressed and SJ became more familiar with it, its attentional aspects were changed. Instead of staff informing SJ that he was wet, he would be asked for a token immediately following any episode of incontinence and then asked why it had been taken from him. In this way, in addition to directing his attention to his body state, he was also encouraged to introspect and self-verbalize that he had been incontinent.

After 27 weeks, the programme was discontinued. During treatment, a significant downward trend in the weekly frequency of incontinence was found, ($C = 0.542$; $Z = 3.301$; $p < .01$), whilst the mean rate of incontinence fell from 14.5 to 3.39 per week. This improvement was still evident 34 weeks later when a follow-up assessment was made of his incontinence. Analysis of variance by ranks showed an overall difference between group means ($H = 31.28$; $df = 2$; $p < .01$). Whilst the mean weekly frequency of incontinence for both the response cost and follow-up phases were significantly lower than that for the token system ($q = 11.11$; $p < .01$; $q = 13.47$; $p < .01$), no difference was found between the last two stages ($q = 2.36$), substantiating the visual impression from Figure 10.4 that treatment effects had been maintained. Staff reported that SJ remained continent of urine during the day, the recordings reflecting only occasional nocturnal incontinence.

Figure 10.4. Patient SJ. Reduction in the daily frequency of urinary incontinence following the introduction and eventual withdrawal of a response-cost programme.

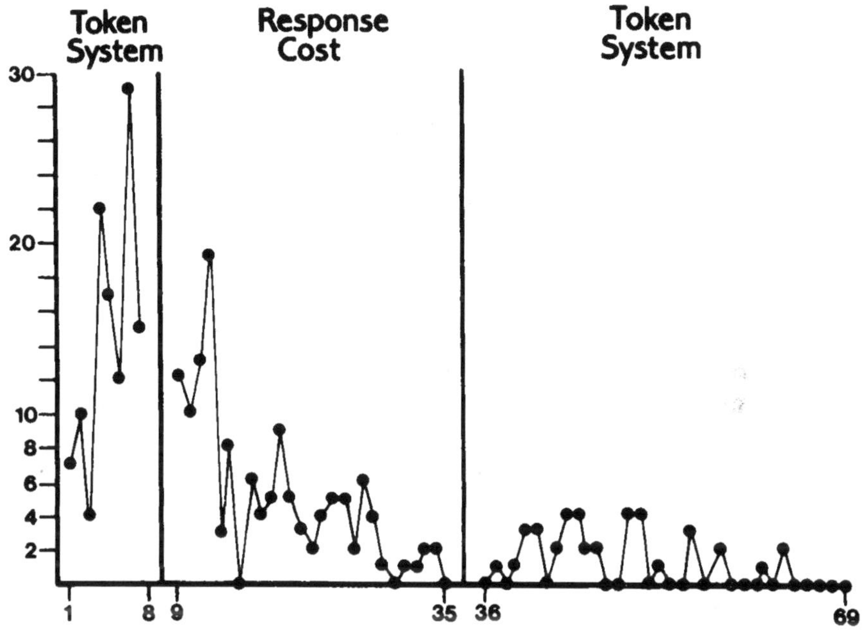

Case Four

In this final case, two techniques will be presented which, when used together, facilitate generalization and maintenance through modification of both behaviour and its verbal mediators following withdrawal of the intervention. The subject, AB, was a 36-year-old female who had contracted herpes simplex encephalitis nine months before admission. She consequently developed a number of psychosocial and behavioural disorders which could not be successfully managed in the community or the hospital resources available in her area.

Behaviour on admission was characterized by gross impulsivity and lack of control. These chiefly took the form of sexual disinhibition, stealing and intrusiveness, together with garrulous, rambling, flighty and repetitive speech. Neuropsychological assessment estimated her pre-morbid level of intellectual functioning as falling within the 'High Average' range. Her current profile was characterized by multiple cognitive handicaps, especially severe verbal and non-verbal memory impairment. Her performance on a range of tests reported to be sensitive to frontal lobe functioning was also very poor, especially with regard to her problem-solving and organizational skills. A concrete and perseverative style of thinking was also very evident.

Within a few weeks of admission, the majority of AB's psychosocial and behavioural disorders were being effectively managed by the token system. However, staff reported that aspects of her social behaviour continued to interfere with rehabilitation, mainly because she consistently repeated verbal phrases in the form of inane questions, instructions she had been given or demands for food. These phrases would be repeated to the extent that rehabilitation activities could not continue. Time-sampling observations showed that she made 951 such multiple repetitions over a variety of different situations in just five hours.

A number of different behavioural techniques were used in an attempt to teach AB control over her repetitive speech, none of which resulted in any success. For example, she would be 'timed-out-on-the-spot' by staff who would not respond to her verbal requests if they were made in the form of constantly repeated phrases to avoid reinforcing this behaviour. In addition, she would not earn tokens for 15-minute periods during which repetitive speech had occurred.

Unfortunately, these treatment approaches did not result in AB gaining greater control over her repetitive speech. The high frequency of this behaviour and its disruptive impact on the ward environment necessitated AB being excluded from group activities, and she became unpopular with members of the treatment team who were reluctant to work with her on an individual basis. Although AB had only been in the token system for two weeks, it was decided that the developing antipathy towards her from members of staff merited a special treatment programme.

Three baseline and three treatment conditions formed the basis of a reversal design to evaluate the effectiveness of treatment. Each session was split into 15-minute periods during which a variety of tasks were carried out. During the first week, AB was baselined; the mean frequency of repetitive speech observed over this time was 35.25 per 15-minute period (range = 16 – 49). Response cost was used in the first intervention by giving AB £.50 in one-pence pieces and explaining to her that, at the end of 15 minutes, she could exchange this money for a small chocolate bar, a commodity she found highly rewarding. AB was also told that she could lose money by repeating herself; every time repetition occurred, the therapist intervened and asked what she had just done. When she herself had verbalized that she had repeated herself, she was prompted to hand over a penny. The cost of the chocolate bar was fixed on the basis of the information collected during the first baseline phase. If AB retained a number of pennies equal to, or more than, this target number, she could exchange the money for her reward.

After 24 sessions, treatment was withdrawn and AB was rebaselined. She was found to have gained considerably greater control during these individual sessions, the mean frequency of repetitive speech falling from 35.25 to 6.3 per 15-minute period. After rebaselining, response cost was used again in the second treatment phase.

However, the cost of chocolate was increased in order to see whether this would bring about even greater control over the target behaviour. Whilst the frequency of her repetitive speech again greatly decreased following implementation of the programme, increasing the target level did not bring about greater control during this phase (mean frequency = 6.94 per 15-minute period).

During the last phase of treatment a 'cognitive overlearning' component was added to the response-cost intervention. The technique is based upon the principles of massed practice, and its aim is to reinforce the desired verbal mediator in the patient's mind (Wood, 1987). In AB's case this meant that repetition had two immediate consequences. First, the therapist intervened as before; AB was prompted to self-verbalize that she had just repeated herself and to hand over a penny. Second, she was then encouraged to repeat the statement 'I must not repeat myself' continually for one minute. Whilst this procedure may seem to be antagonistic to the aims of treatment, it had a number of therapeutic advantages. It resulted in AB being able to verbalize more reliably, what the aims of her programme were, that is, it succeeded in reinforcing the desired verbal mediator, and it caused AB to be reluctant to repeat herself in this way, suggesting that forced repetition of the target behaviour led to satiation taking place. The superior treatment effects of the combined response cost/cognitive overlearning intervention were confirmed by subsequently comparing the mean frequency of repetitive speech per 15-minutes from the previous intervention, using response cost alone (6.94) with that in the last phase (3.2).

The interventions had succeeded in greatly reducing the frequency of AB's repetitive speech during individual sessions, but it remained to be demonstrated as to whether treatment gains had generalized to other settings and if they were maintained following withdrawal of the special programme. Figure 10.5 shows the number of tokens not earned each week because of 'poor social skills', which included repetitive speech, over the duration of AB's admission. These recordings, as with CE, provided a crude continuous measure of the frequency of the target behaviour before, during and after implementation of the special programme. A significant downward trend in the weekly frequency of tokens lost occurred during the phase in which the special programme was introduced ($C = 0.415$; $Z = 1.667$; $p < .05$), suggesting that treatment gains were generalizing to situations outside that in which therapy took place. Analysis of variance by ranks showed a significant difference between group means ($H = 8.994$; $df = 2$; $p < .05$). The average number of tokens lost during and after withdrawal of the special programme were both significantly lower than the pre-treatment mean ($q = 13.272$; $p < .01$; $q = 15.304$; $p < .05$). However, there was no significant difference in means between token recordings made whilst the special programme was in operation and after it had been withdrawn ($q = 4.88$), suggesting that treatment gains were maintained for the remaining duration of AB's admission.

Further evidence of maintenance was also confirmed by comparison of pre-, immediate and three month post-intervention baselines with specific observations

Figure 10.5. Patient AB: Reduction in the number of tokens recorded as 'not earned' for poor social skills following the introduction and eventual withdrawal of daily, individual treatment sessions using response-cost and cognitive overlearning.

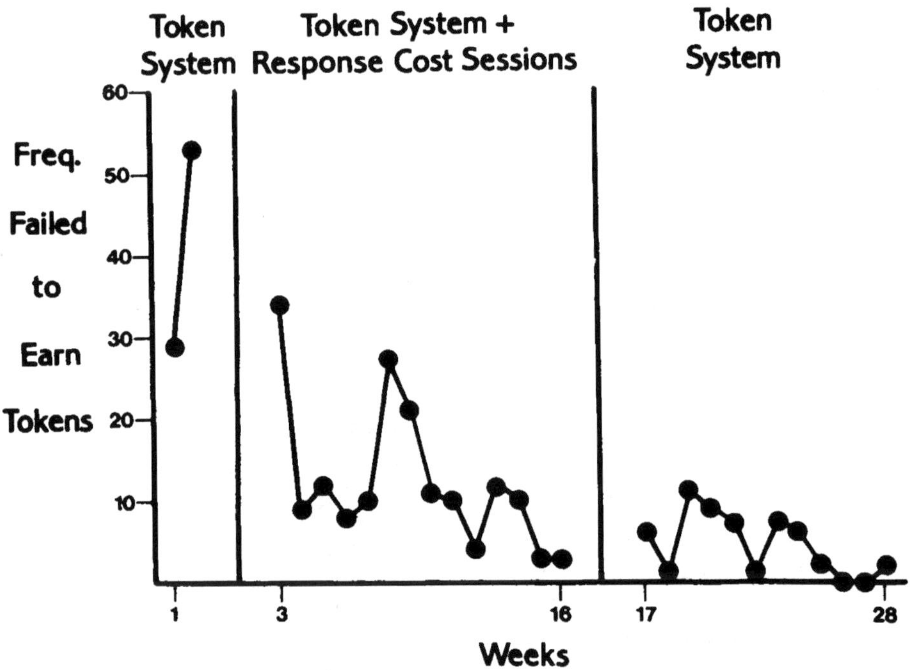

gathered using time-sampling methods (Alderman and Ward, in preparation). Subjective measures of improvement were also reported by staff who developed a great deal of affection for AB. She was included in group activities once again and went from being the most unpopular patient on the ward to the most popular by the time of her discharge.

Discussion

These four case studies illustrate the efficacy of two types of negative punishment procedures with patients who had not responded to treatment methods previously reported to be effective with brain-injured patients. A successful outcome was obtained in the first two patients whose daily behavioural management programme had been replaced by response cost interventions. Both of these patients demonstrated an increase in their ability to tolerate frustration and the frequency of their original target behaviours decreased. In the remaining two case studies, there was clear evidence of treatment gains being maintained following withdrawal of the programme. This occurred when variants of response cost were utilized, both on a sessional basis and as a daily programme in addition to the token economy system. Further within-treatment gains were also made in the case of one patient when a cognitive overlearning component was added.

An explanation is needed to explain why these types of treatment were successful when positive reinforcement and time-out techniques were not. One possible reason has already been mentioned, that the type of technique used here serves to emphasize the patients' own locus of control, thereby involving them more in their own therapy. But there are other reasons why the interventions resulted in superior results. Firstly, this method effected a short-term change in the patients' behaviour because it provided consistent consequences to target behaviours. However, this is hardly unique to this treatment approach because it is a desired property of all behavioural interventions. An additional factor is that response cost programmes rely upon a different contingency schedule compared to many traditional token-payment-based methods. Both human and animal studies have shown repeatedly that whilst rewarding every correct response is a quick method of effecting conditioning, this type of schedule is relatively ineffective in initiating changes which 'resist' extinction (Wood and Burgess, 1988). Yet the response cost programmes described here do seem to lead to changes that last beyond treatment, whereas other partial reinforcement-style treatments do not.

It seems likely that, in addition to providing behavioural consequences, response cost also modifies cognitive schemata in the form of the verbal mediators of behaviour, which regulate or 'gate' the stimulus-response relationship. It is this change which seems likely to be responsible for the maintenance of treatment gains following programme withdrawal. The neuropsychological profiles of the cases described will form the starting point for arguing how this is achieved. All four patients had increased distractibility, specific difficulties monitoring their own performance and gross impairment in their ability to utilize feedback. The response cost programmes enabled a specific, immediate response to be made after their target behaviours in a way that maximized and enhanced the amount of feedback the patient received. This is illustrated in the case of CE who benefited most when feedback was given in its most 'enhanced' version.

In addition, the nature of the feedback itself seems crucial to the modifications of the cognitive schemata which regulate behaviour. Initially, the patient is asked to give a member of staff a token; this will affect the range and availability of reinforcers to which s/he will subsequently have access. However, in addition to this, s/he is then given a brief statement summarizing the reason for token loss. Over time the patient internalizes this information, a process which is facilitated when s/he self-verbalizes, and it forms a new verbal mediator which is then used to modify that behaviour (for further discussion of the mechanisms by which this happens, see Chapter 9).

Evidence that this process occurs was clearly obtained with all four cases.

Subsequent verbal cueing reliably elicited these new verbal mediators in the form of self-statements which were not evident prior to the instigation of the programmes. For example, before her special programme started, AB remained unaware that she made multiple verbal repetitions and of the effect they had on others. In contrast, during the period following withdrawal of her programme and up to the time of her discharge, she was consistently able to inform an enquirer that she was not to repeat herself and tell them why. In addition, the study of SJ and AB suggests that the acquisition of new, appropriate verbal mediators can be facilitated more quickly by gradually fading out staff-given, direct verbal feedback and replacing it with a prompt for the patient to give the reason as to why a token has been lost. This procedure promotes reflection and internalization of new self-statements leading to more rapid changes in cognitive schemata.

Another reason for the success of response cost might be that the nature of this verbal feedback allows the programme to compensate for poor executive functioning that has resulted from the patient's frontal lobe damage by focusing attention and selecting the relevant information from the environment on the patient's behalf. This is directly comparable with the success of self-instructional training in the treatment of impulsive and aggressive behaviours reported by Lowe and Higson (1981). The response cost approach can, therefore, be said to constitute an 'ameliorative' strategy to compensate for impairment of frontal lobe functioning.

As well as enhancing feedback through the delivery of behavioural consequences and modifying underlying cognitive schemata, response cost may be particularly effective for another reason. It is an 'active' as opposed to a 'passive' form of treatment. Rather than simply being done to the patient, they have to play an active role by handing over tokens and eliciting more appropriate self-statements. This 'active' element to treatment may imply that procedural learning takes place and that this is necessary in order to facilitate acquisition of the new self-statements through declarative learning. Compare this, for example, with the failure of the various time-out programmes described in some of our cases which, whilst derived from the same principle of negative punishment, still result in treatment failure. One significant difference between the programmes is that the patient does not play an active role in the latter. It may be that response-cost programmes either place less reliance upon declarative aspects of learning or, conversely, enhance the procedural aspects in comparison with other methods. This, then, would lead to greater chance of treatment success since it is well known that procedural learning is relatively spared in those with memory problems (and all our patients had such impairments). Fixed-interval, token payment schedules place considerable emphasis, for their effectiveness, upon declarative or episodic memory. As discussed above, it seems commonsensical that it would be easier for patients to learn prosocial behaviour from a token system when they can remember each time they earn (or fail to earn) a token and why it was that they earned (or failed). Response-cost programmes rely less upon this declarative memory aspect for their effectiveness.

Finally, AB was found to benefit when a cognitive overlearning element was added to the response cost programme. Here, it was used with the patient who had the most severe frontal dysfunction after some control had been achieved over the target behaviour using response cost. This would suggest that cognitive overlearning in addition to response-cost may enhance the relationship between behaviour and its consequences, which will help patients with very severe impairment of their ability to make discriminations in their environment and utilize feedback effectively.

Acknowledgements

The authors would like to thank the staff of the Kemsley Head Injury Rehabilitation Unit, St Andrew's Hospital, Northampton, UK, without whose support and cooperation the programmes described here could not have been carried out. Particular thanks are due to Heather Youngson, Claire Grant and Tony Ward and to Doreen Baxter for neuropsychological assessment data. Finally, many thanks to Dr Martyn Rose for permission to report patients under his care.

Appendix 1

(1) Criteria for cognitive impairment index scores

Measure	*Criteria*	*Score*
Intellectual	NART-FSIQ discrepency up to 10 points[1]	0
Impairment	10–20 points	1
	20–30 points	2
	> 30 points	3
Perception	No perception tests[2] below 5%ile	0
	Up to 2 tests below 5%ile	1
	3 tests below 5%ile	2
	4 tests below 5%ile	3
Memory	No memory tests[3] below 5%ile	0
	Mean percentile of tests 5-25%ile range	1
	Mean percentile of tests 1-5%ile range	2
	Mean percentile of tests below 1%ile	3

Frontal Functioning	Unimpaired on any tests[4]	0
	Impaired on up to 3 tests	1
	Impaired on all tests	2
	Impaired on all tests plus at least one gross behavioural sign, e.g. perseveration, gross lack of insight, confabulation, etc.	3

(2) Criteria for behaviour disorder criteria index

Up to nine staff complete the Unit's Behaviour Rating Scale (BRS) for each patient within their first six weeks of admission. The BRS lists 145 undesirable behaviours, grouped into categories; each item is rated by staff on a nine-point likert scale. Raw scores then undergo computer analyses and are converted into a single mean percentage score for each item; the higher the score, the more severe the behaviour. The computer automatically lists the top five items. The BRS can be found in full in Wood (1987), pp. 179–186.

For the purpose of this analysis, the authors took the top five items for each patient and classified them as either 'positive', 'negative' or other 'psychosocial' behaviour disorders. A mean percentage score was then obtained for each of the three categories, and this was then rated, as below, for use in the group analyses:

Mean percentage score	*Score*
0– 25	0
26– 50	1
51– 75	2
75–100	3

(3) Criteria for ADL/physical problems criteria index

The authors consulted the Occupational Therapist's Six-Week Assessment Report in order to rate the following items from an Independency Scale which is used as part of the pre-admission selection procedure as follows:

Measure	*Criteria*	*Score*
Incontinence	No problem	0
	Night incontinence only	1
	Occasional day urinary and/or faecal incontinence	2
	Incontinent of urine and faeces	3

Mobility	Ambulant without aids in and out of doors	0
	Ambulant indoors with frame or stick or independent in wheelchair	1
	Requires help with outdoor mobility	2
	Requires help to transfer out of chair and/or pushing in wheelchair	3
Feeding	No problems	0
	Requires food to be cut up or a feeding programme	1
	Requires feeding	2
	Naso-gastric tube	3
Washing and dressing	No problems	0
	Requires verbal prompts only	1
	Requires physical assistance of one person	2
	Requires physical assistance of two persons	3

1 The National Adult Reading Test (Nelson and O'Connell, 1978); The Wechsler Adult Intelligence Scale (Wechsler, 1955).
2 Fragmented Letters, Silhouette Objects (Warrington and James, 1988); Dot Counting, Dot Centre (Warrington and Taylor, 1973).
3 Recognition Memory for Words and Faces (Warrington, 1984); Camden A Triple Choice Recognition Memory for Simple Pictures (Warrington, personal communication); Story Recall, Immediate and Delayed (Wechsler, 1945; Coughlan and Hollows, 1985); List Learning (Rey, 1964; Coughlan and Hollows, 1985); Complex Figure, Immediate and Delayed Recall (Osterreith and Rey, 1944; Coughlan and Hollows, 1985).
4 Weigl-Goldstein-Scheerer Colour-Form Sorting Task (Weigl, 1941); Modified Wisconsin Card Sorting Task (Nelson, 1976); Verbal Fluency (Miller, 1984); Bilateral Hand Movements (Luria, 1966); Proverb Interpretation (Luria, 1966); Cognitive Estimates (Shallice and Evans, 1978).

References

ALDERMAN, N. and WARD, A. 'Reduction of repetitive speech using response cost and cognitive overlearning and the dysexecutive syndrome'. (In preparation).

BAER, D., WOLF, M. and RISLEY, T., 1968, 'Some current dimensions of applied behaviour analysis'. *Journal of Applied Behaviour Analysis*, 1, 91–7.

BECK, A., 1976, *Cognitive therapy and emotional disorders* (New York: International Universities Press).

BELMONT, J. and BUTTERFIELD E., 1977, 'The instructional approach to developmental cognitive research'. In R. Kail and J. Hagen (Eds) *Perspectives on the development of memory and cognition* (New Jersey: Lawrence Erlbaum).

COUGHLAN, A. K. and HOLLOWS, S. E., 1985, *The adult memory and information processing battery* (Leeds: St James's University Hospital).

EAMES, P. G. and WOOD, R. Ll., 1985a, 'Rehabilitation after severe brain injury: A special unit approach to behaviour disorders'. *International Rehabilitation Medicine*, **7**, 130–3.

EAMES, P G. and WOOD, R Ll. 1985b, 'Rehabilitation after severe brain injury: a follow-up study of a behaviour modification approach'. *Journal of Neurology, Neurosurgery and Psychiatry*, **48**, 613–9.

ELLIS, A., 1962, *Reason and emotion in psychotherapy* (New York: Lyle Stuart Press).

JONES, R. R., VAUGHT, R. S. and WEINROTT, M., 1977, 'Time-series analysis in operant research'. *Journal of Applied Behaviour Analysis*, **10**, 151–66.

JONES R. T., OLLENDICK, T. H. and SHINSKE F. K., 1989, 'The role of behavioural versus cognitive variables in skill acquisition'. *Behaviour Therapy*, **20**, 293–302.

KEELEY, S., SHEMBERG, K. and CARBONELL, J., 1976, 'Operant clinical intervention: Behaviour management or beyond? Where are the data'. *Behaviour Therapy*, **7**, 292–305.

LEPPER, M. R., GEENE, D. and NISBETT, R. E., 1973, 'Undermining children's intrinsic interest with extrinsic reward: A test of the overjustification hypothesis'. *Journal of Personal and Social Psychology*, **31**, 479–86.

LEVINE, F. M. and FASNACHT, G., 1973, 'Token rewards may lead to token learning'. *American Psychologist*, **29**, 816–21.

LOWE, C. F. and HIGSON, P., 1981 'Self-instructional training and cognitive behaviour modification: A behavioural analysis'. In G. Davey (Ed.) *Applications of conditioning theory* (London: Methuen).

LOWE, C. F., HIGSON, P. J., BENTALL, R. P. and DEAN, P., 1979, 'Self-instructional training in schizophrenics: specific and generalised effectiveness'. *Paper presented at the Ninth European Congress of Behaviour Therapy, Paris.*

LURIA, A. R., 1966, *Higher cortical functions in man*, translated by B. Haigh (New York: Plenum Press).

MCLAUGHLIN, T. F., MABEE, W. S., BYRAM, B. J. and REITER, S. M., 1987, 'Effects of academic positive practice and response cost on writing legibility of behaviourally disordered and learning-disabled junior high school students. *Journal of Child and Adolescent Psychotherapy*, **4**, 216–21.

MEICHENBAUM, D., 1977, *Cognitive behaviour modification: An integrative approach* (New York: Plenum Press).

MEICHENBAUM, D. and CAMERON, J., 1973 'Training schizophrenics to talk to themselves: A means of developing attentional controls'. *Behaviour Therapy*, **4**, 515–34.

MILLER, E., 1984, 'Verbal fluency as a function of a measure of verbal intelligence and in relation to different types of cerebral pathology'. *British Journal of Clinical Psychology*, **23**, 52–7.

NELSON, H.E., 1976, 'A modified card sorting test sensitive to frontal lobe deficits'. *Cortex*, **12**, 313–24.

NELSON, H.E. and O'CONNELL, A., 1978, 'Dementia: The estimation of pre-morbid intelligence levels using the new adult reading test'. *Cortex*, **14**, 234–44.

OGILVIE, L. and PRIOR, M., 1982, 'Behaviour modification and the overjustification effect'. *Behavioural Psychotherapy*, **10**, 26–39.

OSTERREITH, P. and REY, A., 1944, 'Le test de copie d'une figure complexe'. *Archives de Psychologie*, **30**, 206–356.

PRIGITANO, G. P., 1985, *Neuropsychological rehabilitation after brain injury* (Baltimore: The Johns Hopkins Press Ltd).

PRIGITANO, G. P., FORDYCE, D. J., ZEINER, H. K., ROUECHE, J. R., PEPPING, M. and WOOD, B. C., 1984, 'Neuropsychological rehabilitation after closed head injury in young adults'. *Journal of Neurology, Neurosurgery and Psychiatry*, **47**, 505–13.

REY, A., 1964, *L'examen clinique en psychologie* (Paris: Presses Universitaires de France).

SHALLICE, T. and EVANS, M. E., 1978, 'The involvement of the frontal lobes in cognitive estimation'. *Cortex*, **14**, 294–303.

STERN, J. M., 1985, 'The quality of the psychotherapeutic process in brain-injured patients'. *Scandinavian Journal of Rehabilitation Medicine,* Supplement **12**, 42–3.

TEUBER, H. L. 1964, 'The riddle of frontal lobe functioning in man'. In J. M. Warren and K. Albert (Eds) *The frontal granular cortex and behaviour* (New York: McGraw-Hill).

TYRON, W. W., 1982, 'A simplified time-series analysis for evaluating treatment interventions'. *Journal of Applied Behaviour Analysis*, **15**, 423–9.

WARRINGTON, E. K., 1984, *Recognition memory test* (Windsor, Berks: NFER-Nelson Publishing Co. Ltd.).

WARRINGTON, E. K. and TAYLOR, A. M., 1973, 'The contribution of the right parietal lobe to object recognition'. *Cortex*, **9**, 152–64.

WARRINGTON, E. K. and JAMES, M. 1988, 'Visual apperceptive agnosia: A clinico-anatomical study of three cases'. *Cortex*, **24**, 13–32.

WECHSLER, D., 1945 'A standardised memory scale for clinical use'. *The Journal of Psychology*, **19**, 87–95.

WECHSLER, D., 1955, *Wechsler Adult Intelligence Scale* (New York: Psychological Corporation).

WEIGL, E., 1941, 'On the psychology of so-called processes of abstraction'. *Journal of Abnormal and Social Psychology*, **36**, 3–33.

WOOD, R. Ll., 1984, 'Behaviour disorders following severe brain injury: Their presentation and management'. In D. N. Brooks (Ed.) *Closed head injury: Psychological, social and family consequences* (Oxford: Oxford University Press).

WOOD, R. Ll., 1987, *Brain Injury Rehabilitation: A Neurobehavioural approach* (London: Croom Helm).

WOOD, R. Ll., 1988a, 'Management of behaviour disorders in a day treatment setting'. *Journal of Head Trauma Rehabilitation*, **3**, 53–61.

WOOD, R. Ll., 1988b, Clinical constraints affecting human conditioning. In G. Davey and C. Cullen (Eds) *Human operant conditioning and behaviour modification* (Chichester: John Wiley and Sons Ltd.).

WOOD, R. Ll., 1988c 'Attention disorders in brain injury rehabilitation'. *Journal of Learning Disabilities*, **21**, 327–51.

WOOD, R. Ll. and EAMES, P. G., 1981, 'Applications of behaviour modification in the rehabilitation of traumatically brain injured patients'. In G. Davey (Ed.) *Applications of conditioning theory* (London: Methuen).

WOOD, R. Ll. and BURGESS, P. W., 1988, 'The psychological management of behaviour disorders following brain injury'. In I. Fussey and G. M. Giles (Eds) *Rehabilitation of the severely brain injured adult: A practical approach* (London: Croom Helm).

WULFSOHN, D. and BARLING, J., 1978, 'Behavioural treatment of trichotillomania in an eleven year old girl'. *Psychology Reports*, **42**, 1171–4.

Chapter 11

Behavioral Learning Therapies for the Traumatically Brain-Injured Patient

C. A. Hopewell, W. H. Burke, M. Weslowski and R. Zawlocki

Many rehabilitation practitioners are now discovering that learning and behavioral principles may be applied to the challenge presented by 'cognitive rehabilitation'. This follows a decade during which practitioners failed to understand the necessity of behavioral analysis when trying to validate cognitive rehabilitation techniques. As a result, several faulty assumptions have been established within the rehabilitation community, one of the most erroneous being that cognitive rehabilitation results in some type of global improvement in the patient's condition. Of course, families really interpret this as the promise that their relative will 'get smarter', following which they will behave normally, and that cognitive difficulties will be either eliminated or ameliorated. Such an error is exemplified by assertions such as the following passage by Bracy (1985): 'The key, I think, is that Cognitive Rehabilitation has as its goal the reattainment (sic) of basic mental abilities or the acquisition of compensation skills for those mental abilities that cannot be retrained. Teaching daily living skills, educational information and other such skills is much needed with many patients, but these activities are not Cognitive Rehabilitation' (p. 2).

Such a faulty assumption contains at least three errors: Firstly, 'cognition' is erroneously separated from 'behavior', with the subsequent failure to realize that thoughts *are* behaviors, viz. covert verbally mediated behaviors. Secondly, mistaken treatment goals are pursued due to a faulty functional analysis of the barriers to rehabilitation. Although few would quarrel with goals of 'the acquisition of compensation skills for those mental abilities that cannot be retrained', in reality many therapists and, especially families, expect global mental improvement rather than the domain-specific acquisition of functional skills. This generally translates into simply 'memory retraining', or similar classroom-type activities which supposedly result in a global cognitive improvement, an error which is often due to this faulty functional analysis. And thirdly, a less stringent test of validity is generally applied than would be permissible with an adequate functional analysis of behavior and the resultant demonstrated behavioral validity of any given rehabilitation technique. For example, psychologists continue to debate the possibility of measurement of the 'reattainment of basic mental abilities'. If they are so difficult, or even impossible to measure, how could one ever realistically hope to validate such abilities?

Functional Analysis of the Barriers to Rehabilitation

Just as a functional analysis of behavior must be accomplished before the introduction of any learning paradigm, a functional analysis of the deficits encountered by the neuropsychologically impaired individual also must be performed. Rather than engaging in global 'cognitive rehabilitation', an appropriate domain-specific behavioral goal, such as making a bed or completing a social interaction without aggression, must be selected, and a functional analysis of the barriers precluding the successful making of beds or interaction must be performed. Only then can we hope both to specify a behavioral intervention as well as demonstrate its validity.

The current chapter will, therefore, review our assertion that (1) the actual and not the superficially perceived nature of the neuropsychological dysfunction or rehabilitation barriers should lead directly to a specific treatment strategy and (2) barriers to rehabilitation have often been identified which, in reality, are not the most formidable obstacles encountered. An argument will be pursued that only a proper, behavioral, functional analysis of rehabilitation barriers will give us the data needed to design specific treatment approaches. And, finally, the issue of generalization will be discussed.

Our experience leads us to assert that this type of analysis strongly suggests that cognitive remediation programs should be geared towards the executive and interpersonal deficits exhibited by the traumatically brain-injured (TBI) survivor. The analysis also suggests the overall paradigm which can be applied for the shaping of a particular behavior and also provides for the monitoring and any necessary adjustment to the conditions of learning. This chapter, therefore, may be to some extent viewed as a functional analysis of the cognitive behavioral deficits of the TBI survivor, a demonstration of the application of domain-specific retraining principles and a summary of the validity demonstration of a number of training projects. In order to illustrate these processes, a hospital-based outpatient as well as a residential post-acute program have been selected.

Memory Dysfunction as a Barrier to Rehabilitation

The cognitive, behavioral and personality consequences of TBI have been well documented and extensively researched in recent years (Prigatano, 1986; Ben–Yishay *et al.*, 1987; Prigatano *et al.*, 1987; Thomsen, 1987; Wood, 1987). However, in actual practice, many rehabilitation programs designed to enhance independence and productivity following TBI continue to focus largely upon memory dysfunction.

A canvassing of rehabilitation professionals at a major head-injury conference (Hopewell, 1987) also suggested that a significant number of rehabilitation therapists continue to view memory deficits as the most crippling of the cognitive dysfunctions, often specifically rating these disorders as creating more difficulty for the survivor than interpersonal or decision-making deficits. Hopewell's sample consisted of 45 rehabilitation therapists comprising a variety of professional disciplines, including nursing, occupational therapy, physical therapy, rehabilitation counselling, speech/language pathology and psychology. Of this group, 20% of the professionals rated memory impairment as the single most debilitating cognitive function, and 22% rated memory impairment as the second most crippling cognitive symptom seen after TBI. Therefore, 42% of the sample ranked memory deficits as among the two primary symptoms of TBI.

Compounding this frequent emphasis upon memory dysfunction as a primary rehabilitation barrier are the common and significant misconceptions families hold regarding TBI in general and memory dysfunction in particular (Gouvier *et al.*, 1988). Similarly, Michael Oddy and colleagues (1985) found that head-injured survivors generally complain of memory problems, most likely reinforcing this view of 'memory disorders' as the most disabling of the cognitive symptoms. And yet, how many patients would be expected to complain that 'I can't get along with people', 'I can't make decisions', or 'my judgement is bad'?

This state of affairs has very immediate and practical implications for the design of cognitive remediation programs. If memory impairment is considered to be the most important symptom to be addressed, treatment programs will necessarily be designed with the goal of memory improvement in mind. While laudable, this almost certainly leads to a relative neglect of the executive and interpersonal disorders.

The initiation of the cognitive remediation program at a hospital-based outpatient clinic may be considered as a typical example of such thinking. The program was originally based on a number of 'cognitive remediation modules' which were initially designed in the early 1980s. However, in the beginning of the program, these modules were applied in a rigid and inflexible manner, with classroom therapies being given mostly in a model similar to spinal cord services. This was obviously not the intent of the developers of such modules, and yet this represented a stage in the development of a new remediation program by a young staff eager to begin working with TBI survivors.

In the initial training groups, much emphasis was placed on the remediation of patients' 'memory disorders', with a concomitant reliance upon computers and memory training. As staff gained experience and were able to observe clients directly on job trials, the emotional and behavioral deficiencies, which were considerably more important in terms of vocational and community failure, rapidly became apparent. As the program developed and as staff gained experience, memory facilitation was still considered important, but increasing emphasis was placed upon the behavioral training of social and emotional competence within the workplace and the community. Clients moved much earlier into job trials and stayed there longer, and staff eventually spent most of their time training and shaping behavioral competence. The result of this change in program emphasis was a significant improvement in job placement as well as increasingly acceptable patient outcomes for the program.

An analysis of job-trial performances for the first 34 clients served through the program supported our clinical impression that memory dysfunction by itself rarely (actually never) accounted for vocational failure and that emotional and behavioral competence was much more critical for success. Standard rating forms were used by the vocational coordinator, with behavioral samples taken on a fixed interval schedule. Results of these samplings were combined with standard rating forms used by job supervisors. The results of these analyses indicated the following rankings, from those symptoms most related to job-trial failure to those least responsible:

1 Poor judgement/self-monitoring
2 Can't get along with others/psychomotor retardation (equal rating)
3 Defective problem solving and organizational skills
4 Erratic attendance
5 Defective memory/poor stress tolerance (equal rating)

With data such as these, staff were able to see empirically that memory dysfunction *per se* was rarely related to job-trial failure and quickly modified the overall program to address executive and behavioral dysfunctions.

Executive Dysfunctions as Barriers to Rehabilitation

Impairment of the higher cerebral functions or the executive system (initiation, planning, problem solving, self-regulation) has received little attention in the literature, and yet these are the very functions which we consider to interfere most significantly with independent and productive functioning (Lezak, 1983; Prigatano, 1986; Thomsen, 1987). The executive functions of the human brain are mostly, although not exclusively, associated with the frontal lobes, areas which are easily damaged in TBI (Stuss, 1987). Indeed, data from the programs presented here indicate that rehabilitation failure is almost always associated, at least to some degree, with executive and interpersonal difficulties.

Executive functioning is described as the ability to engage in independent, purposeful, self-directed and self-serving behavior (Luria, 1966, 1973; Lezak, 1983). To differentiate the executive system from cognitive functioning, Lezak (1983) noted that cognitive impairment usually implies a specific functional deficit, while executive function affects all aspects of one's life.

Deficits in executive functions are often not immediately apparent in casual conversation. Frequently, persons with disorders of executive function appear cognitively intact (Vogenthaler, 1987). Such patients generally perform well on neurological, as well as neuropsychological, examination, especially when provided with a structured setting (Lezak, 1982, 1983; Prigatano, 1986; Vogenthaler, 1987). Students, in particular, may function adequately in school settings as these are highly structured. The seriousness of the executive deficits become apparent only after graduation when the (former) students subsequently fail to make a successful transition to the roles required of them as adults. At this point, the young adult's inability to direct and regulate behavior seriously interferes with community adjustment.

Disorders of executive function are generally manifested by emotional lability, irritability, rigidity, apathy, defective behavioral initiation, carelessness, poor judgement and inappropriate social behavior. Lezak (1983) has described the problem as a serious impairment in the starting, switching and stopping of behavior. This results in a decrease in spontaneous behavior, productivity, initiative and self-control, while at the same time increasing perseveration, impulsiveness and disinhibition. Executive function can be conceptualized as consisting of four primary areas (Lezak, 1983):

1 Formulating goals
2 Planning/problem solving
3 Carrying out the plan
4 Effective performance.

Luria (1973) stated that all human activity begins with an intention directed toward a goal. When our ability to conceptualize our desires and needs before acting is impaired, the result is impulsive action with little thought of the potential consequences or automatic and perseverative responses to environmental stimuli. The individual with executive dysfunction is often unable to formulate goals. It just does not occur to the patient to do anything, and this results in an inability to initiate action. Many clients with executive dysfunction are capable of performing a task but will not engage in the activity unless directed in a step-by-step manner.

Planning requires an ability to generate alternatives, consider the consequences of those alternatives, make an appropriate choice and develop a framework or cognitive map to direct the activity. In addition, the capacity to sustain attention and to view oneself and the environment objectively are critical to effective planning and problem solving (Goldstein, 1942; Lezak, 1983; Prigatano, 1986). The inability to initiate a plan is often described as a decrease or absence of motivation. The client is referred to as lazy, emotionally disturbed or malingering (Lezak, 1978, 1983) when, in fact, the individual lacks the ability to identify the sequential steps to plan an activity. These individuals are often impulsive when solving problems. They act immediately without analyzing options and often select the same option, regardless of the problem at hand. They perseverate and apply the same poor solution that leads to further failure. These individuals are virtually immobilized by their inability to plan and effectively solve problems.

Translating an intention or plan into a productive and purposeful activity requires the ability to initiate, switch and stop action in an orderly fashion. The lack of initiative is a frequent complaint from families of patients. The TBI survivors must be told what to do because they lack the cognitive skills to know how or when to carry out goal-directed activity (Prigatano, 1986). On neuropsychological examinations, Prigatano (1986) notes that these individuals demonstrate deficits in abstract reasoning. The cognitive skills required to carry out complex action are not present. In structured settings, they do what they are told but again become immobilized when left to self-direction.

To interact successfully with the environment an individual requires the ability to self-correct and self-regulate behavior. Individuals with executive dysfunction often do not perceive their mistakes, are impaired in the processing of social cues (Jackson and Hopewell, 1988) and thus do nothing to correct their behavior. They can often discuss their errors but still do nothing to remedy them. These individuals frequently lack awareness of their strengths and deficits, resulting in unrealistic self-appraisals, which is demonstrated in their failure to perceive performance errors. They fail to perceive or to understand social cues and are therefore unable to be self-critical (Lezak, 1983; Luria, 1966). Such deficits make it difficult for these patients to profit from experience (Lezak, 1978). Frequently, TBI survivors will misinterpret social situations and feedback and do not understand the consequences of their behavior. This decreased ability to self-regulate behavior often results in socially inappropriate remarks and actions, a condition often referred to as 'disinhibition syndrome'.

The disinhibited TBI survivor will act before thinking. Such patients often express exactly what they think, regardless of the appropriateness of the situation, are frequently demanding and are noncompliant with rules or schedules. The appearance of aggressive outbursts is simply the end result of a chain of behaviors which begins with poor perception of social cues and is maintained and exacerbated by poor judgement, faulty behavioral goal-direction and defective monitoring and self-correction.

An individual's inability to formulate goals, develop plans, carry out those plans and monitor and regulate goal-directed behavior will result in certain failure in the community. Impairments of these higher cerebral functions almost always result in the the TBI survivor being judged as incompetent to live or work in the community. In addition, these deficits often lead to social isolation and a lack of social support systems as friends and family become less tolerant of the individual's behavior (Brooks, 1984). The present challenge in head injury rehabilitation is to develop effective strategies to enhance executive system functioning, thus making community living and gainful employment a realistic goal for these individuals. Since executive dysfunction results in difficulty in interpersonal relationships, we have focused our treatment primarily upon social competence training and, secondarily, upon functional activity training and generalization skills.

Social Competence Training

Methods of Training

To meet the challenge presented by remediation of executive and personality dysfunction by means of behavioral intervention, a series of training steps was developed and a residential program for severe TBI survivors was implemented. Functional analyses of behavioral deficits were performed by an evaluation team; training strategies were applied, and behavioral interventions validated. The subsequent description of the training program illustrates these interventions.

The following steps are offered as a sequence in both individual and group sessions:

1 The trainer should first present the control technique in a didactic manner and then model the implementation.

2 Simulate an actual conflict incident so that the client can practice each alternative response to a given stimulus (behavioral rehearsal).

3 Use peer models and actual authority figures in these practice role-playing sessions to enhance generalization of skills by providing closer approximations to actual stimuli.

4 Use the 'barb' technique, which provides unplanned, intensive, aversive stimulation and enactment of powerful situations, such as encounters with police officers. This should only be instituted after the client has learned to handle mild stimuli.

The 'barb' technique entails the gradual presentation of specific provocative statements to the client, while decreasing warnings or prompts to 'get ready'. For example, a client who reliably responds with anger to statements about 'his mother' would receive these provocations repeatedly in order to inoculate him to the intensity of this provoking stimulus and enable him to display increasing self-control.

Clients usually enjoy role-playing, conflict situations, but at times, certain teaching aids may be necessary. The trainers or other group members may need to coach or prompt a client during role plays. Some impulsive clients also require extra visual cues in order to decide which coping strategy to employ and when to implement that strategy. Flashcards presented by the trainer during role plays provide a cueing procedure that prompts the client to review an alternative response repertoire.

Sequential worksheets are also useful in helping a client understand the antecedent, response and consequence components of a given situation.

At this point, one could begin to videotape the role play and replay it to the clients. During the feedback, clients are asked to identify the problem-solving steps and to rate each other's performance as being aggressive, appropriately assertive or passive. Videotaping is helpful in such a process, although we suggest that a specific sequence be followed. First, a very positive tape section is selected and viewed in private by only the client and the therapist. This allows reinforcement, clarification of communication and prevents, or at least minimizes, embarrassment. Next, more problematic sections are viewed alone by client and therapist. Subsequently, positive sections are viewed by members of the group, and lastly, problematic vignettes are viewed and commented upon by the therapy group. A variant which both maintains the interest of the clients and provides training is to use film or videotape clips of emotional scenes from well-known movies, such as the farewell scene from *Casablanca* (Paul Deutsch, personal communication).

Finally, transfer of training must be programmed in any social competence training program. Treatment techniques that enhance generalization of behavior change include homework assignments, prompting the use of self-control skills in a variety of problem situations, e.g. academic, recreational, dating and family situations.

These homework assignments require the client to practice each skill between training sessions and to document this practice in some fashion. For example, the clients may be directed to generate three contingency statements incorporated into the thinking-ahead procedure and to use these statements in three problem situations. If clients continue to self-monitor social situations, these new responses can readily be recorded. Other homework assignments include twice-weekly practice of relaxation, observation of another's social cues, listing of coping statements to use before a conflict situation or the use of the 'broken record' technique in a peer and a family situation. Completion of such concrete assignments has been demonstrated to facilitate transfer of training to natural environments (Feindler *et al.*, 1986).

It is also useful to establish simple cues for self-control, such as 'keep cool' stickers placed on a notebook or a pocketbook easily transferred across environments. *In vivo* role plays, in which persons provoking anger in the client are prompted in order to reinforce increased self-control as well as follow-up booster sessions, should also aid long-term maintenance of behavior change. Furthermore, each client in the training program should receive systematic preparation for non-reinforcement or punishment of increased self-control. Changes in clients as a result of this training program may very well not be supported in a natural environment and may, in fact, result in increased social inappropriateness by others. Preparatory role plays and the application of relevant coping statements will serve to strengthen the individual's self-regulatory responses in these situations.

Role plays in which a client, responding in a controlled manner, ignores the teasing of a peer and in return is ridiculed by other clients for being a 'wimp' should be conducted toward the end of training. Self-statements relative to the client's increased self-control and reprisals of other clients' teasing will be instrumental in maintaining appropriate responses in such situations. Other potential problem situations involve loss of 'macho' status, increased hostility from others, loss of property, physical danger, teasing, ridicule and failure to obtain desired outcomes or reinforcers immediately. Preparing the client to deal with these sometimes harsh punishers through behavioral rehearsal and self-evaluative statements will certainly help to promote generalization and maintenance of training.

Some clients may be reluctant to participate in the program and to change ways of responding. It is critical to have clients voluntarily consent to participate in treatment and to involve them in the planning of in-session role-plays and homework assignments. This initial commitment may be prompted through a discussion of the negative consequences for out-of-control behavior. The examples of short-term and long-term punishers, such as frequent school detentions, suspensions, extra assignments, loss of privileges, possible incarceration, not getting dates or repeated court contacts, may prompt a desire to control behavior.

The potential reduction of aggressive behavior provides the primary source of resistance. For certain cultures and environments, aggression may be adaptive. It may be helpful to 'sell' social competence training as a way to increase self-control, control of others and personal power.

Impulsive clients are often the targets of others' manipulation or teasing, since they respond quickly and reliably to provocation. The notion of being 'harder to get' or of having self-control and detachment can be presented as an enhancement to the client's powerful self-image. Finally, resistance and lack of cooperation may be circumvented by providing some tangible reinforcers for participation in training sessions and completion of homework assignments. Free time, leaving early, learning to work the videotape equipment or roles as actors in the role-played scenes are all potential reinforcers that can be employed to maintain attention to and encourage participation in the group.

Session Content

The protocols by which social competence training was conducted in this investigation called for 12 sessions, two sessions per week. Sessions were conducted individually or in groups of no more than four clients. The content of each session is delineated below:

Session one

The introductory session includes a discussion of the program rationale and nature of the training program. Some impulse delay techniques (e.g. taking deep breaths, counting backward and pleasant imagery) are introduced. The use of time-delay techniques are role played in situations in which the client feels uncomfortable. Homework is generally assigned after each session.

Session two

Self-monitoring is introduced. A special sheet is given to all clients so that they can get an accurate picture of how they handle various conflict situations between sessions. The sheet provides identification of antecedents provoking the behavior, as well as consequent events. The sheet also provides a self-rating of the way conflict situations are handled. Staff are provided with these sheets so that if a client enters a situation where the sheet should have been used but was not, the staff member can give the client the recording sheet and prompt him or her to fill it out.

Session three

Based on the self-recording sheets filled out since the last session, the client is instructed in the identification of those situation variables (both indirect/direct and covert/overt) that generally trigger inappropriate responses. Although deep muscle relaxation may not be an appropriate response in most social situations, some clients who evidence anxiety and agitation readily respond to increasing their control of physiological arousal. A number of relaxation techniques are practiced.

Session four

Problem-solving strategies are introduced, and such training aids the client in identifying the problem situation, enumerating and evaluating alternative solutions. Each problem-solving skill (problem specification, enumerating alternative responses, listing consequences for each response and rank ordering alternatives, implementing an alternative and evaluating the outcome) is presented verbally to the client with accompanying examples from typical work and family social situations. Verbal rehearsal of these skills, accompanied by prompting analysis of numerous relevant problem situations and the identification of each component step, teaches the client to conceptualize problems in this sequenced manner and to use these skills to guide overt responding.

Sessions five and six

Clients' rights and rights of others are discussed and assertion techniques are introduced. If a possible skill deficiency in assertion and problem solving is assumed, then appropriate verbal and non-verbal assertive responses designed to replace inappropriate responding must be taught concurrently with self-control skills. Observations during role playing and videotape feedback of brief conflict scenes help to identify the successes and deficiencies in the verbal and non-verbal components of assertive and aggressive responding. Through behavior rehearsal of conflict scenes, behaviors, such as direct eye contact, appropriate gestures, modulated tone of voice and request for another's behavior change, replace inappropriate behaviors, such as staring, threatening gestures, a harsh tone and demands. A reduction in the use of threatening body posture or in voice volume, for example, may result in others perceiving a client as socially competent and as providing fewer provoking stimuli.

Techniques, such as the 'broken record', which involves calm repetition of the client's original request or assertion until the problem is solved; 'fogging', which entails agreement with another's direct criticism in such a manner as to confuse the other; and 'minimal effective response', which entails a gradual escalation of assertive demands beginning with the least forceful and ending with a direct command, can all be modelled and practiced through role plays of interpersonal conflicts along with videotape feedback. Teaching common assertion techniques detailed in other sources will broaden a client's repertoire and enable him or her to obtain desirable reinforcers in a more appropriate manner.

Sessions seven and eight

The client is trained in self-instruction with specific focus on the use of reminders, such as 'stop and think', 'I am going to ignore this guy and keep my cool', and 'chill out', to guide behavior, for self-control and to remember certain things. The client is prompted to generate a list of reminders that could be used in various social situations. The therapist models appropriate ways of using the technique and then role play them with the client. Training begins with the therapist and client using overt statements, then whispering these statements and then finally using the statements covertly. Overall, a self-instruction sequence seems most effective if it (1) includes the inhibition of the first impulsive response of the client, (2) enumerates and guides the selection of alternative responses to provoking stimuli and (3) connects the verbalizations with subsequent behavior.

Some clients require visual cues, such as self-statements on index cards or specific signals from the therapist, in the early stages of covert rehearsal of the self-instruction procedure. A six-step coping strategy is as follows: (1) Recognition of problem situations in one's history, (2) preparation for such events through self-instruction to remain calm, (3) continuation of self-instruction to remain calm when actually confronting the problem, (4) use of autonomic responses as cues to employ coping skills to reduce the intensity of feeling (e.g. relaxation, backward counting, pleasant imagery), (5) exhibition of an assertive response and (6) self-reinforcement for effectively handling the situation.

Sessions nine and ten

The 'thinking-ahead procedure', which involves the use of self-instructions and problem solving to estimate future negative consequences for inappropriate behavior in conflict situations, is introduced. First, an outline must be made of a range of predictable punishers for an inappropriate behavior, from least to most severe. Next, the client is given self-contingency statements, such as 'if I (misbehave) now, then I will get (future negative consequences)', and is asked to complete the statement by inserting a frequent inappropriate behavior and one of the negative consequences resulting from it.

After practicing the generation of these contingency statements, generalizations to specific social situations are then made explicit. The therapist can prompt recollection of recent problem situations in which the client exhibited a specific inappropriate response and received a specific negative consequence. Some imagery training designed to increase attention to actual parameters of the eventual punishing stimulus may also be helpful in these sessions.

Session eleven

Self-evaluation training is introduced. Basically, self-evaluation responses are reminders which occur after a problem situation and provide immediate feedback on behavior occurring during a given problem situation. Self-recording sheets from the clients and various coping statements used by the client before, during and after both the solved and unresolved problem situations are discussed and role played.

Session twelve

The procedures taught during the program are reviewed. The therapist may use a question and answer format along with role playing. This session may be repeated with individuals or small groups as often as is deemed necessary.

Validity of the Training Program

To measure the impact of social competence training alone, we measured five pre-/post-test measures, four prosocial behaviors and five inappropriate behaviors over a period of 35 weeks. The pre-/post-dependent measures were:

1 A videotaped 44-item test of social competence (Freedman *et al.*, 1978)
2 The Matching Familiar Figures Test
3 Latency to complete the Matching Familiar Figures Test
4 The Porteus Maze Test
5 The latency to complete the Porteus Maze Test.

The only one of these dependent measures to show significance from the pre-test to the post-test was in the Porteus Maze Test ($t = 2.55$, $df = 11, 1$; $p < .05$), perhaps again demonstrating the difficulty in achieving or measuring any global cognitive changes.

The functional behavioral measurements demonstrated much more clearly the effect of the training period. Inspection of the data collected daily for the four prosocial behaviors (accepting criticism, accepting 'no' for an answer, ignoring peer misbehavior, disagreeing appropriately) and five inappropriate behaviors (physical aggression, threats, unauthorized absences, teasing, inappropriate contact) showed a general trend of increasing of prosocial and decreasing of inappropriate behavior over the 35-week period.

Figure 11.1 shows that during the six-week baseline, there was an average of 36.4 occurrences of inappropriate behavior and an average of 22.7 occurrences of prosocial behavior among the seven clients monitored. Maladaptive behavior decreased to a mean of 24.2 per week during training, while prosocial behaviors decreased to a mean of 19.3 per week. During the eleven-week follow-up period, prosocial behaviors increased to a mean of 31.3 per week and inappropriate behaviors decreased to a mean of 2.7 per week. The data in Figure 11.1 show that there was an unequivocal effect on behavior as a result of social competence training, and that these effects were maintained well beyond the training period; there was a significant decrease in inappropriate behavior and a substantial increase in prosocial behavior on an ongoing basis.

On the surface, why should clients demonstrate an initial decrease in both inappropriate and prosocial behaviors and then, apparently paradoxically, show evidence of a continuing decline in inappropriate behavior while prosocial actions become more frequent? While such a phenomenon needs further investigation, it may be that a substantial decrease in inappropriate behavior may be all that the client can manage at the beginning of training and that other behavioral changes may be simply 'too much to handle' at the time of program initiation. Also, the development of prosocial behavior is very much dependent upon a decrease in inappropriate behaviors,

Figure 11.1 Mean frequencies of inappropriate and prosocial behaviors.

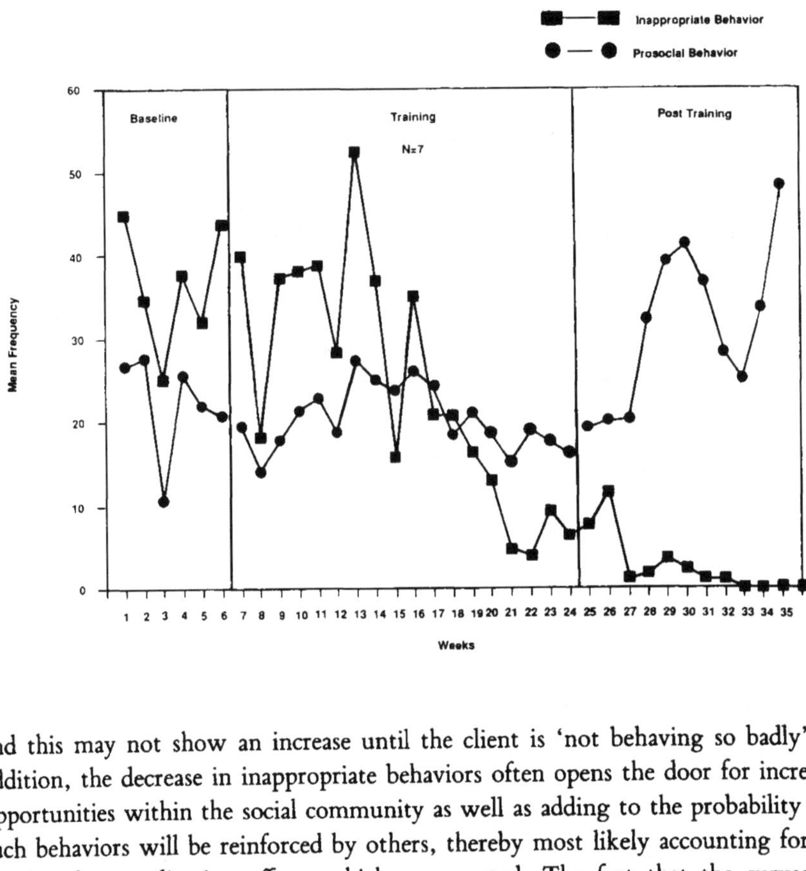

and this may not show an increase until the client is 'not behaving so badly'. In addition, the decrease in inappropriate behaviors often opens the door for increased opportunities within the social community as well as adding to the probability that such behaviors will be reinforced by others, thereby most likely accounting for the continued generalization effects which were noted. The fact that the curves for prosocial and inappropriate behaviors begin to separate in a significant sense at about week 20 may also suggest that training needs to be continued for a certain critical time period, and that failure of training may occur if therapy is terminated too quickly, or if the client or trainer 'give up too soon'.

The failure to find significant differences in the pre-/post-test measures while the behavioral charting clearly indicates improvement and generalization in a number of domain-specific behaviors, again supports the assertion that pertinent behavioral goals rather than the reacquisition of basic mental abilities are generally the targets of choice for rehabilitation programs dealing with TBI survivors.

Functional Activities Training

Should social and emotional competence training stop with the formal therapeutic approach, and reinforcement subsequently be automatically expected from the social community? Difficulties with executive and interpersonal functioning form at least part of the basis for a remediation approach known as Functional Activities Training (Lewis *et al.*, 1987). The Social Competence Training Program, as outlined above, leads naturally into a Functional Activities Program for clients who are able to participate. In this type of training, little emphasis is placed on 'classroom' therapies. Instead, a variety of functional activities are coordinated with an interdisciplinary staff and several trainees. For example, a functional activity may involve the production of a variety of flower boxes for sale or use in a town beautification project. Although the activity may have a vocational component, it should be emphasized that this is not primarily an occupational project, nor is it a supported employment setting. Rather, staff identify problem behaviors which present barriers to the completion of the functional activity and continually train social, emotional and executive competence in a naturalistic setting. The repeated overlearning of such functions helps to generalize competence as survivors move into real employment, supported employment or community activities.

In conjunction with the theorem that 'idle hands the Devil's playground make', Functional Activities Training also provides a powerful reciprocal inhibition paradigm in which engagement in the functional activity automatically inhibits inappropriate behavior. We have found that identification of the salient barriers to rehabilitation through a functional analysis of behavior and behavioral paradigms, such as those described along with a Functional Activities Training approach, have resulted in a significantly improved outcome to the cognitive retraining of our TBI survivors. At the same time, this approach offers the only way in which behavioral change may be adequately measured and training methods validated.

Summary

Learning theorists well know that principles of learning may not only be naturally applied to the problems faced by survivors of traumatic brain injury, but that such applications are inevitable. They would also assert that such a scientific application of behavioral methodology is the only way in which the validity of any given technique of cognitive remediation can be validated. The failure to understand this necessity has led to several faulty assumptions within the rehabilitation community. First, 'cognition' is erroneously separated from 'behavior'. Secondly, mistaken treatment goals are pursued due to a faulty functional analysis of the barriers to rehabilitation. And thirdly, less stringent tests of validity are generally applied than would be permissible with an adequate functional analysis of behavior and a resultant demonstrated behavioral validity of any given rehabilitation technique.

Our experience at this point strongly suggests that cognitive remediation programs should be geared toward the executive and interpersonal deficits exhibited by the TBI survivor and that domain-specific skills be addressed. This chapter, therefore, may be viewed as a functional analysis of the cognitive behavioral deficits of the TBI survivor, a demonstration of the application of domain-specific retraining principles and a summary of the valid demonstrations of a number of training projects.

References

BEN-YISHAY, SILVER, S. M., PIASETSKY, E. and RATTOCK, J., 1987, 'Relationship between employability and vocational outcome after intensive holistic cognitive rehabilitation'. *Journal of Head Trauma Rehabilitation*, **2**, 35–48.

BRACY, O., 1985, *Cognitive Rehabilitation*, **3**(5), 2.

BROOKS, D. N. (Ed.), 1984, *Closed head injury: Psychological social and family consequences* (Oxford: Oxford University Press).

FEINDLER, E. L., ECTON, R. B., KINGSLEY, D. and DUBEY, D. R., 1986, 'Group anger-control training for institutionalized psychiatric male adolescents'. *Behavior Therapy*, **17**, (2), 109–24.

FREEDMAN, B. J., ROSENTHAL, L., DONAHOE, C. P., SCHLUNDT, D. G. and MCFALL, R. M., 1978, 'A social-behavioral analysis of skill deficits in delinquent and nondelinquent adolescent boys'. *Journal of Consulting and Clinical Psychology*, **46**, 1448–62.

GOLDSTEIN, K., 1942, *After effects of brain injury in war* (New York: Grune and Stratton).

GOUVIER, W. D., PRESTHOLD, P. H. and WARNER, M. S., 1988, 'A survey of common misconceptions about head injury and recovery'. *Archives of Clinical Neuropsychology*, **3**, 331–43.

JACKSON, H. F. and HOPEWELL, C. A., 1988, 'Personality and emotional disorders following brain injury'. Presented at the *3rd Annual Symposium on Advances in Head Injury Rehabilitation, Dallas, Texas*.

LEWIS, F. D., BURKE, W. H. and CARILLO, R., 1987, 'Model for rehabilitation of head injured adults in the post acute setting'. *Journal of Applied Rehabilitation Counselling*, **18**(2), 39–45.

LEZAK, M. D., 1978, 'Living with the characterologically altered brain injured patient'. *Journal of Clinical Psychiatry*, **39**(7), 592–8.

LEZAK, M. D., 1982, 'The problem of assessing executive function'. *International Journal of Psychology*, **17**, 281–97.

LEZAK, M. D., 1983, *Neuropsychological assessment*, 2nd Ed. (New York: Oxford University Press).

LURIA, A. R., 1966, *Higher cortical functions in man* (New York: Basic Books).

LURIA, A. R., 1973, *The working brain: An introduction to neuropsychology* (New York: Basic Books).

ODDY, M., HUMPHREY, M. and UTTLEY, D., 1978, 'Stresses upon the relatives of head injury patients'. *British Journal of Psychiatry*, **133**, 507–13.

ODDY, M., COUGHLAN, T., TYERMAN, A. and JENKINS, D., 1985, 'Social adjustment after closed head injury: A further follow-up seven years after injury'. *Journal of Neurology, Neurosurgery and Psychiatry*, **48**, 564–8.

PRIGATANO, G. P., 1986, *Neuropsychological rehabilitation after brain injury* (Baltimore: Johns Hopkins University Press).

PRIGATANO, G. P., 1987, 'Personality and psychosocial consequences after brain injury'. In M. Meier, A. Benton and L. Diller (Eds.), *Neuropsychological rehabilitation* (New York: Guilford Press).

STUSS, D. T., 1987, 'The neuropsychology of the frontal lobes'. *BNI Quart.*, **3**(1), 28–33.

THOMSEN, I. V., 1987, 'Late psychosocial outcome in severe blunt head trauma'. *Brain Injury*, **1**(2), 131–43.

VOGENTHALER, D. R., 1987, 'An overview of head injury: its consequences and rehabilitation'. *Brain Injury*, **1**, 113–27.

WOOD, R. L., 1987, *Brain injury rehabilitation, a neurobehavioral approach* (Rockville, Maryland: Aspen Publishers).

PART 6
CONCLUDING REMARKS

Chapter 12

Evaluating the Status of Cognitive Rehabilitation

I. Fussey

The preface to this volume offered what, in our opinion, are the minimal criteria for any clinical discipline of cognitive rehabilitation. These criteria seem a useful way of evaluating the status of cognitive rehabilitation at this time because while the chapters in this volume attempt to meet these criteria, the general approach to cognitive rehabilitation remains fragmented and there remains some confusion over exactly what cognitive rehabilitation is.

The danger with the phrase 'cognitive rehabilitation' is that it gives a misleading picture as to the target of the intervention. To attempt to rehabilitate 'cognition' is to approach a highly complex set of interactions, the nature of which, even in the normally functioning brain, is still unclear. It appears far more useful to consider the target of rehabilitation as the skill or activity to be developed and construct a rehabilitation programme in the light of what is known about the individual's injury, and therefore optimum learning style. This would appear to be in agreement with Butler and Namerow (1988) who advocate a skills training approach and criticize cognitive remediation on the grounds that its general efficacy has not been demonstrated.

Sohlberg and Mateer (1989) suggest that the aim of cognitive rehabilitation is to provide 'therapy methods that actually retrain or alleviate problems caused by deficits in attention, visual processing, language, memory, reasoning/problem solving and executive functions' (p. 4). They follow Goldstein and Ruthven (1983) in proposing that the aim should be to provide rational rehabilitation in that methods should take account of brain–behaviour relationships and address specific goals which, in turn, should be amenable to research or outcome studies. It may be argued that one should be even more explicit when considering the specific aims and suggest that they have some ecological validity for the patient, thus avoiding too narrow a focus when formulating goals (for example, learning word lists or associations, a practice still widely accepted but quite inadequate as far as life skills are concerned). In summary, the aims of cognitive rehabilitation should be to retrain or alleviate the problems arising from the cognitive legacy of the injury, in terms of the constraints upon thinking and activities of daily living.

There appear to be two emerging schools of thought in the field of cognitive rehabilitation. On the one hand we have Mateer and co-workers (e.g. Sohlberg and Mateer, 1987; Mateer *et al.*, Chapter 4, this volume) training information-processing skills that underlie cognitive processes, that is, they approach rehabilitation at the substrate or foundations of cognition. On the other hand, we have Diller and Gordon (1981) and others (e.g. Gross and Schutz, 1986; Wood, 1987) proposing models which concentrate on defining a behaviour to be acquired and then using skills-building techniques to achieve that aim. While approaching cognitive rehabilitation differently, these schools of thought are similar in that they are both using procedural learning to achieve their goals. It may be useful here to clarify the distinction between procedural learning and declarative learning. Procedural learning forms the basis of any learned physical activity in which a skill is acquired slowly through practice or rehearsal. Procedural learning specifies the conditions under which an action or behaviour pattern is elicited. Declarative learning, however, describes relationships between events in the individual's world and tries to improve understanding by increasing awareness of these event relationships (see Wood, 1990, for a detailed description).

In so far as a declarative approach to learning provides an important framework for understanding principles, acquiring information and applying knowledge, one may question why both the main schools of thought in cognitive rehabilitation noted above are not applying what appears to be the learning paradigm with the greatest potential for learning new skills and generalization. One answer would appear to lie in the fact that both schools describe cognitive rehabilitation with severe cases and therefore recognize that the choice of learning paradigm is dependent upon the nature of the brain injury. Even so, there are workers in the field of cognitive rehabilitation using declarative learning. For example, Prigatano *et al.* (1984) described a rehabilitation programme for young adults with closed head injury in which the major themes of treatment included increased awareness and acceptance of the injury and residual deficits, together with intensive cognitive retraining of selected residual deficits. In some respects, a treatment programme that aims to increase awareness and 'insight' is using cognitive therapy and therefore relying heavily on intact frontal lobes, in the same way that Cicerone (1989) used psychotherapeutic interventions with traumatically brain-injured patients. The description, cognitive therapy, is used here advisedly to highlight the danger of taking terms from various disciplines and using them out of the appropriate context, for as Sohlberg and Mateer (1989) pointed out, labels, such as cognitive therapy and cognitive rehabilitation, are used interchangeably by some professionals, but to others they denote quite different principles.

Clinical psychologists especially will be aware of the historical division between cognitive therapy and behaviour therapy, that is, to either change the way patients think or to change the way they behave; unfortunately, the division creates an illusion of choice between the two. However, Ellis (1984) argued that humans are so uniquely involved in cognitive processes that they continually use them to instigate or change their emotional and behavioural reactions. When they feel and behave, they almost always have some thoughts about their feelings and actions; and these thoughts lead them to have other feelings, and possibly, further behaviours. Dryden (1984) followed Ellis (1962) in believing that the outward display of behaviour cannot be considered separately from intrinsic actions, such as sensing, thinking and emotional experience. Furthermore, he considered that the most efficient way of effecting lasting behavioural change is for people to change their thinking. However, if the concepts of cognitive therapy are to be introduced into a model of cognitive rehabilitation, it is questionable whether the severely brain injured can utilize the technique if, as would appear from neuropsychological evidence, they cannot control their thinking. Even so, those familiar with Ellis' work will see the similarities between the emphasis he placed upon thinking and its relationship with behaviour, and the work of Luria (1961) involving verbal mediation of behaviour.

It is suggested that verbal regulation or verbal self-regulation, can be used to assist cognitive processing following brain injury. We also know from the work of Ellis that cognitive self-statements are used to govern the relationships between an outside stimulus and a behavioural response. It is interesting to note that verbal self-regulation used in cognitive rehabilitation after brain injury has a parallel in the assessment of cognitive 'self-statements' used in other therapeutic areas, notably the treatment of anxiety or depressive disorders. In this area, one of the difficulties in restructuring cognitive self-statements is the apparent difficulty people have in recognizing not only the nature but the very existence of the self-statement. In the same way that the brain-injured individual is asked to verbalize the instruction to govern behaviour (or suppress behaviour), then so, too, in cognitive therapy the individual is required to verbalize the restructured self-statement. Is this perhaps too complex an aim for the severely brain injured? However, the chapters by Burgess and Alderman (Chapter 9) and Alderman and Burgess (Chapter 10) suggest that, if used appropriately, such approaches may have merit.

We can distinguish three different ways in which the concept of cognition is used; namely, as a cognitive event, as cognitive processes and as cognitive structures. Cognitive events refer to conscious, identifiable thoughts and images. Meichenbaum (1977) described such cognitive events as a form of internal dialogue that takes place when the automaticity of one's behaviour is interrupted. When considering this, however, it is obvious that individuals do not go about talking to themselves. Their behaviour is apparently automatic, although under certain conditions, conscious processes can come into play. For example, when individuals have to act in uncertain or novel situations, they tend to talk to themselves.

As Goldfried *et al.* (1974) have indicated, because of the habitual nature of one's expectations and beliefs, it is likely that thinking processes become automatic and seemingly involuntary, like most over-learned acts. The principles of therapy would be to help an individual become aware of such thought processes and increase the likelihood that, in future, s/he will notice and change the internal dialogue in order to effect behavioural change. Again, problems of control and lack of insight would appear to be incompatible with a cognitive rehabilitation process that relies heavily upon insight and awareness, especially in the severely brain injured.

In many cases, the individual's cognitive events may be symbolic as well as verbal. As we have already suggested, the nature and content of such cognitive events can influence how one both feels and behaves. Sarason (1975) suggested that individuals can report a variety of self-defeating or interfering thoughts and feelings, and he furthermore believed that engaging in such self-defeating thoughts and feelings is likely to lead to less than optimal performance, further increasing a possibly already high level of behavioural dysfunction.

A second way in which the concept of cognition is used considers cognitive processes. This refers to the way we unconsciously process information, and such processes shape mental representations and schemata. Personal knowledge of such cognitive processes and the ability to control them represent meta-cognition, which provides an interface between that which is normally out of conscious awareness and that which is accessible to assessment, research and training.

Cognitive structures can be thought of as schemata that are implicit or operate at an unconscious level, are highly interdependent and probably hierarchically arranged. They are mental organizations of experience that influence the way information is processed and the way behaviour is organized. Cognitive structures may engender cognitive and affective processes and events and may in turn be developed or modified by ongoing processes and events.

The complexity of cognitive processes may be just one reason why many people offer behavioural approaches to brain-injury rehabilitation as the most effective form of intervention. Behavioural or learning theory does indeed offer a structure for rehabilitation with emphasis placed on measurable and reproducible techniques. Behavioural techniques cover a wide range of possible strategies and are problem-orientated, although, as Fussey and Giles (1988) suggested, a complex interaction of many types of learning are probably present in the acquisition of most types of learned behaviour in man. Even so, although the specifics of an intervention will depend upon the type of learning thought to predominate, in general terms it is felt that behavioural techniques aid the mapping of relationships between events occurring in the environment (Mackintosh, 1983).

It is clear that brain injury causes changes in the nature of human cognition, a phenomenon we describe as a cognitive deficit in one or more areas of cognition. However, given that cognition is generally inferred from behaviour, even in the normally functioning brain, then our definition of cognitive deficit is inferred from behavioural or performance deficit. Unfortunately, there is no necessary correlation between brain-behaviour relationships established in the normal brain and those which operate after brain injury.

If we consider rehabilitation as a process of learning, where learning is defined as behavioural change leading to restored functional independence, then we have, as our guide to understand this process, the scientific principles of cognitive psychology and behavioural psychology. An important factor in cognitive rehabilitation must, therefore, be an understanding of normal cognition (including normal learning) elaborated by an analysis of cognitive pathology of cognition and its implications for rehabilitation. This is close to Powell's (1981) belief that the state of the damaged brain is of fundamental importance in assessing how best to facilitate learning in the patient. He emphasized the importance of considering the triad of behaviour, cognition and neurophysiology, a combination later referred to by Wilson (1989) as a basis for cognitive rehabilitation.

In assessing the evidence for cognitive rehabilitation as it stands at present, we see that the work of Sohlberg and Mateer, in providing attention-process training, is reasonably effective in producing improvements on various neuropsychological measures (Sohlberg and Mateer, 1987). To a limited extent these improvements suggest gains in living status and vocational outcome; while these gains cannot be attributed solely to the training, the observed functional changes correlated in time with improvements in cognitive performance as measured by tests.

The proponents of skills building (Malec, 1983; Wood, 1987) can also claim to show improvements, and like Sohlberg and Mateer, base their claims on the effectiveness of a procedural approach to cognitive rehabilitation. Booker and Schacter (1988) used a procedural approach to train complex learning, and Wilson (1989) reported a number of studies which all take procedural learning as the paradigm of choice when faced with memory problems. The reason for this becomes clear when we see that there is no evidence for the effectiveness of declarative learning techniques (using social outcome as the criterion for change) in cases of severe brain injury.

The status of cognitive rehabilitation must take into account the effectiveness of its various approaches, and to some extent this volume has tried to assess the 'state of the art' in as wide a variety of methods as possible. However, for a full evaluation of cognitive rehabilitation procedures, see Ruff *et al.* (1990). They strongly emphasize the importance of the relationship between specific treatment goals and functioning in everyday life, often not apparent in the studies they review, and in many areas note the lack of evidence for a theoretical framework. Sohlberg and Mateer (1989) observe that the measurement of treatment efficacy is at an embryonic stage, an embarrassing indictment of a discipline which can draw on a tradition of research paradigms for evaluating clinical procedures (c.f. Hersen and Barlow, 1976).

Let us consider the contributions to this volume bearing in mind that authors were asked to provide outcome data rather than anecdotal or unstructured observations to demonstrate a method of cognitive rehabilitation appropriate to the type of brain injury, with evidence of generalization to real-life skills or activities.

In the rehabilitation of attention disorders, Ponsford (Chapter 3) demonstrates no gains to everyday life from computer-training procedures and suggests a focus on domain-specific problems, utilizing a skills-building paradigm. Gray (Chapter 2) also finds improvement on psychometric tests but notes that the conditions for generalization are unknown, whereas Mateer *et al.* (Chapter 4) argue that generalization should never be left to chance, but should be 'planned for, trained for, and evaluated' (p. 91). They further point to the benefit of individual programmes and a focus on functional outcomes.

With regard to memory rehabilitation, the chapters by Deelman *et al.* (Chapter 6) and Finset and Andresen (Chapter 5) indicate a move towards the use of ecological memory tasks and strive to help patients develop insight into their problems with acceptance of the deficits and increase their awareness of intact skills (suggesting some optimism for a declarative approach in less severely damaged individuals). It is interesting to note that although Deelman and his colleagues are working with severely brain-injured patients, the severity of their cognitive disability varied, allowing them to utilize some of the techniques of cognitive therapy. While their results are encouraging, it appears that many of the gains could be attributed to improved psychosocial adjustment, which is admitted, but difficult to quantify. Finset and Andresen also note the difficulties in assessing the contribution of programme-specific, as opposed to non-specific recovery of function.

The approach to the rehabilitation of reasoning and problem-solving difficulties is similar to the approach of Mateer *et al.* (Chapter 4), and Ponsford (Chapter 3) in that it addresses a basic component of cognitive functioning. Von Cramon and Matthes–von Cramon (Chapter 8) focus specifically on those deficits associated with frontal lobe damage, whereas Evyatar and colleagues (Chapter 7) present methods that can be applied with no regard for the site of brain injury. With frontal lobe patients, the former authors feel that tasks in training should be ecologically relevant and are preferable to non-specific computer tasks. The latter authors present an alternative view and demonstrate improvements both on psychometric tests and in vocational placement. However, they also note that their programme cannot be considered the sole cause of the improvements but should be seen as a valid contribution to a general programme of cognitive rehabilitation.

In the section considering cognitive approaches to the rehabilitation of behavioural disorders, we find a useful synthesis of cognition, cognitive restructuring and behavioural methodology, addressing specific skills deficits. Burgess and Alderman (Chapter 9) specifically approach a substrate of cognition, namely, the functions carried out by frontal lobes. They apply techniques of procedural learning but incorporate cognitive therapy techniques, such as 'cognitive restructuring', aimed at modifying cognitions. They see cognitive restructuring as the 'active ingredient in the modification of a "thought schema" ', even when used with patients with demonstrable frontal lobe involvement. Regardless of this, they note limited generalization, which they see as compatible with frontal lobe damage not allowing the extraction of general principles to be applied in any situation. Alderman and Burgess (Chapter 10) more explicitly note that, in practice, as the severity of the injury increases, then the usefulness of psychotherapy methods declines. Be that as it may, even with a group of severely damaged patients, they still use the principles of cognitive-behaviour modification (Meichenbaum, 1977).

Hopewell and his colleagues (Chapter 11) state their views unequivocally by asserting that 'behavioural methodology is the only way in which the validity of any given technique of cognitive remediation can be validated.' They aim for domain-specific behavioural goals with considerable ecological validity, such as making a bed. With such goals, it becomes easy to assess the effectiveness of treatment. They pose a useful question in asking who judges the effectiveness of cognitive rehabilitation and give the example that, while many professionals feel that memory problems are most significant in terms of outcome, many employers complain more of executive and behavioural dysfunction. With this knowledge, Hopewell and his coworkers propose that cognitive remediation programmes should predominantly aim at executive and interpersonal deficits, through domain-specific skills that underlie these problems. However, although strongly advocating behavioural methodology, they use a number of techniques from cognitive therapy, including the 'inoculation' of patients to provocative stimuli to develop self-control and asking them to generate three contingency statements to subsequently use in problem situations.

All the chapters contained within this volume describe research by professionals whose commitment to cognitive rehabilitation is equalled by a desire to establish a scientific basis for their methods. Their findings take us further towards a greater understanding of the potential for cognitive rehabilitation as well as its limitations, while improving the lot of their patients and, possibly more importantly, the patients' carers. However, the broad cross-section of cognitive rehabilitation contained in this volume reflects the diversity of approaches contained within that description, and in many respects it still remains an 'umbrella' term, often giving respectability to pseudo-scientific techniques applied to the brain injured in the hope of achieving indeterminate aims with no way of assessing effectiveness, either of the technique or its subsequent generalization to activities of daily living.

This problem can largely be avoided if we direct cognitive rehabilitation towards improving functional skills. Under such conditions, treatment methods would have to consider both normal cognition and how brain injury has affected normal cognition in order to be in a position to provide rehabilitation which has the restitution of a particular functional skill as its goal. To achieve this, cognitive rehabilitation may have to employ methods that are appropriate for the most effective style of learning for any given individual, while preserving the conceptual integrity of a cognitive learning process. However, the efficacy of cognitive rehabilitation can only be measured in so far as it translates into behaviour, a view supported by Kreutzer *et al.* (1989) who state that '. . . ultimately judgements regarding treatment efficacy should be based on improvements in daily living skills' (p. 128).

It seems that the historical, and possibly unhelpful, distinction between cognitive therapy and behavioural therapy can now be considered unnecessary. We see that cognition is a processing system facilitating behaviour and strongly mediated by language. It is known that frontal involvement has a direct effect on the use of language as a mediator of behaviour. We therefore see that, in the normally functioning brain, some of the language-based interventions, such as those found in cognitive therapy, can be quite effective if the frontal lobes are performing adequately. It may be that in less severe head injuries, verbal regulation can still be appropriate, but as one proceeds to more severe injury with extensive frontal lobe impairment, language-based interventions may not be effective.

From this we deduce that some techniques of cognitive rehabilitation are more appropriate to mild rather than severe brain injury, as the work of Mateer *et al.* (Chapter 4) implies, and so we cannot completely exclude cognitive therapy approaches in a model of cognitive rehabilitation that encompasses both ends of the spectrum of severity.

The criteria outlined in the preface of this volume for cognitive rehabilitation procedures are demanding, although justifiable, when one considers that what has been described as cognitive rehabilitation to date has been sadly lacking in terms of a theoretical base and a built-in research methodology that allows for the evaluation of efficacy, or otherwise, of the various treatment approaches. At one extreme of brain injury disability, there seems little opportunity for using verbally-based cognitive rehabilitation in that severe cases respond best to a structured behavioural approach, although, no doubt, cognitive changes are taking place. However, such cognitive changes can only be inferred from the emergence of new behaviour. At the other extreme, where brain injury is mild, then rehabilitation approaches aimed at alleviating a specific cognitive deficit can be more usefully applied, although improvements in neuropsychological test scores of, memory, for example, cannot be taken as evidence of efficacy unless changes in activities of daily living are also seen.

The status of cognitive rehabilitation has been uncertain, because of the limited criteria adopted by professionals to evaluate methods and outcome of treatment. Recently, however, the concepts of attention and information processing have been recognized as important factors in the design of treatment programmes, and the evidence from this volume shows that combining these basic systems into a framework of treatment, utilizing principles from cognitive psychology and behavioural psychology applied to ecologically relevant skills, allows an evaluation of treatment efficacy which enhances the future status of cognitive rehabilitation as an important contribution to the spectrum of services available to the survivors of brain injury.

References

BOOKER, J. D. and SCHACTER, D. L., 1988, 'Towards a cognitive neuropsychology of complex learning'. In J. M. Williams and C. J. Long (Eds.), *Cognitive approaches to neuropsychology* (New York: Plenum Press).

BUTLER, R. W. and NAMEROW, N. S., 1988, 'Cognitive retraining and brain injury rehabilitation: A critical review'. *Journal of Neurological Rehabilitation*, **2**, 97–101.

CICERONE, K. D., 1989, 'Psychotherapeutic interventions with traumatically brain-injured patients'. *Rehabilitation Psychology*, **34**, 105–14.

DILLER, L. and GORDON, W. A., 1981, 'Rehabilitation and clinical neuropsychology'. In S. B. Fiskov and T. J. Boll (Eds.), *Handbook of clinical neuropsychology* (New York: John Wiley).

DRYDEN, W., 1984, *Rational-emotive therapy-fundamentals and innovations* (London: Croom Helm).

ELLIS, A., 1962, *Reason and emotion in psychotherapy* (New York: Lyle Stewart).

ELLIS, A., 1984, *Rational-emotive therapy and cognitive behavior therapy* (New York: Springer).

FUSSEY, I. and GILES, G. M., 1988, *Rehabilitation of the severely brain injured adult — A practical approach* (London: Croom Helm).

GOLDFRIED, M., DECENTECEO, E. and WEINBERG, L., 1974, 'Systematic reactional restructuring as a self-control technique'. *Behavior Therapy*, **5**, 247–54.

GOLDSTEIN, G. and RUTHVEN, L., 1983, *Rehabilitation of the brain-damaged adult* (New York: Plenum Press).

GROSS, Y. and SCHUTZ, L. E., 1986, 'Intervention models in neuropsychology'. In B. Uzell and Y. Gross (Eds.), *Clinical neuropsychology of intervention* (Boston: Martinus Nijhoff).

HERSEN, M. and BARLOW, D. H., 1976, *Single case experimental designs: Strategies for studying behavior change* (New York: Pergamon Press).

KREUTZER, J. S., GORDON, W. A. and WEHMAN, P., 1989, 'Cognitive remediation following traumatic brain injury'. *Rehabilitation Psychology*, **34**(2), 117–30.

LURIA, A. R., 1961, *The role of speech in regulation of normal and abnormal behaviour* (Oxford: Pergamon Press).

MACKINTOSH, N. J., 1983, *Conditioning and associate learning* (Oxford: Oxford University Press).

MALEC, J., 1983, 'Training the brain injured client in behavioral self-management skills'. In R. Edelstein and E. C. Couture (Eds.), *Behavioral assessment and treatment of the traumatically brain damaged* (New York: Plenum Press).

MEICHENBAUM, D., 1977, *Cognitive-behavior modification — an integrative approach* (New York: Plenum Press).

POWELL, G. E., 1981, *Brain function therapy* (Gower, Aldershot, Hants.).

PRIGATANO, G. P., FORDYCE, D. J., ZEINER, H. K., ROUECHE, J. R., PEPPING, M. and WOOD, B. C., 1984, 'Neuropsychological rehabilitation after closed head injury in young adults'. *Journal of Neurology, Neurosurgery and Psychiatry*, **47**, 505–13.

RUFF, R. M., NEIMAN, H. I. and TROSTER, A. I., 1990, 'Effectiveness of behavioral management in rehabilitation: Cognitive procedures'. In R. Ll. Wood (Ed.), *Neurobehavioural sequelae of traumatic brain injury* (London: Chapman Hall).

SARASON, I., 1975, 'Anxiety and self-preoccupation'. In I. Sarason and C. Spielberger (Eds.), *Stress and anxiety*, Vol. 2 (Washington, DC: Hemisphere Press).

SOHLBERG, M. M. and MATEER, C., 1987, 'Effectiveness of an attention retraining program'. *Journal of Clinical and Experimental Neuropsychology*, **9**(2), 117–30.

SOHLBERG, M. M. and MATEER, C., 1989, *Introduction to cognitive rehabilitation — theory and practice* (New York: The Guilford Press).

WILSON, B., 1989, 'Models of cognitive rehabilitation'. In R. Ll. Wood and P. Eames (Eds.), *Models of brain injury rehabilitation* (London: Chapman Hall).

WOOD, R. Ll., 1987, *Brain injury rehabilitation: A neurobehavioural approach* (London: Croom Helm).

WOOD, R. Ll., 1990, 'A neurobehavioural paradigm for brain injury rehabilitation'. In R. Ll. Wood (Ed.), *Neurobehavioural Sequelae of Traumatic Brain Injury* (London: Chapman Hall).

Author Index

Subject Index